MEDICAL RECORDS

RECORDS

AND THE

LAW

THIRD EDITION

MEDICAL RECORDS

AND THE

LAW

THIRD EDITION

William H. Roach, Jr., J.D.
Gardner, Carton & Douglas
Chicago, Illinois

and

The Aspen Health Law and Compliance Center
Jane Coyle Garwood
Cynthia Conner, LL.L.
Kara Kinney Cartwright, J.D.
Susan Kole, J.D.
Jennifer Forsyth, J.D.

JONES AND BARTLETT PUBLISHERS
Sudbury, Massachusetts
BOSTON   TORONTO   LONDON   SINGAPORE

World Headquarters
Jones and Bartlett Publishers
40 Tall Pine Drive
Sudbury, MA 01776
978-443-5000
info@jbpub.com
www.jbpub.com

Jones and Bartlett Publishers Canada
2406 Nikanna Road
Mississauga, ON L5C 2W6
CANADA

Jones and Bartlett Publishers International
Barb House, Barb Mews
London W6 7PA
UK

This publication is designed to provide accurate and authoritative information in regard to the Subject Matter covered. It is sold with the understanding that the publisher is not engaged in rendering legal, accounting, or other professional service. If legal advice or other expert assistance is required, the service of a competent professional person should be sought. (From a Declaration of Principles jointly adopted by a Committee of the American Bar Association and a Committee of Publishers and Associations.)

Production Credits
Chief Executive Officer: Clayton Jones
Chief Operating Officer: Don W. Jones, Jr.
Executive V.P. & Publisher: Robert W. Holland, Jr.
V.P., Sales and Marketing: William Kane
Acquisitions Editor: David Cella
Manufacturing Buyer: Amy Bacus

Library of Congress Cataloging-in-Publication Data

Roach, William H.
Medical records and the law / William H. Roach, Jr. and the Aspen Health Law and Compliance Center. —3rd ed.
p. cm.
Rev. ed. of : Medical records and the law / William H. Roach, Jr. . . . [et al]. 2nd ed. 1994.
Includes bibliographical references and index.
ISBN 0-7637-2598-6
1. Medical records—Law and legislation—United States. I. Aspen Health Law and Compliance Center. II. Medical records and the law. III. Title.
KF3827.R4R63 1998
44.73'041—dc21
98-25735
CIP

Printed in the United States of America
07 06 05 04   10 9 8 7 6 5 4 3 2

Table of Contents

Preface

The role that medical record information plays in the delivery of health care services has expanded significantly over the past five years, as managed care continues to dominate the delivery of health care services and advances in computer technology allow for widespread access and integration of this type of data. These two trends have had and will continue to have a profound impact on the traditional legal issues affecting the collection, maintenance and access to medical record information. Freestanding hospitals and solo physicians are no longer the focus of the law of medical records, and the very concept of a a "medical record" is increasingly patient-centered, as health care services are delivered by network providers under health insurance plans. The need to offer multiprovider access has created an impetus for the electronic conversion of records but also raises new and serious security conerns. The legal issues relating to patient information must now be examined in a variety of settings, as accreditation standards and legistlative requirements expand to cover new players in the health care delivery system, including networks and managed care organizations. Finally, the importance of complete and accurate medical record information has grown dramatically as a result of aggressive enforcement of fraud and abuse laws and as proper documentation becomes a key component of any successful corporate compliance program.

The second edition of *Medical Records and the Law,* published in 1994, acknowledged these trends, but the full impact of the changes they would bring to the field of health information management was not manifest. This third edition of *Medical Records and the Law* recognizes the consolidation of these trends, and refocuses its analysis of the legal issues affecting health information management to consider new methods of delivering health care services, the role of a variety of health care providers, the different uses made of health data, and the heightened confidentiality concerns that have arisen in this environment. New topics that address legal issues associated with these trends have been added to the book, including the impact of managed care on health information management, medical record ownership issues in a managed care environment, required disclosures by managed care organizations, information management accreditation standards for networks, MCOs and other providers, the role of medical record documentation in corporate compliance programs, fraud and abuse investigations, telemedicine and telemedical records, electronic claims prociessing, e-mail, the Internet and other confidentiality issues.

The integration of health information into sophisticated computer systems to provide links between providers, payers, employers, vendors and other support organizations while protecting the traditional role of medical information on the delivery of clinical services remains one of the most daunting challenges for the health care industry. This third edition of the highly acclaimed *Medical Records and the Law* contains valuable and practical information that will assist attorneys and health care professionals in meeting this challenge.

Acknowledgments

The Aspen Health Law and Compliance Center is grateful to every member of its staff for the patience and dedication they brought to creating a third edition of *Medical Records and the Law* that would live up to the distinguished reputation of the first two editions of this book. The Center's staff attorneys, Cynthia Conner, Kara Kinney Cartwright, Susan Kole, and Jennifer Forsyth each made significant contributions to the book through their writing and research efforts. Dawn Dorman, the Center's research assistant, also provided precious help in verifying citations and compiling a glossary. Finally, we are also grateful to Lenda Hill, Managing Editor, who kept us on schedule and once again made us look good in print.

Introduction to the American Legal System

Chapter Objectives

- Distinguish between public and private law, civil and criminal law, and tort and contract actions.
- Discuss how the federal constitution delineates governmental authority.
- Identify the two specific procedural protections the due process clause generally requires and when they are required.
- Discuss the concept of equal protection.
- Give examples of the rights encompassed by the constitutional right to privacy.
- Explain what happens when local, state, and federal law overlap.
- Give examples of administrative agencies, describing their source of authority and how they regulate the public.
- Discuss how courts make law, defining the principles of stare decisis and res judicata.
- Name the three branches of government and outline the responsibilities of each.
- Distinguish between trial courts, appeals courts, and supreme courts.
- Explain the relationship between state and federal courts.

INTRODUCTION

The law affects many of the judgments that health record administrators, health professionals, and technical staff members must make each day. Their decisions may have significant potential legal consequences. Since it is impractical, if not impossible, to obtain professional legal advice before making every decision, medical records administrators, technicians, and indeed all health care providers who collect patient-related data must develop an understanding of the medical records law so they will be able to exercise judgment consistent with applicable law and to identify problems that require expert legal counsel.

This chapter sets forth general information about law, including the mechanics of the American legal system and the roles of the branches of government in creating, administering, and enforcing it.

THE NATURE OF LAW

According to most definitions, law is, in essence, a system of principles and processes by which people who live in a society deal with their disputes and problems, seeking to solve or settle them without resort to force. Law governs the relationships among private individuals, organizations, and government. Through law, society establishes standards of behavior and the means to enforce those standards. Law that deals with the relationships between private parties is called private law; public law deals with the relationships between private parties and government. As society has become more complex, the scope of public law has broadened and the regulation of private persons and institutions has become more pervasive.

Private law is concerned with the recognition and enforcement of the rights and duties of private individuals and organizations. Legal actions between private parties are of two types: tort and contract. In a tort action, one party asserts that wrongful conduct on the part of the other party has caused harm, and seeks compensation for the harm suffered. In a contract action, one party asserts that, in failing to fulfill an obligation, the other party has breached a contract, and the injured party seeks either compensation or performance of the obligations as a remedy.

An important part of public law is criminal law, which proscribes conduct considered injurious to the public order and provides for punishment of those found to have engaged in such conduct. Public law consists also of an enormous variety of regulations designed to advance societal objectives by requiring private individuals and organizations to follow specified courses of action in connection with their activities. While there are criminal penalties for those who do not abide by the regulations, the primary purpose of public law is to secure compliance with and attain the goals of the law, not to punish offenders.

The formulation of public policy concerning health care has thrust hospitals into the arena of legislative debate about containment of health care costs, quality of care, medical device safety, research involving human subjects, confidentiality of patient information, labor relations, employment policies, facility safety, and other important issues. The object of public law at both the federal and state level is to deal with societal problems of a broad nature.

Law serves as a guide to conduct. Most disputes or controversies that are covered by legal principles or rules are resolved without resort to the courts. Thus, each party's awareness of the law and of the relative likelihood of success in court affects its willingness to modify its original position and reach a compromise acceptable to both sides.

SOURCES OF LAW

The four primary sources of law are federal and state constitutions, federal and state statutes, the decisions and rules of administrative agencies, and the decisions of the courts.

The Constitution

The Constitution of the United States is the supreme law of the land. It establishes the general organization of the federal government, grants certain powers to the federal government, and places certain limits on what the federal and state governments may do.

The Constitution establishes and grants certain powers to the three branches of the federal government—legislative, executive, and judicial. The Constitution also is a grant of power from the states to the federal government. The federal government has only the powers granted to it by the Constitution. These powers are both express and implied. The express powers include, for example, the power to collect taxes, declare war, and regulate interstate commerce. The Constitution also grants the federal government broad implied powers to enact laws "necessary and proper" for exercising its other powers. When the federal government establishes law, within the scope of its powers, that law is supreme. All conflicting state and local laws are invalid.

The Constitution also places certain limits on what the federal and state governments may do. The most famous limits on federal power are the first ten amendments to the Constitution—the Bill of Rights. The basic rights protected by the Bill of Rights include the right to free speech, free exercise of religion, freedom from unreasonable searches and seizures, trial by jury, and the right not to be deprived of life, liberty, or property without due process of law. State powers are limited by the Fourteenth Amendment, as follows: ". . . nor shall any state deprive any person of life, liberty or property, without due process of law; nor deny to any person within its jurisdiction the equal protection of the laws." These clauses of the Fourteenth Amendment frequently are referred to as the due process clause and the equal protection clause. The right to privacy is another constitutional limitation on both state and federal governmental power that frequently affects hospitals and health care professionals.

Due Process of Law

The due process clause imposes restrictions and duties only on state action, not on private action. Actions by state and local governmental agencies, including public hospitals, are considered to be state actions and must comply with due process requirements. Actions by private individuals at the behest of the state also can be subject to the requirements. In the past, private hospitals were considered to be engaged in state action when they were regulated or partly funded by governmental agencies. Today it is rare for private hospitals to be considered engaged in state action on that basis.

The due process clause applies to state actions that deprive a person of "life, liberty or property." In that context, a position or a particular status can be considered property. For example, a physician's appointment to the medical staff of a public hospital and a hospital's institutional licensure by the state are considered property rights. Thus, in the first example, the public hospital must provide due process to the medical staff applicant, while in the second the state and local governmental agencies provide due process to the hospital.

The process that is due varies somewhat depending on the situation. Due process consists primarily of two elements: (1) the rules being applied must be reasonable and not vague or arbitrary; and (2) fair procedures must be followed in enforcing the rules. Two fundamental procedural protections must be offered: (1) notice of the proposed action and (2) an opportunity to present evidence as to why the disputed action should not be taken. The phrase "due process" in the Fourteenth Amendment also has been interpreted by the United States Supreme Court to include nearly all of the rights in the Bill of Rights. Thus, state governments may not infringe on those rights.

Equal Protection of the Laws

The equal protection clause also restricts state action. The concept of equal protection is intended to ensure that like persons are treated in like fashion. As a result, the equal protection clause is concerned with the legitimacy of the classification used to distinguish persons for various legal purposes. The determination of whether a particular difference between persons can justify a particular difference in rules or procedures can be difficult. In general, courts require that the government agency justify the difference with a rational reason. The major exception to this standard is the strict scrutiny courts apply to distinctions based on particular "suspect classifications," such as race.

Right of Privacy

In *Griswold v. Connecticut,*[1] the United States Supreme Court recognized a constitutional right of privacy. The Court has ruled that the right of privacy limits governmental authority to regulate contraception, abortion, and other decisions affecting reproduction. Several state courts have ruled that the right of privacy permits terminally ill patients and those acting on their behalf to choose to withhold or withdraw medical treatment.[2] In the area of health care information, the unauthorized disclosure of confidential patient information can also give rise to a claim for invasion of privacy based on the federal constitutional right of privacy, although it is more common to see such claims based on the common law. (For a more detailed discussion of invasion of privacy claims for the improper disclo-

---

[1]Griswold v. Connecticut, 381 U.S. 479 (1965).

[2]*See, e.g.*, Satz v. Perlmutter, 379 So. 2d 359 (Fla. 1980).

sure of medical records, see Chapter 10, DISCOVERY AND ADMISSIBILITY OF MEDICAL RECORDS.)

State Constitutions

Each state also has its own constitution. The state constitution establishes the organization of the state government, grants certain powers to the state government, and places certain limits on what the state government may do.

Statutes

Another major source of law is statutory law, which is the law enacted by a legislature. Legislative bodies include the United States Congress, state legislatures, and local legislative entities, such as city councils and county boards of supervisors. Congress has only the powers delegated by the Constitution, but those powers have been interpreted broadly. State legislatures have all powers not denied by the United States Constitution, by federal laws enacted under the authority of the federal government, or by their state constitutions. Local legislative bodies have only those powers granted by the state. Through statutes or constitutional amendments, some states have granted local governments broad powers authorizing home rule.

When federal and state law conflict, valid federal law supersedes. In some cases, federal law may preempt an entire area of law, so that state law is superseded even if it is not in direct conflict. In some law, such as bankruptcy law, Congress explicitly preempts dual state regulation. In other areas of the law, the courts find that preemption is implied from the aim and pervasiveness of the federal scheme, the need for uniformity, and the likelihood that state regulation would obstruct the full goals of the federal action. In the area of health care law, one of the most frequently applied preemption provisions can be found in the Employee Retirement Income Security Act of 1974 (ERISA). Designed to achieve uniformity in the regulation of health care benefits, ERISA's preemption provisions determine whether state law claims will be heard in state or federal court and what damages are available.

When state law and local government rules conflict, valid state law supersedes. In some cases, state law may preempt an entire area of law, so that local law is superseded even if it is not in direct conflict. For example, in *Robin v. Incorporated Village of Hempstead*,[3] the court ruled that New York had preempted the regulation of abortions. Therefore, additional regulation by local authorities was prohibited.

Medical records law is still largely governed by state legislation and regulation, which cover a variety of issues. Provisions relating to health care information can be found in health care information confidentiality statutes, health care provider licensure laws, communicable diseases legislation, child and elder abuse legislation, peer review legislation, and in statutes governing the dying process.

Decisions and Rules of Administrative Agencies

The decisions and rules of administrative agencies are other sources of law. Legislatures have delegated to numerous administrative agencies the responsibility and power to implement various laws. The delegated powers include the quasi-legislative power to adopt regulations and the quasi-judicial power to decide how the statutes and regulations apply to individual situations. The legislature has delegated this authority because it does not have the time or expertise to address the complex issues involved in many areas that it believes need to be regulated.

Administrative agencies that have been invested with these powers include the Food and Drug Administration (FDA), the National Labor Relations Board (NLRB), and the Internal Revenue Service (IRS). The FDA promulgates regulations and applies them to individual determinations involving the manufacture, marketing, and advertising of foods, drugs, cosmetics, and medical devices. The NLRB decides how national labor law applies to individual disputes. The IRS promulgates and applies regulations to individual disputes concerning federal taxation.

Many administrative agencies, such as the NLRB, seek to achieve some consistency in their decisions by following the position they adopted in previous cases involving similar matters. That is similar to the way the courts develop the common law, discussed later in this chapter. When dealing with these agencies, it is important to review the body of law that has evolved from their previous decisions.

Administrative rules and regulations are valid only to the extent that they are within the scope of the authority granted by legislation to the

---

[3]Robin v. Incorporated Village of Hempstead, 285 N.E.2d 285 (N.Y. 1972).

agency that has issued them. The Constitution also limits delegation by the legislature. The legislature must retain ultimate responsibility and authority by specifying what regulations the administrative body may make. In the past, courts often declared delegations to be unconstitutional unless there was considerable specificity. Today the courts interpret the Constitution as permitting much broader delegation, but the general area of law still must be specified.

Congress and many state legislatures have passed administrative procedure acts. These specify the procedures administrative agencies must follow in promulgating rules or reaching decisions in contested cases, unless an overriding law specifies different procedures. Generally, these laws provide that most proposed rules be published to allow individuals an opportunity to comment before the rules are finalized. Many federal agencies must publish both proposed and final rules in the Federal Register. Many states have comparable publications of the proposed and final rules of state agencies. Those involved with hospitals should monitor proposed and final rules through these publications, other publications, or their professional or hospital associations. Administrative agencies often rely on this comment process to learn, from the public and from the affected industries, of the potential implications of agency proposals.

Court Decisions

The judicial decision is the fourth source of law. In the process of deciding individual cases, the courts interpret statutes and regulations, determine whether specific statutes and regulations are permitted by state or federal constitution, and create the common law when deciding cases not controlled by statutes, regulations, or a constitution.

Disagreements over the application of statutes or regulations to specific situations arise frequently. In some situations, an administrative agency has the initial authority to decide how the law shall be applied. That agency's decision usually can be appealed to the courts. However, courts generally defer to the decisions of administrative agencies in discretionary matters and limit their review to whether the delegation to the agency was constitutional and whether the agency acted within its authority, followed proper procedures, had a substantial basis for its decision, and acted without arbitrariness or discrimination.

Whether or not an administrative agency is involved, the court still may have to interpret the statute or regulation or decide which of two or more conflicting statutes or regulations apply. Courts have developed several rules for interpretation of statutes. In some states, a statute specifies rules of interpretation. These rules or statutes are designed to help determine the intent of the legislature in passing the law.

The courts also determine whether specific statutes or regulations violate the Constitution. All legislation and regulations must be consistent with the Constitution. The case of *Marbury v. Madison*[4] established the power of the courts to declare legislation invalid when it is unconstitutional.

Many of the legal principles and rules applied by the courts in the United States are the product of the common law developed in England and, subsequently, in the United States. The term "common law" is applied to the body of principles that evolves from court decisions resolving controversies. Common law continually is being adapted and expanded. During the Colonial period, English common law applied uniformly. After the American Revolution, each state provided for the adoption of part or all of the then existing English common law. All subsequent common law in the United States has been developed on a state basis, so common law may differ from state to state.

Statutory law has been enacted to restate many legal rules and principles that initially were established by the courts as part of the common law. However, many issues, especially those pertaining to disputes in private law, still are decided according to common law. Common law in a state may be changed by enactment of legislation modifying it or by later court decisions that establish new and different common law.

In deciding specific controversies, courts for the most part adhere to the doctrine of *stare decisis*, which frequently is described as following precedent. By referring to similar cases decided previously and applying the same rules and principles, a court arrives at the same ruling in the current case as in the preceding one. However, slight differences in the situations presented may provide a basis for recognizing distinctions between precedent and the current case. Even when such differences are absent, a court may conclude that a particular common law rule no longer is in accord with the needs of society and may depart from precedent.

One clear example of this departure from precedent in the law affecting hospitals was the reconsideration and elimination in nearly every state of the principle of charitable immunity, which had provided nonprofit hospitals with virtual freedom from liability for harm to patients resulting from

---

[4]Marbury v. Madison, 5 U.S. (1 Cranch) 137 (1803).

wrongful conduct. In state after state over a period of 30 years, courts found justification to overrule precedents that had provided immunity and, thereby, to allow suits against nonprofit hospitals.

Another doctrine that courts follow to avoid duplicative litigation and conflicting decisions is *res judicata*, which means a thing or matter settled by judgment. When a legal controversy has been decided by a court and no more appeals are available, those involved in the suit may not take the same matters to court again. This is different from *stare decisis* in that *res judicata* applies only to the parties involved in the prior suit and the issues decided in that suit. The application of the doctrine of *res judicata* can be complicated by disagreements over whether specific matters actually were decided in the prior case.

GOVERNMENTAL ORGANIZATION AND FUNCTION

This section focuses on the structure of the three branches of government—the legislative, executive, and judicial branches—and the manner in which their functions interrelate. In a simplified summary of the functions of the three branches, the legislature makes the laws, the executive branch enforces the laws, and the judiciary interprets the laws. The three branches of government exist under a vital concept in the constitutional framework of the United States government and of the various state governments: the separation of powers. Essentially, separation of powers means that no one of the three branches of government is clearly dominant over the other two; however, in the exercise of its functions, each may affect and limit the activities, functions, and powers of the others.

The concept of separation of powers, which may be referred to as a system of checks and balances, is illustrated by the involvement of the three branches in the federal legislative process. Specifically, when a bill to create a statute is enacted by Congress and signed by the President, a representative of the executive branch, it becomes law. If the President should veto the bill, a two-thirds vote of each house of Congress can override the veto. Finally, the President can prevent a bill from becoming law by not taking any action while Congress is in session. Thus, by his veto the President can prevent a bill from becoming law temporarily and possibly prevent it from becoming law at all if later sessions of Congress do not act favorably on it. A bill that has become law ultimately may be declared invalid by the United States Supreme Court, an agency of the judicial branch of government, if the Court decides that the law is in violation of the Constitution.

Another example of the relationship among the branches of government involves the selection of federal court judges. Individuals nominated by the President for appointment to the federal judiciary, including the United States Supreme Court, must be approved by the United States Senate. Thus, over time, both the executive and legislative branches can affect the composition of the judicial branch of government.

In addition, while a Supreme Court decision may be final with regard to the specific controversy before the Court, Congress and the President may generate revised legislation to replace the law previously held unconstitutional. The processes for amending the Constitution, while complex and often time-consuming, also can serve as a method for offsetting or overriding a Supreme Court decision.

Each of the three branches of government has a different primary function. The function of the legislative branch is to enact laws. This process may involve creating new legislation or amending or repealing existing legislation. It is the legislature's responsibility to determine the nature and extent of the need for new laws and for changes in existing laws. By means of a committee system, legislative proposals are assigned or referred for study to committees with specific areas of concern or interest. The committees conduct investigations and hold hearings, at which interested persons may present their views, in order to assist the committee members in their consideration of the bills. Some bills eventually reach the full legislative body where, after consideration and debate, they may be either approved or rejected. The Congress and every state legislature except Nebraska consist of two houses. (Nebraska has only one house.) Both houses must pass identical versions of a legislative proposal before it can be presented to the chief executive.

The primary function of the executive branch is to enforce and administer the law. However, the chief executive, either the governor of a state or the President of the United States, has a role in the creation of law through the power either to approve or to veto a legislative proposal. If the chief executive accepts the bill through the constitutionally established process, it becomes a statute, a part of the enacted law. If the chief executive vetoes the bill, it can become law only if the process for overriding the veto by the legislature is successful.

The executive branch of government is organized into departments. The departments have responsibilities for different areas of public affairs and each enforces the law within its assigned area of responsibility. Much of the federal law affecting or pertaining to hospitals is administered by the

Department of Health and Human Services. In most states there are separate departments with responsibility over health and welfare matters, and those departments administer and enforce most laws pertaining to hospitals. Other departments and government agencies also affect hospital affairs, however. On the federal level, for example, laws relating to wages and hours of employment are enforced by the Department of Labor. The federal Department of Justice is also a key player in enforcing health care fraud and abuse prohibitions.

The judicial branch of government is responsible for adjudicating and resolving disputes in accordance with law. Many types of disputes involving hospitals go before the courts. For example, suits against hospitals by patients seeking compensation for harm allegedly suffered as the result of wrongful conduct by hospital personnel are decided by the courts. Hospitals resort to the courts to challenge exercises of authority by government agencies and departments, to have legislation concerning hospitals declared invalid, to collect unpaid hospital bills, and to enforce contracts.

Although many disputes and controversies are resolved without resort to the courts, in many situations there is no way to end a controversy without submitting to the adjudicatory process of the courts. A dispute taken before a court is decided in accordance with the applicable law; this application of the law is the essence of the judicial process.

ORGANIZATION OF THE COURT SYSTEM

It is necessary to understand the structure of the court system to understand the effect of court decisions as precedents and to understand the judicial branch of government. There are more than 50 court systems in the United States, including the federal court system, each state's court system, the District of Columbia court system, and those of Puerto Rico and the territories. These courts do not all reach the same decisions on specific issues. Frequently, a majority approach and several minority approaches exist on each issue. Thus, careful review is necessary to determine which court's decisions apply to an individual hospital and, if no decisions are specifically applicable, to predict which approach the courts are likely to adopt.

The federal court system and many state court systems have three levels of courts—trial courts, intermediate courts of appeal, and a supreme court. Some states have no intermediate courts of appeal.

State Court System

The trial courts in some states are divided into special courts that deal with specific issues, such as family courts, juvenile courts, probate courts, and limited courts that deal only with lesser crimes, such as misdemeanors, or with civil cases involving limited amounts of money. Each state has trial courts of general jurisdiction that may decide all disputes not assigned to other courts or disputes barred from the courts by valid federal or state law.

At the trial court level, the applicable law is determined and the evidence is assessed to determine the facts. The applicable law then is applied to those facts. It is the judge's role to determine what the law is. If there is a jury, the judge instructs the jury as to the law, and the jury determines the facts and applies the law. If there is no jury, the judge also determines the facts. In either case, the determination of the facts must be based on the evidence properly admitted during the trial, so the facts as heard by the decision maker may not necessarily be what actually happened.

In some cases, everyone agrees on the facts and the only issues presented to the court concern what the law is. In other cases, everyone agrees what the law is, but there is disagreement over the facts. To determine the facts for purposes of deciding the case, the credibility of the witnesses and the weight to be given other evidence must be determined. Many cases involve both questions of law and questions of fact. The judge has significant control over the trial even when a jury is involved. If the judge finds that insufficient evidence has been presented to establish a factual issue for the jury to resolve, the judge can dismiss the case or, in civil cases, direct the jury to decide the case in a specific way. In civil cases, even after the jury has decided, the judge can rule in favor of the other side.

Most state court systems have an intermediate appellate court. Usually, this court decides only appeals from trial court decisions. In some states, there are a few issues that can be taken directly to the intermediate appellate court. When an appellate court decides an appeal, it does not accept additional evidence. It uses the evidence presented in the record from the trial court. Appellate courts almost always accept the determination of the facts by the jury or judge in the trial court because they saw the witnesses and therefore can judge their credibility more accurately. Usually, the appellate court bases its decision on whether proper procedures were followed in the trial court and whether the trial court properly interpreted the law. However, an appellate court occasionally will find that a jury verdict is so clearly contrary to the evidence that it will either reverse the decision or order a new trial.

Each state has a single court at the highest level, usually called the supreme court. In some states the name is different. For example, in New York the highest court is the Court of Appeals, while trial courts are called supreme courts. The highest level court in each state decides appeals from the intermediate appellate courts or, in states without such courts, from trial courts. The highest level court frequently has other duties, including adopting rules of procedure for the state court system and determining who may practice law in the state, which includes disciplining lawyers for improper conduct.

Federal Court System

The federal court system has a structure similar to state court systems. The federal trial courts are the United States district courts and special purpose courts, such as the Court of Claims, which hears certain claims against the United States. Federal trial courts are fundamentally different from state trial courts because the federal courts have limited jurisdiction. A federal suit must involve either a question of federal law or a dispute between citizens of different states. In many cases, the controversy must involve at least $10,000. Federal questions include cases involving possible violations of federal law or of rights under the United States Constitution. When a federal trial court decides a controversy between citizens of different states, it is acting under what is called its diversity jurisdiction, using federal court procedures but applying the law of the applicable state.

Sometimes federal trial courts will decline to decide state law questions until they have been ruled on by a state court. That is called abstention. It is designed to leave states' issues for state courts and to minimize the workload of the federal courts. Federal courts generally will not abstain when there also are important federal questions not affected by the state law question. Some states have procedures by which the federal courts can ask a state court directly to decide a particular question of state law when it is important to the decision of a case before the federal court.

Appeals from the federal trial courts go to a United States court of appeals. The United States is divided into 12 areas, called circuits, numbered 1 through 11, plus the District of Columbia circuit court.

The highest court in the United States is the United States Supreme Court, which decides appeals from the United States courts of appeals. Decisions of the highest state courts also may be appealed to the United States Supreme Court if they involve federal laws or the United States Constitution. When the courts of appeals or the highest state courts decline to review a lower court decision, the decision sometimes can be appealed directly to the United States Supreme Court.

The United States Supreme Court has the authority to decline to review most cases. With only a few exceptions, a request for review is made by filing a petition for a *writ of certiorari*. If the Supreme Court grants *certiorari*, the record for the lower court decision is transmitted to the Supreme Court for review. In most cases, the Supreme Court denies the *writ of certiorari*. Such a denial does not indicate approval of the lower court decision; it merely means the Supreme Court declines to review the decision.

Stare Decisis

The preceding description illustrates the complexity of the court system in the United States. When a court is confronted with an issue, it is bound by the doctrine of *stare decisis* to follow the precedents of higher courts in the same court system that have jurisdiction over the geographic area where the court is located. Each appellate court, including the highest court, generally is bound also to follow the precedents of its own decisions, unless it decides to overrule the precedent due to changing conditions.

Thus, decisions from equal or lower courts or from courts in other court systems do not have to be followed. One exception occurs when a federal court decides a controversy between citizens of different states and must follow the state law as determined by the highest court of the state. Another exception is when a state court decides a controversy involving a federal law or constitutional questions and must follow the decisions of the United States Supreme Court. Another situation that may force a court to alter its prior position is a change in the applicable statutes or regulations by the legislature or an administrative agency.

When a court is confronted with a question that is not answered by applicable statutes or regulations and the question has not been addressed by its court system, the court usually will examine the judicial solutions reached in the other systems to decide the new issue. When a court decides to reexamine its position on an issue it has addressed, it often will examine the judicial decisions of the other systems to decide whether to overrule its position. A clear trend in decisions across the country can form a basis for a reasonable legal assessment of how to act even when the courts in a particular area have not decided the issue. However, a court is not bound by decisions in other systems, and it may reach a different conclusion.

Thus, there can be a majority approach to a certain issue that many state court systems follow and several minority approaches that other states follow. State courts show more consistency on some issues than on others. For example, nearly all state courts have completely eliminated charitable immunity. However, while nearly all states require informed consent to medical procedures, many states determine the information that must be provided to patients by reference to what a patient needs to know, while several states make the determination by reference to what other physicians would disclose. A few states have not yet decided what reference to use.

Differences in applicable statutes and regulations between states may force courts in different states to reach different conclusions on certain questions. For example, numerous states have enacted statutes that protect hospital and medical staff review committee records from discovery, although the extent of protection varies. Some statutes provide that such records generally are subject to subpoena, discovery, or disclosure; other statutes state specifically that such committee records, proceedings, and reports are not discoverable or describe such material as confidential or privileged. There also are common exceptions to the nondiscovery statutes, allowing physicians to discover records of staff privilege committees when contesting the termination, suspension, or limitation of their staff privileges. As a result of these variations, courts throughout the country have construed nondiscovery statutes with varying results.

In summary, while it is important to be aware of trends in court decisions across the country, legal advice should be sought before taking actions based on decisions from court systems that have no jurisdiction over the geographic area in which the hospital is located.

2

Medical Records and Managed Care

Chapter Objectives

- Identify the characteristics of the managed care industry that have changed the nature of patient records.
- Describe the changes in medical record standards made in response to the growth of managed care—whether instituted by legislatures, accrediting organizations, or health information managers.
- Compare and contrast the HMO, PPO, EPO, IPA, GPWW, consolidated medical group, PHO, MSO, foundation model IDS, and physician ownership model IDS.
- Define utilization management and utilization review organization.
- Explain the role of patient information with respect to the utilization management process.

THE IMPACT OF MANAGED CARE ON HEALTH INFORMATION MANAGEMENT

As managed care and computerization of information continue to proliferate in the health care delivery system, traditional legal issues affecting the collection, maintenance, and access to medical record information have evolved. The settings in which today's health care system gathers and uses patient-related health care information include individual health care provider offices, ambulatory care centers, health maintenance organizations, home health agencies, hospitals, places of employment, and insurance companies. In addition, this type of information increasingly is being collected and stored electronically. These two trends, increased computer automation and dispersed access to the information, have had and will continue to have a profound effect on the legal issues surrounding health information management.

The traditional approach to studying the legal issues associated with medical records, as was reflected in the two previous editions of this book, has been to consider the hospital's role in creating and maintaining these documents. Indeed, much of the legislation that addresses medical record management focuses on hospitals' responsibilities for ensuring that the information gathered is accurate and complete, and that its confidentiality is protected in accordance with the law. Medical records case law also frequently deals with hospitals as primary players in the delivery of health care services, often involving claims for improper disclosure of information or access to peer review records.

Today, managed care is the dominant form of health insurance coverage in the United States. Increasingly, the hospital's role is simply part of a continuum of care that involves a multitude of providers and payers. A patient may consult many health care providers, including primary care physicians, specialists, hospitals, laboratories, surgical centers, and rehabilitation centers, and each of them will participate in creating a record for that patient. Records containing health care information are held by numerous individuals and entities in different locations, many of which are part of a network of providers established by a managed care plan. The information gathered by these providers needs to be shared for clinical purposes in the interest of optimal care of individual patients. In addition, managed care plans themselves rely heavily on the data gathered in patient records, and accumulate enormous amounts of this kind of information for cost assessment and utilization review purposes. Employers also become part of this data integration and frequently collect and store patient-related information as part of the process of providing health care benefits to their employees and documenting workers' compensation claims.

The penetration of managed care into the health care delivery system has also been an impetus for the computerization of patient information as data networking becomes necessary to link providers, payers, employers, and consumers both regionally and nationally. Many health care reform proposals include recommendations for information system networks that would achieve managed care goals of cutting costs while safeguarding the quality of patient care. The establishment of this type of data-exchange ability, however, has raised significant concerns about protecting the privacy of patient information as the control of any individual provider over the release of the information decreases. Health care reform proposals also factor into their recommendations the growing difficulty of determining who owns and assumes ultimate responsibility for protecting against unauthorized access to medical records in electronic format.

Although reform proposals envision the creation of a health care information trust to be held by the provider for the benefit of the patient, the current state of the law with respect to the issue of ownership of medical records is generally that the health care provider owns the records, which may only be released or accessed in accordance with the law. Some states have begun to respond to the ambiguities that arise in today's managed care setting, where individual providers are in fact employees of larger health care organizations. Florida law, for example, provides that "records owner" refers to any health care practitioner "who generates a medical record after making a physical or mental examination of, or dispensing legend drugs to, any person; any health care practitioner to whom records are transferred by a previous record owner; or any health care practitioner's employer, including but not limited to group practices and staff-model health maintenance organizations, provided the employment contract or agreement between the employer and the health care practitioner designates the employer as the records owner."[1] The Florida statute goes on to list certain practitioners and entities that are not authorized to acquire or own medical records, but are authorized to maintain such documents under their respective licensing statutes (e.g., pharmacies and pharmacists, nursing home administrators, clinical laboratory personnel). Record owners as defined in the Florida statute bear the responsibility of maintaining a register of all disclosures of medical record information to third parties.

In addition, although much of the law relating to health care information is still based on the patient/provider relationship, with legislation in the majority of states imposing on physicians and other licensed health care providers the duty to guard against unauthorized disclosure, state legislatures have had to respond to changes affecting the way health care is

---

[1]*See* FLA. STAT. ch. 455.241.

delivered and recorded. In a minority of states, legislatures have adopted more generic statutes governing health care information. Many states now impose confidentiality requirements on health maintenance organizations[2] (e.g., New York) and numerous other states impose similar obligations on utilization review organizations, insurance institutions, agents, and insurance support organizations.[3] States have also begun regulating the gathering of patient-related information by private peer review organizations, requiring as part of the license application process that an organization submit its policies and procedures governing the confidentiality of medical records information.

Recognized exceptions to patient privacy in mandatory reporting laws relating to child abuse, infectious diseases, or dangers to third parties generally impose a duty to report certain conditions or events on the health care provider who is closest to the patient in the treatment relationship. These statutes have been in effect for many years and many do not contemplate the computerized distribution of patient information that is occurring in today's managed care environment. Increasingly, however, managed care plans are acquiring medical record information that can generate the same duty to disclose information as that imposed on primary health care providers such as the physician or the hospital. Nonprovider entities, such as individual provider associations, utilization review organizations, third-party administrators, or an employer-sponsored health plan, that lawfully access patient care information can be considered "health care providers" for the purposes of mandatory reporting obligations, even though they do not directly deliver health care services to patients. In Maryland, for example, under the state Medical Records Act,[4] the definition of "health care provider" includes health maintenance organizations and the agents, employees, officers, and directors of a health care professional or health care facility. Because many managed care plans would fall within the statutory definition of "health maintenance organization," the agents of these plans who work in claims processing, utilization review, or cost or utilization assessments have duties to disclose patient information under specific circumstances and are protected from liability for good faith actions.[5]

---

[2]*See* TENN. CODE ANN. 56-32-225.

[3]*See, e.g.,* N.Y. INS. LAW § 4905.

[4]MD. CODE ANN., HEALTH-GEN. II, §§ 4-301 through 4-305.

[5]*See* E. J. Krill, *Required Disclosure of Medical Record Information—Applications to Managed Care.* American Bar Association Forum on Health Law, Monograph 3, Health Care Facility Records. Confidentialing, Computerization, and Security, July 1995, pp. 11-26.

Associations that accredit health care organizations and state regulations have also responded to the growing number of entities that collect patient data by elaborating information management standards that apply to the types of health care organizations that have emerged in the managed care environment. The Joint Commission on Accreditation of Healthcare Organizations (Joint Commission) now accredits health care networks and preferred provider organizations (PPOs) and has standards that govern the type of patient-related data they collect. The Joint Commission accreditation standards for health care networks govern information management, and require that a record of health information contain sufficient information to facilitate continuity of care among the components of the network.[6] The Joint Commission PPO Accreditation Manual also addresses information management, requiring preferred provider organizations to determine appropriate levels of security and confidentiality of data and information while at the same time ensuring that it has adequate capability to integrate and interpret data from various sources.[7] The National Committee for Quality Assurance (NCQA) accredits managed care organizations, and has elaborated specific medical record standards that apply to this type of organization.[8]

For these reasons, when studying the legal issues associated with this topic it is no longer appropriate to focus on the hospital's role in creating and maintaining medical records. Increasingly, the law governing medical records must consider the roles of a variety of players in respecting a multitude of standards that define ownership, content, access, reporting, and retention issues. To facilitate this approach, this chapter will provide an overview of some of the organizations that are involved in some significant aspect of collecting, using, maintaining, and distributing patient-related information in the managed care setting. Throughout this third edition of *Medical Records and the Law*, examples and explanations will continue to refer to hospitals and physicians in some instances, but will also cite to other specific health care providers or to a more generic category of health care providers where appropriate.

---

[6]JOINT COMMISSION, 1998-2000 COMPREHENSIVE ACCREDITATION MANUAL FOR HEALTH CARE NETWORKS, Standard IM 6.3.

[7]JOINT COMMISSION, 1997 ACCREDITATION MANUAL FOR PREFERRED PROVIDER ORGANIZATIONS, Standards IM 1 through IM 4.

[8]NATIONAL COMMITTEE FOR QUALITY ASSURANCE, 1997 STANDARDS FOR ACCREDITATION OF MANAGED CARE ORGANIZATIONS, Standards MR 1 through MR 4. *See also* NATIONAL COMMITTEE FOR QUALITY ASSURANCE, 1997 STANDARDS FOR THE CERTIFICATION OF PHYSICIAN ORGANIZATIONS, Standards MR 1 through MR 4.

MANAGED CARE ORGANIZATIONS AND RELATED ENTITIES

Managed health care organizations (MCOs), once referred to as alternative delivery systems, now dominate the delivery of health care services in the United States. Although these organizations were reasonably distinct as recently as 1988, the differences between them and traditional insurance companies have become blurred over the last decade.

The following section provides a description of the different types of MCOs and the common acronyms used to represent them. A brief explanation is provided for each type of organization. The section will also provide an overview of the more common forms of integrated delivery systems (IDSs) in today's health care industry.

Health Maintenance Organizations

Health maintenance organizations (HMOs) are organized health care systems that are responsible for both the financing and delivery of a broad range of comprehensive health services to an enrolled population. In many ways, an HMO can be viewed as a combination of health care insurer and health care delivery system. Whereas traditional health care insurance companies are responsible for reimbursing covered individuals for the cost of their health care, HMOs are responsible for providing health care services to their covered members through affiliated providers who are reimbursed under various methods. There are different models of HMOs, including staff, group practice, network, IPA, and direct contract, depending on the nature of the relationship between the HMO and its participating physicians. Frequently, an HMO will set up different relationships with a variety of physician groups. As a result, many HMOs cannot easily be classified as a single model type, although such plans are occasionally referred to as mixed models. The HMO model type description now may be more appropriately used to describe an HMO's relationship with certain segments of its physicians.

Preferred Provider Organizations

Preferred provider organizations (PPOs) are entities through which employer health benefit plans and health insurance carriers contract to purchase health care services for covered beneficiaries from a selected group of participating providers. Typically, providers participating in PPOs agree to abide by utilization management and other procedures implemented by the PPO and agree to accept the PPO's reimbursement structure and payment levels. In return, PPOs often limit the size of their participating provider panels and provide incentives for their covered individuals to use participating providers instead of other providers. In contrast to individuals with traditional HMO coverage, individuals with PPO coverage are permitted to use non-PPO providers, although higher levels of coinsurance or deductibles routinely apply to services provided by the nonparticipating providers.

Exclusive Provider Organizations

Exclusive provider organizations (EPOs) are similar to PPOs in their organization and purpose. Unlike PPOs, however, EPOs limit their beneficiaries to participating providers for all health care services. In other words, beneficiaries covered by an EPO are required to receive all their covered health care services from providers that participate in the EPO. An EPO generally does not cover services received from other providers, although there may be exceptions.

Some EPOs parallel HMOs in that they not only require exclusive use of the EPO provider network but also use a gatekeeper approach to authorizing nonprimary care services. In these cases, the primary difference between an HMO and an EPO is that the former is regulated under HMO laws and regulations whereas the latter is regulated under insurance laws and regulations or the Employee Retirement Income Security Act of 1974 (ERISA), which governs self-insured health insurance plans.[9]

Independent Practice Associations

An independent practice association (IPA) is a legal entity, the members of which are independent physicians who contract with the IPA for the sole purpose of having the IPA contract with one or more HMOs. IPAs are usually not for profit, although that is not an absolute requirement.

In its common incarnation, the IPA negotiates with the HMO for a capitation rate that covers all physician services. The IPA in turn reimburses the member physicians, although not necessarily using capitation. The IPA and its member physicians are at risk for at least some portion of

---

[9]29 U.S.C. §§ 1001 through 1461.

medical costs in that, if the capitation payment is lower than the required reimbursement to the physicians, the member physicians must accept lower income. The usual form of an IPA is as an umbrella organization for physicians in all specialties to participate in managed care. Recently, however, IPAs that represent only a single specialty have emerged.

Group Practice Without Walls

Another type of physician group formation is the group practice without walls (GPWW), representing a more significant step toward the greater integration of physician services. The formation of a GPWW does not require the participation of a hospital and indeed is often formed as a vehicle for physicians to organize without being dependent on a hospital for services or support.

The GPWW comprises private-practice physicians who agree to aggregate their practices into a single legal entity, but the physicians continue to practice medicine in their independent locations. In other words, the physicians appear to be independent from the view of their patients, but from the view of a contracting entity (usually an MCO) they are a single group. The GPWW is owned by the member physicians, and governance is by the physicians. The GPWW may contract with an outside organization to provide business support services, although as a practical matter the practicing physicians may notice little difference in what they are used to receiving.

Consolidated Medical Group

The term "consolidated medical group," or "medical group practice," refers to a traditional structure in which physicians have combined their resources into a true medical group practice. Unlike the GPWW, in which the physicians combine certain assets and risks but remain in their own offices and continue to practice medicine as they always have, the true medical group is consolidated into a few sites and functions in a group setting. In other words, the physicians occupy the same facility or facilities. This results in a good deal of interaction among members of the group and requires common goals and objectives for group success.

Physician/Hospital Organizations

A physician/hospital organization (PHO) is usually a separate business entity, such as a for-profit corporation, that allows a hospital and its physicians to negotiate with third-party payers. In its simplest and most common version, the participating physicians and the hospital develop model contract terms and reimbursement levels, and use those terms to negotiate with MCOs.

Governance of the PHO is typically shared between hospital administrators and physicians.

A PHO represents a first step toward greater integration between a hospital and its medical staff. This type of organization has the advantage of being able to negotiate contracts on behalf of a large group of physicians allied with a hospital. Another advantage of a PHO is its ability to track and use data to manage the delivery system, at least from the standpoints of utilization management and quality assessment. In actuality, however, PHOs frequently fail to deliver any meaningful improvement in contracting ability, because many MCOs already have contracts in place and see little advantage in going through the PHO; therefore, some experts have predicted that PHOs will not be long-term players in the managed care environment.[10]

Management Services Organizations

A management service organization (MSO) represents the evolution of the PHO into an entity that provides more services to the physicians. The MSO not only provides a vehicle for negotiating with MCOs but also provides additional services to support the physician's practice. The physician, however, usually remains an independent private practitioner. MSOs are based around one or more hospitals. The reasons for the MSO's formation are generally the same as for the PHO, and ownership and governance issues are similar to those discussed earlier.

In its simplest form, the MSO operates as a service bureau, providing basic practice support services to member physicians. These services include activities such as billing, collection, administrative support in certain areas, and electronic data interchanges (such as electronic billing). The physician remains an independent practitioner under no legal obligation to use the services of the hospital on an exclusive basis.

---

[10]Ernst & Young, LLP, *Physician/Hospital Organizations: Profile 1995* (Washington, D.C.).

Foundation Model Integrated Delivery System

A foundation model integrated delivery system (IDS) is one in which a tax-exempt organization, frequently a hospital, creates a not-for-profit foundation that purchases and operates physicians' practices. Depending on the applicable law, the foundation is either licensed to practice medicine or is exempt from licensure requirements, and it may employ physicians directly or use hospital funds to purchase the practices directly. The foundation as a subsidiary of a tax-exempt organization combines with other affiliated entities to operate as an integrated health care system. In another model of integrated delivery systems, the foundation is an entity that exists on its own and contracts for services with medical groups and a hospital. The foundation owns and manages the practices, but the physicians become members of a medical group that in turn has an exclusive contract for services with the foundation. The foundation itself is governed by a board that is not dominated by either the hospital or the physicians (physician representation is crucial to the tax-exempt status of the foundation) and includes lay members.

Physician Ownership Model Integrated Delivery System

The physician ownership model refers to a vertically integrated system in which the physicians hold a significant portion of ownership interest of the health care entities that compose the system. In some cases, the physicians own the entire system; in other cases, the physicians own less than 100 percent but more than 51 percent. The physicians' ownership interest is typically through their medical group, so as to avoid problems that could arise under federal fraud and abuse prohibitions. The medical groups play a strong role in the overall management of the system, and the physicians have a clear vested interest in the system's success.

Utilization Review Organizations

Utilization management is an essential element of managed care because it allows a managed care organization to coordinate providers and provider services by monitoring treatment quality, identifying superior and cost-efficient providers, identifying and minimizing inappropriate use of services or facilities, and making medically necessary determinations. Utilization review, the function of evaluating the medical necessity of nonemergency care, is a central element of utilization management that relies heavily on patient-related information. The regulation of utilization review organizations by state legislatures and accreditation associations, including restrictions on the type of medical record information that may be gathered and the uses to which it may be put, has increased significantly over the past decade because of the growing importance of these organizations in managed health care.

As the number and complexity of organizations and enterprises involved in the delivery of health care services increases, so evolves the law of health information management. Medical records professionals, who traditionally have performed highly quantitative and departmentally focused tasks, must now adopt a systems approach to health information management in a managed care environment. Traditional medical records management activities, such as forms control, record content analysis and control, record tracking, release of information monitoring, record storage, and record destruction, are now performed within large and diverse health care enterprises, requiring that decision making and problem solving address the system as a whole. The range of personnel, facilities, and equipment that frequently are connected and supported by an information management system also dictates a more global approach to the subject of medical records and the law.

Although the focus of this book will expand to cover the legal issues involved in managing patient records in a variety of health care settings, the emphasis will continue to be on health information relating to patient care. The control and use of patient-specific data remain the primary areas of concern of today's health information managers, and are still the source of the most significant legal issues in this field.

3

Medical Record Requirements

Chapter Objectives

- Identify the governmental and private entities that establish medical records requirements.
- List the types of information contained in a patient record.
- Explain why it is important for a record to be complete and accurate.
- Give examples of the information state law may require in a medical record.
- Discuss the role of HCFA with regard to medical record content and retention.
- Describe how private associations address medical record content and retention, giving examples of the information associations require.
- List the sources of law governing medical record retention, providing examples of state law requirements.
- Define statute of limitations and discuss how a statute of limitations affects record retention practices.
- Explain how medical research and storage space impact medical record retention.
- Give examples of court cases illustrating the importance of medical record retention.
- Recommend considerations for medical record destruction policy.

RECORDS THAT MUST BE KEPT

Health care providers must maintain a record for each of their patients. This requirement is imposed by state licensure laws and regulations, accreditation standards, professional association guidelines, and conditions of participation in federal reimbursement programs. Judicial opinions have reinforced the requirement that health care providers develop and implement proper recordkeeping procedures, by imposing liability for the failure to maintain a proper record. Policies concerning medical records should therefore address the relevant standards of the health care organization or provider concerned and clearly set forth criteria relating to the types of information to be included in each record, the length of time each record must be kept, and the proper methods for final destruction of records.

A patient's medical record consists of four types of data: (1) personal, (2) financial, (3) social, and (4) medical.[1] Personal information usually is obtained upon admission or first visit to the provider, and will include name, birth date, sex, marital status, next of kin, occupation, identification of physicians, and other items needed for specific patient identification. Financial data include the names of the patient's employer and health insurance company, types of insurance and insurance policy numbers, Medicare and Medicaid numbers, if any, and other information that will enable the health care provider to bill for its services. Social data may include the patient's race and ethnic background, family relationships, community activities, and lifestyle. It also includes any court orders or other directions concerning the patient, and additional information related to the patient's position in society that may indicate a need for special confidentiality protection.

Medical data form the patient's clinical record, a continuously maintained history of the treatment provided in the hospital. These data include the patient's chief complaint, medical and family histories, results of physical examinations, planned course of treatment, physicians' diagnosis and therapeutic orders, evidence of informed consent, clinical observations, progress notes, consultation reports, nursing notes, reports and results of all procedures and tests including pathology and clinical laboratory tests and examinations,[2] operative record, radiology and nuclear medicine examinations and treatment, anesthesia records, and other re-

---

[1] *See* K. Waters and G. Murphy, *Medical Records in Health Information* (Gaithersburg, Md.: Aspen Publishers, Inc., 1975), 39-95.

ports generated during the patient's treatment. Medical data also may include information obtained from outside sources, such as diagnostic tests performed at another facility or laboratory.

The medical record may be written, typed, or computer-generated. Regardless of its form, the medical record should be a complete, accurate, and current account of the history, condition, and treatment of the patient and the results of the individual's hospitalization or outpatient treatment. The computerized record can expand the information network concerning a patient, enhancing completeness and accuracy as well as immediate availability of the record to authorized personnel. However, computerized medical records present special concerns, which are addressed in Chapter 13.

The importance of a complete and accurate medical record to the quality of care rendered to a patient is obvious. The medical record is used not only to document chronologically the care rendered to the patient, but also to plan and evaluate treatment and to enhance communication among the patient's physician and other treating health care professionals. In addition, medical records must be complete and accurate because of the heavy reliance on this information for scientific research, utilization management, and peer review purposes.

Medical records are important legal documents for both the health care provider and the patient. The most important legal function of medical records is to provide essential evidence in professional negligence actions brought by patients against the health care providers who treated them. Because these actions often are litigated two to five years after a patient received the treatment in question, the medical record frequently is the only detailed record of what actually occurred. The individual health care providers who participated in the patient's treatment may not be available to testify or may not remember important details of the case. A properly created record enables an individual provider or facility to reconstruct the patient's course of treatment and to show whether the care provided was acceptable under the circumstances.[3]

---

[2]*See* Laubach v. Franklin Square Hosp., 556 A.2d 682 (1989), holding that fetal monitor tracings are part of the medical record.

[3]*See, e.g.,* Foley v. Flushing Hosp. and Medical Ctr., 359 N.Y.S.2d 113 (1974), where an infant plaintiff's medical records provided evidence sufficient to prevent dismissal of a malpractice suit.

CONTENT REQUIREMENTS

The requirements that health care practitioners and organizations create and maintain medical records for the patients they treat is found in state and federal statutes and regulations, municipal codes, and accreditation standards. In some state statutes, a general definition of "medical records" provides guidance on what the records should contain. In Colorado, for example, legislation defines "medical record" as a "record of services pertaining to medical and health care, which are performed at the direction of a physician or other licensed health care provider on behalf of a patient by . . . health care personnel" including "such diagnostic documentation as X-rays, electrocardiograms, electroencephalograms, and other test results."[4] The Nevada statute defines health care records as "any written reports, notes, orders, photographs, X-rays, or other recorded data or information whether maintained in written, electronic or other form which is received or produced by a provider of health care, or any person employed by him, and contains information relating to the medical history, examinations, diagnosis or treatment of the patient."[5] In a few states, hospital-licensing statutes set forth the minimum record requirements. The Florida statute is illustrative:

> Each hospital . . . shall require the use of a system of problem-oriented medical records for its patients, which system shall include the following elements: basic client data collection; a listing of the patient's problems; the initial plan with diagnostic and therapeutic orders as appropriate for each problem identified; and progress notes, including a discharge summary.[6]

The Tennessee statute simply refers to standards prescribed by the hospital licensing board.[7]

For the vast majority of states, however, the regulatory agencies for hospitals as well as for other health care providers have jurisdiction to establish detailed requirements on medical record content. The rules and regulations have the effect of law.

The regulations issued by these agencies cover a variety of health care providers and types of medical information. In Alabama, for instance, the

---

[4]*See* COLO. REV. STAT. § 18-4-412.

[5]NEV. REV. STAT. § 629.021.

[6]FLA. STAT. § 395.3015.

[7]TENN. CODE ANN. § 68-11-303.

State Board of Health enunciates minimum content requirements for different hospital records, including admission, medical and surgical, obstetrical, and newborn.[8] That state also has content requirements for nursing home medical records. California regulations on record content requirements for acute care hospitals distinguish between inpatient and outpatient medical records as well as between records generated by other facilities, including intermediate care facilities, home health agencies, and adult day care centers.[9] Oregon regulations provide general requirements for the contents of medical records and add specific requirements for surgical, obstetrical, emergency department, outpatient, and clinic records.[10]

The Illinois hospital licensing regulation illustrates the detailed record content requirements found in many states:

> For each patient there shall be an adequate, accurate, timely, and complete medical record. Minimum requirements for medical record content are as follows: patient identification and admission information; history of patient as to chief complaints, present illness and pertinent past history, family history, and social history; physical examination report; provisional diagnosis; diagnostic and therapeutic reports on laboratory test results, X-ray findings, any surgical procedure performed, any pathological examination, any consultation, and any other diagnostic or therapeutic procedure performed; orders and progress notes made by the attending physician and when applicable by other members of the medical staff and allied health personnel; observation notes and vital sign charting made by nursing personnel; and conclusions as to the primary and any associated diagnosis, brief clinical resume, disposition at discharge to include instructions and/or medications and any autopsy findings on a hospital death.[11]

A few states, however, have regulations that specify only broad areas of information required in a medical record.[12] The Hawaii regulations provide that the "medical records shall clearly and accurately document a patient's identity, the diagnosis of the patient's illness, treatment, orders by

---

[8]ALA. ADMIN. CODE r. 420-5-7.07.

[9]CAL. CODE REGS. tit. 22, §§ 70749(o), 70527, 73423, & 73439.

[10]OR. ADMIN. R. 333-505.050.

[11]ILL. ADMIN. CODE tit. 77, § 250.1510(b)(2).

[12]See, e.g., CONN. AGENCIES REGS. § 19-13-D3(d).

medical staff, observations, and conclusion concerning the patient."[13] Iowa has a very general requirement that medical records be "accurate and complete" and signed by the attending physician.[14] Other states simply adopt the accreditation requirements of the Joint Commission on Accreditation of Healthcare Organizations (Joint Commission)[15] or Medicare conditions of participation requirements as the minimum state standard for medical records.[16]

Health care providers seeking to participate in federal reimbursement programs must satisfy federal regulations governing conditions of participation in those programs, which also impose record maintenance requirements. Regulations issued by the Health Care Financing Administration (HCFA) require specific categories of health care providers to maintain a clinical record for every patient who receives care and services, requiring in general that these records be maintained in accordance with professional standards, promptly completed and properly filed and retained.[17]

In addition, the HCFA regulations on the conditions of participation for some types of health care providers also impose specific content requirements. Conditions of participation for hospitals, for example, provide that all records must contain the following information as appropriate:

1. evidence of a physician examination, including a health history, performed no more than 7 days prior to admission or within 48 hours after admission;
2. admitting diagnosis;
3. results of all consultative evaluations of the patient and appropriate findings by clinical and other staff involved in the care of the patient;
4. documentation of complications, hospital-acquired infections, and unfavorable reactions to drugs and anesthesia;
5. properly executed informed consent forms for procedures and treatments specified by the medical staff, or by federal or state law if applicable, to require written patient consent;

---

[13]Haw. Admin. Rules § 11-93-21.

[14]Iowa Admin. Code r. 481-51.6.

[15]*See, e.g.,* R.I. Regs Code r.14090 007 § 25.7; Rules and Regulations for the Licensure of Hospitals in Va. § 12 VAC 5-410-370.

[16]*See, e.g.,* Mass. Regs. Code tit. 105, § 130.200.

[17]*See, e.g.,* 42 C.F.R. § 482.24 (hospitals), 42 C.F.R. § 418.74 (hospices), and 42 C.F.R. § 484.48 (home health agencies). HCFA Conditions of Participation for health maintenance organizations require the organization to maintain a medical recordkeeping system that accumulates pertinent information relating to Medicare enrollees and makes this information available to appropriate professionals. *See* 42 C.F.R. § 417.418.

6. all practitioners' orders, nursing notes, reports of a treatment, medication records, radiology and laboratory reports, vital signs, and other information necessary to monitor the patient's condition;
7. discharge summary with outcome of hospitalization, disposition of case, and provisions for follow-up care;
8. final diagnosis with completion of medical records within 30 days following discharge.[18]

Associations that accredit various health care organizations frequently impose maintenance standards for clinical records. For example, the Joint Commission's information management standards for managed care plans, integrated delivery networks, and provider-sponsored organizations require that the health information record contain sufficient information to identify the patient, justify the diagnosis, treatment, or services, provide written documentation of the chronology and results of treatment, and facilitate continuity of care among the components of the health care system.[19] The Joint Commission's intent statement for this standard delineates the content of the health record, including member identification, diagnoses, plan of care, medical history, appropriate physical examinations, immunization and screening status, documentation and results of treatments, procedures and tests, referrals or transfers to other practitioners, and evidence of known advance directives.[20] The Joint Commission's standards of accreditation for home health care has detailed content requirements for the records generated in the delivery of this type of service, specifying that home care records must contain the patient's height and weight, dietary restrictions, notations relating to the home's suitability for the services provided, and documentation of patient and family education. A home care record must also contain the names of other individuals and organizations involved in the patient's care.[21] The Joint Commission's standards for hospitals have a general content requirement similar to the one imposed on health care networks.[22] In addition, the standards require

---

[18]42 C.F.R. § 482.24(c)(2).

[19]JOINT COMMISSION, 1998-2000 COMPREHENSIVE ACCREDITATION MANUAL FOR HEALTH CARE NETWORKS, Standard IM 6.3.

[20]JOINT COMMISSION, 1998-2000 COMPREHENSIVE ACCREDITATION MANUAL FOR HEALTH CARE NETWORKS, Standards, Scoring and Aggregations Rules, IM 6.2 and 6.3.

[21]JOINT COMMISSION, 1997-1998 COMPREHENSIVE ACCREDITATION MANUAL FOR HOME CARE, Standards 9.1 through 9.25.1.

[22]JOINT COMMISSION, 1998 COMPREHENSIVE ACCREDITATION MANUAL FOR HOSPITALS, Standard IM 7.2.

that medical records thoroughly document operative or other procedures and the use of anesthesia[23] and include specific information when a patient is treated in the hospital emergency department.[24]

Whether or not specific statutory or regulatory guidelines apply, hospitals and other health care organizations or providers should adopt formal written policies concerning the content of medical records. The policy may be a detailed list of data required, or may reference other guidelines, such as state statutes, regulations, or pertinent accreditation standards. Generally, detailed policies require closer periodic review to be kept current, while broad policies remain applicable as circumstance and practice change. The policies should balance the need for providing enough specificity to guide medical records clinical practitioners and the organization's staff against the desire to avoid continual policy revisions.

To maintain the currency of their medical record policies, health care providers should keep abreast of state, federal, and accreditation association requirements relating to medical records. State and national health information associations often publish changes in the applicable law and accreditation standards. All health care institutions should develop reliable ways of monitoring new laws and regulations, and communicating any changes to medical records practitioners and clinical personnel responsible for making entries in records and to the individuals responsible for making policy recommendations concerning medical record content.

In particular, this latter group of individuals should understand the various functions of the medical record and their interrelationships, as well as how those functions are affected by the nature of the specific institution and by current legislative, regulatory, and licensing requirements. Creating an effective record content policy requires the involvement of a variety of disciplines within an organization and of providers who deliver care from networks or facilities outside the organization. Policymakers must be willing to find ways to make practical adjustments to medical record content. In doing so, they should strike a balance among the administrative, financial, and other demands placed upon the medical record and the record's basic patient care function.

---

[23]Joint Commission, 1998 Comprehensive Accreditation Manual for Hospitals, Standard IM 7.3.

[24]Joint Commission, 1998 Comprehensive Accreditation Manual for Hospitals, Standards IM 7.5. through 7.5.3.

RECORD RETENTION REQUIREMENTS

In determining how long to retain medical records, a health care facility should consider applicable federal or state laws and regulations, and sound administrative policy and medical practice. The nature of the facility and the resources available to maintain documents for an extended period of time also will influence its retention policy. Achieving a practical and workable medical record retention policy becomes more difficult in an era of cost containment and reduced financial resources.

Numerous factors need to be considered in establishing a retention policy. First and foremost, a retention policy must respect the applicable statutory and regulatory requirements. Other factors to be considered in defining a retention policy are statutes of limitations and potential future litigation, requirements of the provider's malpractice insurer, the need for records information in medical research and teaching, storage capabilities, cost of microfilming, computerization and other long-term storage methods, and recommendations of provider-specific health care associations. The minimum standard for compliance with respect to retention is that enunciated in the applicable statutes and regulations. A health care provider may establish a retention period longer than the one dictated by statutory or regulatory requirements, however, where it becomes prudent for other considerations to do so.

Statutory and Regulatory Concerns

Medicare conditions of participation require hospitals to retain the original record or a legally reproduced form for a period of at least five years.[25] State statutes and regulations also impose specific retention requirements on medical records.[26] In most jurisdictions, record retention requirements, like content requirements, appear in regulations issued by the state licensing agency. Many jurisdictions also have special retention provisions for certain portions of a patient's record (such as X-rays, graphic data, and discharge summaries), special procedures for records of patients who are minors, and other provisions for records pertaining to deceased persons.

A few states impose extended retention requirements. In Connecticut, for example, a hospital must preserve patient records for a minimum of 25

---

[25]42 C.F.R. § 482.24.

[26]*See, e.g.,* ALASKA STAT. §18.20.085; IND. CODE § 16-397-1; LA. REV. STAT. ANN. § 40:2144; MISS. CODE ANN. § 41-9-69; TENN. CODE ANN. § 68-11-305.

years[27] and in Alabama for at least 22 years.[28] New Jersey requires a discharge summary to be kept for each patient for 20 years that includes a recapitulation of the significant findings and events that occurred during hospitalization and a statement concerning the patient's condition at discharge.[29] The original medical record must be kept for at least ten years.

Most of the remaining states establish a shorter minimum time for preserving the entire patient record. About half of them require at least a ten-year preservation period, while the rest prescribe some number less than ten. Arizona requires patient medical records to be readily retrievable for at least three years and many other states prescribe a minimum of five or seven years.[30]

In some cases, licensing regulations identify no particular number of years to maintain patient records. Instead, the rules refer to other sources of law to define the minimum requirements of record retention, such as the state statute of limitations for malpractice claims as the minimum retention period,[31] the conditions of participation for federal reimbursement programs,[32] or guidelines set by the American Hospital Association.[33]

A few states provide that records may be kept for a minimum number of years plus an additional period determined by the hospital. This additional time could serve the hospital's needs for "clinical, educational, statistical, or administrative purposes,"[34] or extend for as long as the record has "research, legal, or medical value."[35] Of course, hospitals and other health care facilities in any state may retain records beyond the period prescribed by statute or regulation if clinical, legal, or patient care policies indicate such a need. At least one state's regulations specify that nothing in the law should be construed to prohibit retention beyond the period prescribed.[36]

---

[27]CONN. AGENCIES REGS. § 19-13-D3(d)(6).

[28]ALA. ADMIN. CODE r. 420-5-7.07(1)(c).

[29]N.J. REV. STAT. § 26:8-5 and N.J. ADMIN. CODE tit. 8, § 43G-15.2(g). *See also* Ark. Rules and Regulations for Hospitals and Related Institutions, § 601(Y); KAN. ADMIN. REGS. 28-34-9a(d).

[30]ARIZ. COMP. R. & REGS. R9-10-221(F). States that have five year retention periods include Kentucky and Oklahoma. States that have seven year retention periods include Pennsylvania and Indiana.

[31]*See, e.g.,* IOWA ADMIN. Code r. 641-51.6(1).

[32]*See* MICH. ADMIN. CODE r. 325.1021(4).

[33]*See, e.g.,* ILL. ADMIN. CODE tit. 77, § 250.1510(d).

[34]MO. CODE REGS. ANN. tit. 19, § 30-20.021(3)(D)(15).

[35]N.D. ADMIN. CODE § 33-07-01.1-20(1)(6)(3).

[36]MONT. ADMIN. R. 16.32.328(5) (1989).

In addition to the general retention requirements described above, Medicare conditions of participation and several states have special statutory or regulatory provisions governing how long a hospital should maintain specific portions of a patient's record, such as X-rays, scans, and clinical laboratory reports.[37] Health care facilities also must comply with retention laws on vital statistics, including records of births and deaths.[38]

Many states prescribe special retention requirements for records of patients who were minors at the time of treatment, usually requiring that these records be kept. These requirements usually indicate that hospitals must keep records until the patient reaches majority plus some additional time, or until the expiration of the general retention requirement, whichever is longer.[39] The prescribed extension ranges from one to ten years beyond the age of majority.

A few states also address the issue of deceased patients' records. These regulations allow the facility to destroy records of a deceased patient before the expiration of the general retention requirement. The general retention period for hospital medical records in Oklahoma, for instance, is five years after the patient was last seen, or at least three years beyond the patient's death.[40]

Statutes of Limitations

Another key factor in establishing a record retention policy is the statute of limitations on contract and tort actions. A statute of limitations is a period of time established by statute, measured in years, within which a party may bring a lawsuit. The time periods vary with the cause of action (e.g., contract, tort, or real estate).

Except in the case of minors' records, retaining the record for the limitations period would not impose a burden since limitation periods generally are shorter than the period the record would be retained for medical reasons. If the statute of limitations were used as a guide, the medical record of a minor would be kept until the patient reaches the age of majority plus the period of the statute. For example, in a state where the age of

---

[37]*See, e.g.,* 42 C.F.R. § 482.26(d)(2); ALASKA STAT. § 18.20.085; CAL. CODE REGS. tit. 22, § 70751(c); IDAHO CODE § 39-1394(b).

[38]*See, e.g.,* Rules and Regulations for the Licensure of Hospitals in Virginia § 12 VAC 5-410-370(H).

[39]*See, e.g.,* California and Virginia.

[40]Okla. Hospital Standards § 310-667-19-14 (a).

majority is 21 and the statute of limitations for torts is two years, the retention period for a newborn's record would be 23 years; in states in which the age of majority is 18, and the statute of limitations for torts is two years, the retention period for a newborn's record would be 20 years. While the possibility of an infant's waiting until majority to bring suit is slight, it can happen.[41] Although most suits by minors are brought soon after the accident causing the injury, a health care provider is protected best if it retains records until the minor reaches majority and for an additional time equal to the applicable state statute of limitations on tort actions.

Medical Research and Storage Space Considerations

If a hospital or other medical facility engages in extensive medical research, especially retrospective investigations that require detailed medical record data, the institution may wish to establish a long retention period. Moreover, if the medical research conducted in the hospital involves experimental or innovative patient care procedures, the facility is well advised to retain its medical records for at least 75 years.

Another major consideration for a hospital in establishing a retention policy is its capability to store a large number of records. Available space, expansion rates, the endurance of the paper and folders used, the cost of microfilming, and storage safety requirements all affect the institution's ability to retain records. Some space savings may be achieved by microfilming records or storing them on optical disks or in computer media, but microfilming can raise other administrative problems. For example, members of the medical staff might object to the restrictions on the availability of particular records for purposes of research and review, generating additional costs for reading and printing equipment. Some states implicitly or explicitly authorize the microfilming of records.[42]

Where state law and regulations do not specifically authorize microfilming, health care facilities nonetheless may microfilm their medical records and destroy the original records in accordance with law or regulations governing record destruction.

A health care facility may microfilm its records itself, provided it has the proper staff and equipment, or it may send its records to an outside contract service to be filmed. If a contract service is selected, it should be

---

[41]*See, e.g.,* Bettigole v. Deiner, 124 A.2d 265 (Md. Ct. App. 1956).

[42]*See, e.g.,* Ga. Rules & Regulations for Hospitals § 290-5-6.11(h); Idaho Code § 39-1394(a); La. Rev. Stat. Ann. § 40:2144(E) & (F); Mass. Ann. Laws ch. 111, § 70; N.J. Rev. Stat. § 26:8-5.

bound by a written agreement that specifies, among other things, the method of record transfer, the method of reproduction, the quality and cost of the service, the time within which the service will be performed, safeguards against breach of confidentiality, indemnification for loss resulting from the contractor's improper release of information or loss of records, and procedures for destroying the original records.

A health care facility also might consider storing its records in computers. Before deciding on this method of recordkeeping, however, it should consult applicable laws governing licensure, accreditation, federal conditions of participation, and all rules of evidence on the admissibility of copies of business records and patient records at trial. (For a detailed discussion of computerized patient records, see Chapter 13 COMPUTERIZED MEDICAL RECORDS.)

Association Guidelines

The American Health Information Management Association (AHIMA) has adopted a policy that recommends retaining patient health information for the following minimum time periods:

Patient health records (adults)	10 years after most recent encounter
Patient health records (minors)	Age of majority plus statute of limitations
Diagnostic images	5 years
Disease index	10 years
Fetal heart monitor records	10 years after infant reaches majority
Master patient index	Permanently
Operative index	10 years
Physician index	10 years
Register of births	Permanently
Register of deaths	Permanently
Register of surgical procedures	Permanently[43]

---

[43]American Health Information Management Association, Practice Guidelines for Managing Health Information, Retention of Health Information.

Developing a Record Retention Policy

In the final analysis, no blanket record retention rule can be devised. The length of time medical records should be retained after they no longer are needed for medical and administrative purposes should be determined by the facility's administration with the advice of legal counsel, taking into account all factors, including the feasibility and cost of microfilming, the availability and cost of storage space, and the possible future need for such records, as well as the legal considerations arising from lawsuits. In most professional negligence actions against a health care facility or provider, the defendant must show that the care provided was consistent with accepted medical practice at the time and was reasonable under the circumstances. Medical records usually are essential to the defense of such actions. Although courts generally reject the existence of a responsibility by one party to preserve evidence or records for another party's potential suit in the absence of some special relationship or contractual duty between the parties,[44] several courts have recognized a hospital's duty to maintain patient records as a matter of statute or regulation.[45]

Specifically, in cases where the plaintiff had insufficient evidence to pursue a malpractice suit against a hospital because the hospital was unable to produce the patient's record, courts have found the facility liable for this independent act of negligence or have ruled that the plaintiff states a cause of action in negligence.

In one case,[46] a Florida court ruled that a hospital may be sued for its failure to make and maintain patient medical records because state law imposes a duty to make, maintain, and furnish such records to a patient or personal representative upon request. A woman whose husband died during the administration of anesthesia before surgery sued the hospital for negligence. She could not present expert testimony necessary to establish medical malpractice, however, because the anesthesiology records of her husband's treatment could not be located. The appeals court found that a hospital's duty to make and maintain medical records is imposed by state administrative regulations, and that state law further requires that copies of records be provided to patients at their request. The woman was entitled to sue the hospital for negligently breaching these duties, the court con-

---

[44]*See* Panich v. Iron Wood Products Corp., 445 N.W.2d 795 (Mich. Ct. App. 1989); Koplin v. Rosel Well Perforators, Inc., 734 P.2d 1177 (D. Kan. 1987).

[45]*See, e.g.*, Fox v. Cohen, 406 N.E.2d 178 (1980).

[46]*See* Bondu v. Gurvich, 473 So. 2d 1307 (Fla. Dist. Ct. App. 1984). *See also* Thomas v. United States, 660 F. Supp. 216 (D.D.C. 1987).

cluded, because the hospital otherwise "stands to benefit that the prospect of successful litigation against it has disappeared along with the crucial evidence."

An Illinois appeals court also ruled that state legislation governing the retention of X-rays creates the right to sue a hospital for its failure to keep X-rays.[47] The court noted that state law requires hospitals to retain X-rays as part of their regularly maintained records for a period of five years. The statute clearly seeks to protect the property rights of persons involved in litigation, the court declared. According to the court, violating a statute that is designed to protect either property or human life is evidence of negligence.

A patient may not be entitled to sue a hospital for its failure to comply with records retention legislation, however, unless the individual also proves damages and a causal connection with the injuries sustained. In one case,[48] a court dismissed a negligence action against a hospital for failing to preserve all the X-rays taken of a patient. A Medical Malpractice Review Panel had rejected a malpractice complaint after considering only the X-rays still available. The court stated that the patient had failed to show any damages resulting from the alleged negligence of the hospital and dismissed the suit. Similarly, in the Illinois case discussed above,[49] the court ruled that the plaintiff was entitled to sue the hospital for violating the retention statute, but that to succeed, he would have to prove that the violation resulted in the dismissal of his suit against other health care providers.

DESTRUCTION OF THE RECORD

Upon expiration of the medical records retention period, or after the record has been copied onto microfilm or computer or converted to other machine-readable form, the record usually may be destroyed. In some states, the method of medical record destruction is controlled by statute and regulation. The Tennessee statute states:

> Upon retirement of the record as provided in [this section], the record or any part thereof retired shall be destroyed by burning, shredding, or other effective method in keeping with the confi-

---

[47]Rodgers v. St. Mary's Hosp., 556 N.E.2d 913 (Ill. App. Ct. 1990).

[48]*See* Hryniak v. Nathan Littauer Hosp. Assoc., 446 N.Y.S.2d 558 (App. Div. 1982).

[49]Rodgers v. St. Mary's Hosp., 556 N.E. 2d 913 (Ill. App. Ct. 1990).

dential nature of its contents. Destruction of such records must be made in the ordinary course of business and no record shall be destroyed on an individual basis.[50]

Other states require that an abstract of any pertinent data in the medical record be created before destroying the record.[51] Health care facilities that deliver their medical records to a commercial enterprise for destruction should do so pursuant to a written agreement that sets forth safeguards similar to those discussed for microfilming agreements, including the method of destruction, safeguards against breach of confidentiality, indemnification provisions, and certification that the records have been destroyed properly. Similarly, health care providers that destroy their own records also must establish procedures to protect the confidentiality of record information and ensure that records are destroyed completely. The employee responsible for record destruction should certify that the records have been destroyed properly. Whether the records are destroyed commercially or by the facility itself, certificates of destruction should be retained permanently as evidence of disposal.

A health care facility's medical records policies should include provisions governing destruction of records, and these provisions should be applied uniformly. Failure to apply such a policy uniformly or a violation of policy can lead to a damaging inference by a jury in a negligence suit that if the records were available, they would show that the patient did not receive adequate care.[52]

[50]TENN. CODE ANN. § 68-11-305(c). *See also* IDAHO CODE § 39-1394(d).

[51]MISS. CODE ANN. § 41-9-75.

[52]Carr v. St. Paul Fire Ins. Co., 384 F. Supp. 821 (W.D. Ark. 1974).

4

Medical Record Entries

Chapter Objectives

- Illustrate how legibility and accuracy are important to the quality of medical records.
- Give examples of how poor legibility can create difficulties for a health care provider in defending against a claim of poor medical care.
- Explain how inaccurate or incomplete entries can impact claims review and the payment for services.
- Discuss the standards that govern the completeness, accuracy and legibility of medical records.
- Define what timeliness means with respect to medical record entries and the consequences of failing to comply with this standard.
- Distinguish between authorship and countersignatures of medical record entries.
- Explain why authentication is a key element of medical record security and what standards apply to how and when records are authenticated.
- Define auto-authentication and recommend safeguards for auto-authentication systems.
- Discuss how verbal orders affect the quality of medical record entries and what specific policies should be in place to govern how these orders are received and recorded.

- List the types of errors that occur in medical record entries and proper procedures for correcting or altering a medical record.

INTRODUCTION

The quality of a patient record depends largely on the individuals making record entries. All health care practitioners and others who write in patient records must understand the importance of creating legible, complete, and accurate records and the legal and medical implications of failing to do so. Because a medical record enables health care professionals to plan and evaluate a patient's treatment and ensures continuity of care among multiple providers, the quality of care a patient receives depends directly on the accuracy and legibility of the information the medical record contains. The increased emphasis on fraud and abuse prevention in the health care industry has further highlighted the importance of proper medical record documentation. The best evidence a health care provider can offer against allegations of false claims and billing is the data contained in the patient records that are under scrutiny. In addition, a health care facility that fails to comply with medical record standards found in federal and state law risks loss of licensure, accreditation, and eligibility to participate in federal reimbursement programs. Finally, health care providers run the risk of increased exposure in the event of a medical malpractice suit if the entries they make to medical records do not accurately describe the patient's condition or the treatment provided.

A health care organization or provider should strive to ensure that the original entries made to medical records are timely and complete. Corrections to records, while perfectly permissible, can create serious problems, especially for a health care provider involved in negligence litigation. Even if the correction improves the accuracy of the record, a correction can generate difficulties if it is improperly made or deteriorates legibility. In addition, any alterations made simply to improve the defense of a lawsuit or to defraud third-party payers can have serious adverse consequences for a health care provider, including the imposition of criminal sanctions. For all these reasons, therefore, a health care provider's medical records policy should address the timeliness and manner for both creating and updating patient records.

LEGIBLE AND COMPLETE MEDICAL RECORD ENTRIES

The medical record often is the single most important document available to health care providers or organizations in the defense of a negligence action and ordinarily is admissible as evidence of what occurred in the care of the patient. (For a discussion of the admissibility of medical records, see Chapter 10, DISCOVERY AND ADMISSIBILITY OF MEDCIAL RECORDS.) Without a legible and complete medical record, a health care provider may be unable to successfully defend against allegations of improper care. In addition, some courts will allow the jury to resolve any ambiguities in a patient's record in favor of the patient.

Medical record entries should be made in clear and concise language that can be understood by all the health care professionals who treat the patient. An ambiguous or illegible record often is worse than no record, because it documents a failure to communicate clearly, and thus has an adverse impact on the quality of care. This is particularly important in a managed care delivery system, such as a health maintenance organization, where services are frequently provided by different providers who rely heavily on the data a medical record contains to fully understand a patient's medical history.

Maintaining a complete record is important not only to comply with licensing and accreditation requirements (for a more detailed discussion relating to these requirements, see Chapter 3, MEDICAL RECORD REQUIREMENTS), but also to enable a health care provider to establish that a patient received adequate care. If a hospital or other health care provider can demonstrate by testimony that, in accordance with its policy and procedures, it regularly keeps complete and accurate records, the absence of certain notations may be used to defend against a claim of negligence. In *Smith v. Rogers Memorial Hospital*,[1] the medical records of a hospital patient did not indicate that the patient had complained of certain symptoms. In this case, however, testimony that the hospital's records were generally reliable was important evidence in rebutting the patient's claim that she had complained of the symptoms and had not received proper care.

Similarly, in *Hurlock v. Park Lane Medical Center*,[2] a physician ordered that the patient be turned in bed every two hours, but the medical record

---

[1]Smith v. Rogers Mem'l Hosp., 382 A.2d 1025 (D.C. Ct. App. 1978), *cert. denied*, 439 U.S. 847 (1978).

[2]Hurlock v. Park Lane Med. Ctr., 709 S.W.2d 872 (Mo. Ct. App. 1985).

did not indicate each time the patient had been turned. The patient argued that the absence of notes was evidence that the nurses negligently had failed to follow the physician's order, causing the patient to develop serious bedsores and necessitating amputation of her leg. Expert testimony established that, while proper nursing practice required notations to be placed in the patient's record, nurses sometimes get very busy and fail to document each action taken for patients such as the plaintiff who require special attention. In such cases, accepted nursing practice places patient care in priority over proper documentation. Without any direct evidence that the hospital nurses had failed to turn the patient as directed, equally plausible inferences about the patient's care arose from the medical record, the court ruled, and dismissed the suit.

Conversely, courts have allowed an inference of negligence where hospital records fail to include certain data, or fail to comport with adequate medical recordkeeping in general. In a California case,[3] an appeals court ruled that a physician's inability to produce his original records relating to a patient's treatment in defense of a malpractice suit created an inference of the physician's consciousness of guilt. In another case,[4] a federal appeals court held that a jury was entitled to find, or at least to infer, negligence from an incomplete medical record where the plaintiff developed eye problems associated with an excessive use of oxygen at birth. Given the absence of documentation about the amount of oxygen actually ordered or administered, the court accepted testimony from the child's father regarding oxygen administration he remembered observing at the hospital. Based on this evidence, the court upheld the jury's finding of negligence.

Other courts, however, have dismissed claims against health care facilities involving incomplete medical records, ruling that a facility cannot be liable for a patient's injuries where the inadequacy of the records does not proximately cause the patient's harm. One case involved a patient under the constant, direct care of an emergency room physician who did not request information about the individual's vital signs before making a diagnosis. The hospital's failure to take and record the patient's vital signs did not proximately cause an exacerbation of the patient's injuries stemming from the physician's misdiagnosis, the court ruled.[5]

---

[3]Thor v. Boska, 113 Cal. Rptr. 296 (Cal. Ct. App. 1974).

[4]Valdon Martinez v. Hosp. Presbiterno, 806 F.2d 1128 (1st Cir. 1986).

[5]Yaney v. McCray Mem'l Hosp., 469 N.E.2d 135 (Ind. Ct. App. 1986).

While some courts have allowed juries to *infer* negligence by health care providers based on reasonable conclusions drawn from incomplete patient records, other courts have gone further, allowing juries to *presume* negligence when records contain significant omissions. A presumption of negligence affects the evidentiary burden of a defendant health care provider to a much greater extent than a mere inference of negligence. In general, a malpractice plaintiff must show each act of negligence with a preponderance of the evidence. If a plaintiff fails to meet this burden, the court will dismiss the suit, even if the facility presents no evidence in its defense. A presumption of negligence shifts the responsibility to the health care provider to prove that it acted properly. This shift in the burden of proof makes defending against a malpractice suit more difficult, especially when medical records documenting the treatment provided are incomplete.[6]

In addition to ensuring the delivery and evidence of adequate patient care, another significant use of medical record information is to facilitate payment for services and claims review. The failure to insert proper notations of care on a patient's chart, therefore, may lead not only to a finding of provider negligence with respect to the patient's medical care but also to difficulties in recovering the financial cost of the care that was provided. This was illustrated in an Arkansas appeals court ruling on the accuracy of a computerized bill containing charges for services and medication that were not reflected in the patient's chart.[7,8] Because the evidence revealed the strong possibility that the bill contained charges for medication not given, services not rendered, procedures not performed, and supplies not delivered, the court ruled that the bill was insufficient to sustain the hospital's claim for the cost of the patient's medical care.

The importance of complete, accurate, and legible medical record documentation has been highlighted recently in conjunction with health care fraud and abuse prevention and the development of corporate compliance programs in many health care facilities. Federal and state legislation impose a complex and expanding array of restrictions on the way health care providers conduct business and structure relationships among themselves,

---

[6]For an interesting discussion on the role medical records play in determining the outcome of a medical malpractice suit, see L. Stevens, "Let the Record Show . . .," *American Medical News*, May 26, 1997, p. 11.

[7]Tracor/MBA v. Baptist Med. Ctr.,780 S.W.2d 26 (Ark. Ct. App. 1989).

[8]*See in particular* 42 U.S.C. §§ 1320a-7a & 1320a-7b.

generally known as fraud and abuse provisions. At the federal level, these provisions are primarily found in the Medicare/Medicaid statute and Stark legislation[9] and are enforced under the auspices of these statutes, the civil False Claims Act,[10] and a number of other federal laws applicable to fraudulent activities.

The reach of federal legislation governing health care fraud and abuse expanded with the enactment of the Health Care Insurance Portability and Accountability Act (HIPAA).[11] The statute creates a new offense of "health care fraud," defined as "knowingly and willfully executing or attempting to execute, a scheme or artifice to defraud any health care benefit program or to obtain, by means of false or fraudulent pretenses, representations or promises, any of the money owned by or under the custody or control of any health care benefit program." Other federal offenses relating to health care fraud created under the new statute include theft or embezzlement, false statements, and obstruction of criminal investigations.

Allegations relating to false claims and fraudulent billing practices are the object of the vast majority of government enforcement initiatives. These practices involve claims for payment under any federal health care program in which the item or service provided to the patient is misrepresented or claims for services or supplies substantially exceed what the patient actually needed. In order to investigate fraud and abuse violations, the Office of the Inspector General (OIG) of the Department of Health and Human Services has broad authority to access the medical records relating to the services that were allegedly misrepresented or falsified in the claims for payment. The information contained in medical records must be complete and accurate, therefore, to allow a health care provider to defend against the potentially devastating sanctions that can arise in these instances. (For a more detailed discussion of the OIG's investigative authority, see "Fraud and Abuse Investigations" in Chapter 8, DOCUMENTATION AND DISCLOSURE: SPECIAL AREAS OF CONCERN).

Statutes, accreditation standards, and professional associations frequently impose standards relating to the legibility, accuracy, and completeness of medical records. Federal conditions of participation in Medicare, for example, require that all entries to hospital records be legi-

---

[9]42 U.S.C. § 1395nn.
[10]31 U.S.C. §§ 3729 through 3733.
[11]Pub. L. No. 104-191.

ble and complete.[12] Conditions of participation for other types of health care providers contain similar standards.[13] State law imposes similar requirements on medical record entries, frequently found in the licensing regulations for specific types of facilities,[14] or in regulations governing the medical records created by a broader category of health care providers.[15] Accreditation standards frequently impose a variation of the completeness and legibility standard found in state laws. Joint Commission on Accreditation of Healthcare Organizations (Joint Commission) standards of accreditation for hospitals, for example, require that data be collected in a timely, economic, and efficient manner using the degree of accuracy and completeness necessary for the data's required use.[16] Joint Commission standards for managed care plans, integrated delivery networks, and provider-sponsored networks require that member health records be periodically reviewed for completeness, accuracy, and timeliness of the information they contain.[17] Principles of medical record documentation developed by a number of professional associations also recommend that a medical record be legible and complete.[18]

To avoid liability and ensure compliance with the numerous laws and standards that govern their operations, therefore, health care facilities must be certain that all staff members clearly document the care provided to patients. In sensitive cases when careful observations are essential, all staff members should record with particular precision their contacts with patients. A health care provider should never compromise its standards of medical record documentation in the interest of efficiency or cost containment.

---

[12]42 C.F.R. § 482.24(c).

[13]*See, e.g.*, 42 C.F.R. § 416.47(b), which requires ambulatory surgical services to maintain a medical record for each patient that is accurate, legible, and promptly completed.

[14]*See, e.g.*, New Jersey Regulations, Hospital Licensing Standards, NJAC 8:43G-15.2(b) and Maine Regulations 10 144 112 §12.E.

[15]*See, e.g.*, Oregon Regulation OAR § 333-505-050.

[16]JOINT COMMISSION, 1998 COMPREHENSIVE ACCREDITATION MANUAL FOR HOSPITALS, Standard IM 3.2.

[17]JOINT COMMISSION, 1998-2000 COMPREHENSIVE ACCREDITATION MANUAL FOR HEALTH CARE NETWORKS, Standard IM 3.2.1.

[18]*See* American Health Information Management Association, Principles of Medical Record Documentation, developed jointly by representatives of the American Health Information Management Association, American Hospital Association, American Managed Care and Review Association, the American Medical Association, the American Medical Peer Review Association, Blue Cross and Blue Shield Association, and the Health Insurance Association of America.

TIMELY MEDICAL RECORD ENTRIES

Medical records not only must be accurate but also must be completed in a timely manner. Entries to the record should be made when the treatment they describe is given or the observations to be documented are made. Specific legislative requirements that entries be made within a certain time following a patient's discharge also exist. Regulations on participation in federal reimbursement programs, for example, require that hospital records be complete within 30 days following the patient's discharge.[19] State licensing regulations for health care facilities also frequently contain specific time frames for completing records.[20] Joint Commission standards of accreditation for a variety of health care organizations also impose timeliness as a standard for gathering medical record data.[21]

A health care facility's bylaws or policies should require staff members to complete patient records within the specified time and should provide an automatic suspension of clinical privileges for those who fail to comply. Usually, the medical records department or health information manager has the responsibility for making sure records are completed within a specific time, and therefore should establish procedures for notifying attending physicians when records are incomplete.

The timeliness of medical record entries is important for many of the same reasons as the standards relating to legibility and completeness. Late entries to medical records mean that the records are in fact incomplete for a period of time, and, like other deficiencies, this can have disastrous consequences in defending against a professional negligence action. In addition, entries that are not contemporaneous with the service provided are less likely to be accurate, and will therefore have less credibility than those made during or immediately after the treatment. If an entry is made after a lawsuit is threatened or filed, it may appear to have been made for self-serving purposes of establishing a defense rather than for documenting the actual treatment rendered.

---

[19]42 C.F.R. § 482.24(c)(2)(viii).

[20]*See, e.g.*, KAN. ADMIN. Regs. § 28-34-9a(f) (1992); Regulations for the Licensure of General and Specialty Hospitals in Maine, 10 144 112 §12.E.7, requiring records of patients discharged to be completed within 15 days after release.

[21]*See, e.g.*, JOINT COMMISSION, 1998-2000 COMPREHENSIVE ACCREDITATION MANUAL FOR HEALTH CARE NETWORKS, Standard IM 3.1, 1998 COMPREHENSIVE ACCREDITATION MANUAL FOR HOSPITALS, Standard IM 7.6, and 1997-98 COMPREHENSIVE ACCREDITATION MANUAL FOR HOME CARE, Standard IM 3.

AUTHORSHIP AND COUNTERSIGNATURES

As the number and types of people making entries in patient medical records increases, especially in a managed care environment, it becomes increasingly important for health care facilities to have policies addressing who may make entries in a record in order to safeguard the quality of patient care and reduce liability exposure.

State law typically does not impose restrictions on the type of professionals who may write entries in the chart—who may do so is generally a matter of policy within a health care facility. Medical record entries are typically authored by the clinical provider who delivers the service to the patient, and as a rule any person providing care to a patient should be permitted to document that care in the individual's medical record, regardless of the person's position within the facility.

It is the responsibility of a health care facility, therefore, to establish policies that require individual practitioners to function within the scope of practice as authorized by state licensing or certification statutes or, in the absence of such statutes, as defined by their professional competence.[22] Facilities should also define the level of record documentation expected of practitioners working in the institution based on the practitioner's licensure, certification, and professional competence. To the extent that a facility permits physician assistants, nurse midwives, podiatrists, dentists, clinical psychologists, and other nonphysician practitioners to provide treatment, it should require them to document their treatment in accordance with its policy.

The entries of certain individuals do, however, require a physician's countersignature. The purpose of countersignatures is to require a professional to review and, if appropriate, indicate approval of action taken by another practitioner. Usually, the person countersigning a record entry is more experienced or has received a higher level of training than the person who made the original entry. In any case, the person required to countersign should be the individual who has the authority to evaluate the entry. Countersignatures should be viewed as a means for carrying out delegated responsibility, rather than as additional paperwork.

---

[22]*See* JOINT COMMISSION, 1998 COMPREHENSIVE ACCREDITATION MANUAL FOR HOSPITALS, Standard IM 7.1.1, which requires that only authorized individuals make entries in medical records. *See also* JOINT COMMISSION, 1997-98 COMPREHENSIVE ACCREDITATION MANUAL FOR HOME CARE, Standard 9.1, to the same effect.

In most hospitals, for example, licensed house staff members may make entries in patient charts, but attending physicians are required to countersign some or all such entries.[23] In addition, when undergraduate medical students and unlicensed house staff members make record entries that show the application of medical judgment, medical diagnosis, prescription of treatment, or any other act defined by applicable state law to be the practice of medicine, these entries should be countersigned by a licensed physician, who may be an attending or a resident physician. In most states, it is a violation of the medical licensure act for anyone to practice medicine without a license unless the individual is practicing under the direct, proximate supervision of a physician licensed to practice in the state. Therefore, without evidence of such supervision, the student or unlicensed resident might be held to have violated state law. The rules governing a physician's countersignature of medical record entries made by other authorized personnel should be set forth in the hospital's medical staff rules and regulations.

Similarly, the entries of undergraduate nursing students should be countersigned by a licensed professional nurse, if such entries document the practice of professional nursing as defined by the state's nursing licensure act. Without evidence of proper supervision, a nursing student practicing professional nursing could be held in violation of the state's nursing licensure act unless the act specifically authorizes nursing student.[24] The nursing licensure acts of some states also authorize graduate nurses who have applied for a license to practice professional nursing for a limited time without a license.[25] Graduate, unlicensed nurses in those states may make entries in medical records without countersignature by a licensed nurse. In states that have no specific allowances for practice by such graduates, however, their entries should be countersigned.

AUTHENTICATION OF RECORDS

The requirement that the physician or other medical practitioner sign the records or a portion thereof exists to ensure authenticity. Authentication is the key element in system reliability and security. Traditionally, authentication was made by handwritten signature. However, numerous reg-

---

[23]*See, e.g.*, Regulations for the Licensure of General and Specialty Hospitals in Maine, ch. XII-I.3; Minimum Standards of Operation for Mississippi Hospitals, § 1709.4.

[25]*See, e.g.*, 225 ILL. COMP. STAT. ANN. 65/4(b).

ulatory and accrediting organizations also contemplate authentication by a rubber stamp or computer key as well.

The Joint Commission accreditation standards for hospitals, for example, require that medical records be authenticated when necessary.[26] At a minimum, entries of histories and physical examinations, operative procedures, consultations, and discharge summaries must be authenticated, but the facility's policy may designate other types of entries that require authentication in accordance with state law and regulations.

Examples of authentication systems that would meet this accreditation standard include:

- computer entries that allow for an online review of the document and entry of a computer code to signify approval
- a procedure in which transcripts are mailed to the author, who reviews the entry and signs and returns a post card indicating that the records have been reviewed and attesting to their accuracy
- a system that allows for review and approval with a single signature of a list of specific unsigned entries in a record, where the list is permanently retained in the record.[27]

Medicare Conditions of Participation require that all entries to a patient's record be authenticated and dated promptly by the person responsible for ordering, providing, or evaluating the service furnished.[28] The author of each entry must be identified and must authenticate the entry. Under those regulations, authentication may include signatures, written initials, or computer entry.

States also permit authentication by rubber stamp or computer key, in addition to the traditional handwritten signature. All of the states that permit this type of authentication impose controls to safeguard against abuse by limiting access to and use of the authenticating devices to the properly authorized individuals. For example, in California, the State Department of Health Services has regulations providing the following:

---

[26]JOINT COMMISSION, 1998 COMPREHENSIVE ACCREDITATION MANUAL FOR HOSPITALS, Standard IM 7.8.

[27]See JOINT COMMISSION, 1998 COMPREHENSIVE ACCREDITATION MANUAL FOR HOSPITALS, Standards, Intents, and Examples for Patient-Specific Data and Information, Example of Evidence of Implementation for IM 7.8.

[28]42 C.F.R. § 482.24(c)(1).

Medical records shall be completed promptly and authenticated or signed by a physician, dentist or podiatrist within two weeks following the patient's discharge. Medical records may be authenticated by a signature stamp or computer key, in lieu of a physician's signature, only when that physician has placed a signed statement in the hospital administrative offices to the effect that he is the only person who:

(1) has possession of the stamp or key.

(2) will use the stamp or key.[29]

Similarly, Arkansas permits physicians to use rubber-stamp signatures if the method is approved in writing by the hospital administrator and the medical records committee, and requires that the stamp be locked in the medical records department when the physician is not using it.[30] Indiana requires that all physicians' orders for medication and treatment be in writing or acceptable computerized form and be signed by hand or computer key by the attending physician within 24 hours.[31]

Some states, however, do not specifically address the substitution of rubber stamps or computers for the physician's handwritten signature, or impose authentication requirements that appear to preclude the use of stamps or computer codes. For example, Alabama requires that entries in the medical record be made in ink or be typewritten and that they be authenticated and signed or initialed by the attending physician.[32] In Arizona, the person responsible for each entry "shall be identified by initials or signature."[33] In Kansas, each clinical entry must be signed or initialed by the attending physician, who must be identified properly in the record.[34] New Jersey requires that all entries be written in ink, dated, and either signed by the recording person or authenticated through the use of a computerized medical records system.[35]

Because applicable law in these states may be ambiguous or conflicting, hospitals seeking to use alternatives to handwritten signatures should con-

---

[29]CAL. CODE REGS. tit. 22, § 70751(g).

[30]Rules and Regulations for Hospitals and Related Institutions in Arkansas, § 0601(I).

[31]IND. ADMIN. CODE tit. 410 r. 9(1)(d).

[32]ALA. ADMIN. CODE r. § 420-5-7-.07(1)(g).

[33]Arizona Hospital Licensing Regulations § R9-10-221(L).

[34]KAN. ADMIN. REGS. 28-34-9a(f).

[35]N.J. ADMIN. CODE tit. 8, § 43G.-15.2(b).

sult with their legal counsel. Although some courts may be willing to accept an expansive definition of the terms "writing" and "signature," no general rule exists that authentication of medical records may be accomplished by any method other than a written signature. If state law requires a handwritten signature for authentication, the institution must provide for such authentication, even if it maintains its records in computers. The only alternative for the institution or state hospital association is to embark on the often long and difficult task of obtaining an amendment of the applicable restrictive state law.

Auto-Authentication

The introduction of computer technology to medical records management has provided opportunities to improve the speed and accuracy of the authentication process. Computerizing medical records, however, has introduced a new risk that the technology will replace rather than supplement the input of practitioners and hospital personnel into this process of verifying the accuracy and completeness of medical records. In particular, these concerns have arisen with respect to the process of auto-authentication, in which a physician authenticates a report by computer code before the report is transcribed. Physicians enter an electronic signature, and agree to review and correct transcripts of electronic medical records within a certain time frame. If no corrections are made by the deadline, the record is deemed complete. While both federal and state authorities allow electronic signatures to replace handwritten ones, they also require that authentication, regardless of the format, attest to the accuracy of the record.[36] To the degree that an auto-authentication system does not allow a physician to make this verification, many regulatory agencies have adopted the position that the authentication requirement is not fulfilled.

Auto-authentication systems frequently contain safeguards that protect some of the essential functions of the authentication process, however. For example, some facilities require physicians to sign an attestation that they will review all records and, unless they request corrections, the medical records department may enter the physician's signature. These attestations may include a provision in which the physician agrees not to dispute the accuracy of any record based on the absence of the doctor's signature on

---

[36]See M. Kadzielski and M. Reynolds, "Legal Review: Auto-authentication of Medical Records Raises Verification Concerns," *Topics in Health Information Management* 14, no. 1 (1993): 77-82.

any document. Such an agreement provides no supporting evidence that a physician actually reviewed the record, however, and therefore does not resolve any concerns regarding the accuracy of the record's contents.

Other facilities allow physicians to authenticate unsigned progress notes in a medical record by signing a statement on a cover page that they are authenticating all progress reports for a particular hospitalization. A separate authentication is required for other types of reports in the file, including operative reports, physical reports, discharge summaries, etc. Because progress reports are authenticated by the physician when they are created, they are more likely to be accurate and complete.

Under another system of auto-authentication of dictated and transcribed reports, a physician receives a copy of all transcribed reports and a periodic list of unsigned and dictated reports. The physician then indicates next to each report on the list whether he or she wants to sign it or authorize auto-authentication of the report. The level of accountability increases in this type of system because the physician receives a copy of each report and individually selects each report for either signature or auto-authentication.

The Joint Commission states that any auto-authentication process that involves attesting to the fact that an entry is complete, correct, and final before transcription does not meet its accreditation standards.[37] A facility should have a system to determine whether the author of an entry acknowledges the entry after it is transcribed, and a quality control system should monitor the process.

The Health Care Financing Administration's (HCFA) Medicare Conditions of Participation require authentication of each entry in a medical record and allow authentication by computer.[38] However, HCFA has indicated that any failure to obtain a physician's signature with respect to the record in its final form constitutes a deficiency in the authentication requirement.[39]

In addition to exposing health care facilities to loss or denial of accreditation, possible sanctions by administrative agencies, and exclusion from the Medicare/Medicaid program, the use of auto-authentication can gen-

---

[37]See JOINT COMMISSION, 1998 COMPREHENSIVE ACCREDITATION MANUAL FOR HOSPITALS, Examples of Evidence of Implementation for IM 7.8.

[38]42 C.F.R. § 482.24(c)(1).

[39]"Vladeck Warns Auto-authentication Will Violate Medicare Conditions," *BNA Health Law Reporter*, Oct. 21, 1993, 1423.

erate difficulties in offering evidence in litigation, particularly malpractice suits. The outcome of such litigation frequently depends on establishing what actually took place. A physician's signature on the medical record gives evidence that the practitioner actually reviewed the record and acknowledged that it represented a complete and accurate record of the patient's course of treatment. Although a signature does not prove conclusively that the physician reviewed the record, it is stronger evidence of such verification than a signature on a separate form authorizing authentication of the record.

Although the introduction of computer technology has enabled hospitals to introduce new methods for facilitating a physician's role in the authentication process, health care institutions should not lose sight of their responsibility in creating accurate and complete medical records. Any computer system that does not require physicians to review reports after they are transcribed is likely to fall short of both federal and state authentication standards, as well as to create serious liability risks for the facility implementing such a system. (For a discussion of computerized medical records, see Chapter 13.)

VERBAL ORDERS

In the course of providing patient care, health care practitioners often deliver orders verbally. Because of the impact that this practice may have on the quality of patient care, it is important for health care facilities to establish standards governing how these orders are received and recorded. Health care facilities should require physicians to deliver their orders in writing, except in situations in which verbal orders are unavoidable. Written orders are preferable to verbal ones because written orders create fewer chances for error.

Hospital licensing regulations in most states require all physician orders to be written in the patient's medical record and authenticated.[40] At least one state requires that verbal orders be transcribed and authenticated by the physician within 24 hours,[41] although other state licensure laws extend the time period for signing verbal orders to 48 hours.[42] Joint Commission standards of accreditation for hospitals state more generally that verbal

---

[40]See, e.g., S.C. CODE ANN. REGS. R. 61-16 § 601.6.

[41]IND. ADMIN. CODE tit. 410, r. 15-1-9(d).

[42]See, e.g., NEB. ADMIN. R. & REGS. tit. 175, ch. 9 § 003.04A5. Hospitals and Related.

orders from authorized individuals must be accepted and transcribed by qualified personnel as defined in the facility's rules and bylaws.[43] Regardless of licensing laws or accreditation standards, health care facilities should require that physicians are responsible for writing their orders in the medical record unless they are not present when the order must be given, and require all verbal orders to be transcribed within a specified time. Policies should also be predicated on the concept that only personnel who are qualified to understand physicians' orders should be authorized to receive and transcribe verbal orders.

CORRECTIONS AND ALTERATIONS

Some medical record entry errors are inevitable. Generally, two kinds of errors occur: (1) minor errors in transcription, spelling, etc., and (2) more significant errors involving test results, physician orders, inadvertently omitted information, and similar substantive entries.

While the majority of states have no specific statutory or regulatory rules concerning altering medical records, some state regulations specify how corrections should be handled. For example, in Arkansas errors in medical records must be corrected by drawing a single line through the incorrect entry, labeling the entry as an error, and initialing and dating it.[44] In Massachusetts, health care facilities may not erase mistakes, use ink eradicators, or remove pages from the record.[45]

In the absence of such regulations, however, health care facilities enunciate clear rules governing corrections. If the correction is a significant one, a senior person designated in the facility's policy should review the correction to determine whether it complies with the institution's guidelines for record amendments. Obvious minor errors, such as spelling, do not require intervention by senior personnel. As a general rule, the person who made the incorrect record entry should correct the entry. If that is not possible, health care practitioners should make only those changes that are within their scope of practice as defined by state licensing and certifi-

---

[43]*See* JOINT COMMISSION, 1998 COMPREHENSIVE ACCREDITATION MANUAL FOR HOSPITALS, Standard IM 7.7.

[44]Rules and Regulations for Hospitals and Related Institutions in Arkansas, § 601 (G). *See also* N.J. ADMIN. CODE tit. 8, § 8:43G-15.2(k) (corrections shall be made by drawing a single line through the error and initialing and dating the correction).

[45]MASS. REGS. CODE tit. 105, § 150.013(B).

cation laws. A registered nurse, for example, should not amend a physician's medication order unless directed to do so by the physician.

The person correcting a charting error in the record should cross out the incorrect entry with a single line, enter the correction, initial the correction, and enter the time and date the correction was made. Mistakes in the record should not be erased or obliterated, because erasures and obliterations could arouse suspicions in the minds of jurors as to the contents of the original entry. A single line drawn through incorrect entries leaves no doubt as to the original information being corrected. Where a correction requires more space than is available near the original entry, the person correcting the record should enter a reference to an addendum to the record and enter the more lengthy correction in the addendum.

Any amendments made at the patient's request should be included in an addendum to the record. The physician also should add an entry to document that the change was made at the request of the patient, who thereafter will bear the burden of explaining the change. A physician who considers the amendment inappropriate should discuss the matter with the patient.

A few states have regulations that address changes or amendments to medical records at the request of parties. In Maryland, legislation requires health care providers to establish a procedure by which an interested person may request an addition or correction to a medical record.[46] If the facility does not make the requested change, it must permit the individual to insert a statement of disagreement in the record, as well as provide a notice of the change or statement of disagreement to every person to whom it previously disclosed inaccurate, incomplete, or disputed information within the preceding six months.[47] New York law also allows a qualified person to challenge the accuracy of information in a medical record. In the event that a facility refuses to amend a record in accordance with the person's request, it must allow the individual to write a statement challenging the accuracy of the record and include the statement as part of the permanent record.[48] In the event of a threatened or actual suit by a patient against a health care provider or facility, no changes should be made in the patient's medical record without first consulting defense counsel. Attempts to alter medical record entries to favor the providers always are in-

---

[46]MD. CODE ANN. Health-Gen. § 4-304(b)(1).

[47]MD. CODE ANN. Health-Gen. §§ 4-304(b)(5)(1) & § 4-304(b)(6)(2).

[48]N.Y. COMP. CODES R. & REGS., 10 NYCRR § 405.10(6).

appropriate and do not necessarily help their defense, particularly if the patient has obtained a copy of the record before the changes were made.

If the patient can show that the record was altered without justification, the credibility of the entire record may be in jeopardy. In a Connecticut case, for example, nurses rewrote an entire section in the medical record of a patient who was injured while hospitalized. The court held in the patient's subsequent negligence action against the hospital that:

> [i]n addition to all the other evidence in the case, the significance of the revised hospital record should not be overlooked. Although the defendant understandably attempts to minimize what was done by characterizing the action as merely one of ordering expanded notes and by attributing it to poor judgment, the trier [of fact] was not required to be so charitable. An allowable inference from the bungled attempt to cover up the staff inadequacies . . . was that *the revision indicated a consciousness of negligence.* [Emphasis added.] The court so charged and the jury could so find.[49]

If a health care facility or provider that is involved in a negligence suit discovers that an original record entry is inaccurate or incomplete, it should request that clarifications or additions to the record be placed in a properly signed and dated addendum to the record.

In addition, deliberately altering a medical record or writing an incorrect record may subject a health care provider to statutory sanctions. In some states, a practitioner who makes a false entry on a medical record is subject to license revocation for unprofessional conduct.[50] In addition, as is discussed above, altering or falsifying a chart for purposes of wrongfully obtaining Medicare or state health care funds is a crime under federal law, and subjects the violator to a substantial fine or imprisonment.[51]

---

[49]Pisel v. Stamford Hosp., 430 A.2d 1 (Conn. 1980).

[50]*See, e.g.,* KY. REV. STAT. ANN. § 311.595(10).

[51]42 U.S.C. § 1320a-7b(a).

5

Documenting Consent to Treatment

Chapter Objectives

- Distinguish between express and implied consent.
- Identify the information that must be disclosed for informed consent.
- Explain what a patient must show to prove causation in a consent case.
- Describe the emergency exception to the informed consent requirement.
- Define the therapeutic privilege and waiver of consent.
- Outline how informed consent applied to criminal suspects and prisoners.
- Identify who can give consent.
- Discuss the effect of refusal of consent.
- Discuss the application of informed consent to minors.
- Distinguish between emancipated minors and mature minors.
- Compare the responsibility for obtaining consent among physicians, other health care providers, facilities, and organizations.
- Outline the requirements for informed consent documentation.
- Distinguish between the different types of consent forms and their uses.
- Discuss how and when consent may be withdrawn.

INTRODUCTION

Health care providers must obtain proper authorization before performing diagnostic or therapeutic procedures on patients.[1] Consent may be express or implied, and may be obtained from the patient or the patient's representative if the patient is incapacitated. In most instances the law requires that the patient be given sufficient information concerning the nature and risks of the recommended and alternative treatments so that the consent given is an informed consent. Generally, if the patient decides not to consent, the examination or procedure cannot be performed. In some circumstances, however, the law overrides the patient's decision and provides authorization for involuntary treatment, such as in emergencies and for compulsory treatment for certain conditions such as mental illness.

The primary responsibility for obtaining informed consent for treatment falls on physicians and other health care practitioners, rather than on a health care institution, facility, or organization such as a hospital, group practice, clinic, health maintenance organization (HMO), or hospice. The law in this area has developed in the hospital context, with courts and statutes generally establishing that hospitals are not liable for failing to obtain a particular patient's informed consent. There are several important exceptions to the general rule, however. Hospitals and other health care insititutions and facilities may be liable for failure to obtain consent from a patient if the unconsented-to procedure is performed by an employee, rather than an independent contractor. As a practical matter, hospitals frequently assist non-employee members of its medical staff by obtaining written confirmation of the patient's consent. Once a hospital or other corporate health care entity assumes this responsibility, it must consistently comply with its own policies and practices or face increased potential for liability. In addition, a corporate health care entity is legally responsible for the adequacy of its organizational consent requirements, policies, and procedures.

Beyond liability to patients, federal, state, and private accreditation requirements mandate that informed consent be obtained and documented. For example, The Medicare Conditions of Participation require properly

---

[1]At least one state court has held that the informed consent requirement applies only to surgical procedures, however. Morgan v. MacPhail 704 A.2d 617 (Pa. 1997) (informed consent not required for injection of steroids).

executed consent forms as part of the medical record.[2] The Joint Commission on Accreditation of Healthcare Organizations (Joint Commission) requires accredited hospitals, as well as hospitals, home care organizations, ambulatory care organizations, and mental health services that are part of accredited networks, to obtain informed consent.[3] Federal and state laws may create a liability risk by prescribing consent procedures in special situations, such as in connection with a clinical study.[4] State laws may also require written consent documentation on a more general basis, as part of regulatory schemes such as health facility or HMO licensure laws and patients' rights statutes. Thus, health care administrators, medical records administrators, and individual health care providers must be familiar with the legal principles on patient consent and the proper documentation of consent.

The consent requirement, the decision-making roles of patients and their representatives, the exceptions to the consent requirement, and the function of the medical record in the patient consent process are discussed in this chapter.

LEGAL THEORIES OF CONSENT

The common law long has recognized the right to be free from harmful or offensive touching. The intentional harmful or offensive touching of another person without authorization is called battery. The earliest medical consent lawsuits arose in England in the eighteenth century. In those early cases, when surgery was done without consent, the courts found the surgeons liable for battery. Modern courts may still find the physicians liable for battery if they do not obtain patient consent.

On the other hand, courts apply a different legal theory when the patient consents to the procedure but does not have sufficient information to make an informed decision. Today, nearly all courts have adopted the position that failure to disclose the necessary information regarding a procedure's risks and benefits does not constitute a battery, but rather constitutes negligence under the informed consent doctrine.

---

[2]42 C.F.R. § 482.24(c).

[3]JOINT COMMISSION, 1998 COMPREHENSIVE ACCREDITATION MANUAL FOR HOSPITALS, Standard RI.1.2.1; 1998-2000 COMPREHENSIVE ACCREDITATION MANUAL FOR HEALTH CARE NETWORKS, Standard RI.2 and appendices for unaccredited organizations.

[4]See, e.g., 45 C.F.R. § 46.

Express and Implied Consent

Consent may be either express or implied. Express consent is consent given by direct words, either orally or in writing. For some procedures, particularly those involving reproduction and testing for sexually transmitted diseases, state laws require express written consent. Otherwise, either oral or written consent can be legally sufficient authorization where express consent is necessary. However, because it often is difficult to prove oral consent should a dispute arise, providers should seek written consent.

Implied consent is consent inferred from the patient's conduct and consent presumed in certain emergencies. When a patient voluntarily submits to a procedure with apparent knowledge of the nature of the procedure, the courts usually will find implied consent. For example, in a famous early consent case[5] the court found that a woman had given her implied consent to being vaccinated by extending her arm and accepting the vaccination without objection. In a 1983 case, a court held that a patient who revoked his express written consent to a surgical procedure, but then silently acquiesced to preoperative medication and submitted to surgery, had given implied consent.[6]

When Is Consent Implied?

Consent is implied in medical emergencies, unless the health care provider has reason to believe that consent would be refused—for example, if the patient previously had refused treatment. This emergency exception to the consent requirement applies when there is an immediate threat to life or health and the patient is incapacitated and cannot give consent. In an early Iowa case,[7] the court found implied consent to the removal of a patient's mangled limb that had been run over in a train accident. The court accepted the physician's determination that the amputation was necessary to save the patient's life. Courts have disagreed on whether pain is enough justification to find implied consent. An early New York decision[8] held pain to be a significant factor in establishing a finding of implied consent, while a South Dakota court ruled that pain was not a

---

[5]O'Brien v. Cunard S.S. Co., 28 N.E. 266 (Mass. 1891).

[6]Busalacchi v. Vogel, 429 So. 2d 217 (La. Ct. App. 1983).

[7]Jackovach v. Yocom, 237 N.W. 444 (Iowa 1931).

[8]Sullivan v. Montgomery, 279 N.Y.S. 575 (N.Y. City Ct. 1935).

sufficient emergency because the danger to the patient's health was not immediate and the patient was conscious and able to make an informed decision.[9] Some states have enacted laws that formalize the emergency exception. In Pennsylvania, for example, no physician or podiatrist may be held liable for failing to obtain consent in an emergency that prevents consulting with the patient.[10] In California, informed consent for even experimental treatments is not necessary if the patient is in a life-threatening situation and unable to give informed consent, and if certain other conditions are met.[11]

Some courts have found implied consent to extensions or modifications of surgical procedures beyond the scope specifically authorized when unexpected conditions arise, and when the extension or modification is necessary to preserve the patient's life. Many surgical consent forms attempt to minimize disagreements regarding the scope of authorization by including explicit authorization of extensions or modifications to preserve the patient's life or health.

Some courts have addressed whether a patient impliedly has authorized the substitution of one practitioner for another. Generally, unless an emergency or other special circumstance occurs, a patient's consent constitutes authorization for a particular practitioner to perform a procedure; deviation from that authorization may invalidate the consent. If the patient refuses to consent to treatment by a certain caregiver, then that caregiver is prohibited from engaging in treatment. Likewise, if the primary physician chooses an assistant to whom the patient objects, that assistant is precluded from participating in the procedure.[12] For example, one court allowed a patient who specifically requested that no male health care provider view or touch her unclothed body during childbirth to pursue a battery claim against a male nurse who attended delivery.[13] The patient's physician had assured her that the male nurse would not see her unclothed.

---

[9]Cunningham v. Yankton Clinic, 262 N.W.2d 508 (S.D. 1978).

[10]40 PA. CONS. STAT. § 1301.811-A.

[11]CAL. HEALTH & SAFETY CODE § 24177.5.

[12]*See, e.g.*, Kenner v. Northern Illinois Med. Ctr., 517 N.E.2d 1137 (Ill. App. Ct. 1987); Johnson v. McMurray, 461 So. 775 (Ala. 1984).

[13]Cohen v. Smith, 648 N.E.2d 329 (Ill. App. Ct. 1995).

Informed Consent

The term informed consent refers to the process in which a patient is apprised of a procedure's risks and benefits, and freely consents to undergo the proposed treatment. Simply requiring the patient to sign a form does not satisfy informed consent requirements, as the form itself serves merely as evidence of the informed consent process. On the other hand, it is important to document consent or the lack of consent. While not legally conclusive, a well-written, properly executed consent form is strong evidence that informed consent was given. Generally, a legally effective consent form must

- be signed voluntarily
- show that the procedure performed was the one to which consent was given
- show that the consenting person understood the nature of the procedure, the risks involved, and the probable consequences

The courts have developed two standards for determining the adequacy of the information the physician has given the patient during the informed consent process: (1) the reasonable physician standard and (2) the reasonable patient standard. In states using the first standard, physicians have a duty to provide the information that a reasonable medical practitioner would offer under the same or similar circumstances.[14]

The second and more modern standard has been adopted by an increasing number of states. Under the reasonable patient standard, the extent of the physician's duty to provide information is determined by the information needs of the patient, rather than by professional practice. Information that is material to the patient's decision must be disclosed. Some states have adopted this standard through legislation. In Pennsylvania, for example, state law requires physicians to inform a patient of the nature of the proposed treatment, the risks associated with the treatment, and the alternatives that a reasonable patient would consider material to the decision whether to undergo treatment.[15]

---

[14]*See, e.g.*, Natanson v. Kline, 350 P.2d 1093 (Kan. 1960).

[15]40 Pa. Cons. Stat. § 1301.811-A.

What Information Must Be Disclosed?

Generally, a physician or other health care provider must disclose the following categories of information to a patient: (1) diagnosis, (2) nature and purpose of the proposed treatment, (3) risks and consequences of the proposed treatment, (4) probability that the proposed treatment will be successful, (5) feasible treatment alternatives, and (6) alternatives and prognosis if the proposed treatment is not given. Although this is the generally accepted list of items that should be discussed, a health care provider should include all information that the provider knows or reasonably should know would be material to the patient's decision-making process.

Most of the cases concerning informed consent involve allegations that the provider failed to reveal sufficient information as to the risks and consequences of the procedure. Not all risks must be disclosed. For example, risks that are very remote and improbable generally can be omitted, as a person in the patient's position would not likely find them material to the consent decision.[16] Similarly, some risks with a very high probability could be considered to be so commonly known that the physician is not required to mention them. If the provider can document that the patient had knowledge of risks and consequences from other sources, such as from a prior course of treatment or from discussions with another health care provider, the patient's consent may be considered informed. Court cases examining what information must be conveyed to patients are highly dependent on the circumstances. Examples follow:

- In an Arizona case, a patient told a physician that preserving his ability to work was crucial in determining a course of treatment.[17] The court ruled that the physician should have informed the patient of the risks that could affect his ability to work.
- A physician treating a minor patient for a concussion should have informed the patient's parents that a computed axial tomography (CAT) scan would reveal bleeding in the brain, even if there was only a 1 percent to 3 percent chance that the patient suffered that condition, according to the Wisconsin Supreme Court.[18]

---

[16]*See, e.g.*, Lemke v. United States, 557 F. Supp. 1205 (D.N.D. 1983).
[17]Hales v. Pittman, 576 P.2d 493 (Ariz. 1978).
[18]Martin v. Richards, 531 N.W.2d 70 (Wis. 1995).

- A physician may not have fulfilled his duty to fully disclose the risks of breast reduction surgery when he warned a patient that scarring could occur, but responded to the patient's questions by telling her that she shouldn't worry and would be happy with the results.[19]
- A physician who did not disclose that his own lack of experience increased the risk that serious impairment could result from aneurysm surgery might be liable, because information that should be revealed to patients is not limited to complications intrinsic to the procedure, the highest court in Wisconsin ruled.[20]
- A Kansas appeals court ruled that a physician who recommended and performed laser surgery as a treatment for a viral wart on the cervix failed to obtain informed consent because he failed to advise the patient of the treatment option of doing nothing.[21]

Patients have also sued when their refusal to consent to treatment was not sufficiently informed. In California, the courts have extended the informed consent doctrine to require informed refusal. In the California case that established this concept, the court ruled that a physician could be liable for a patient's death from cancer of the cervix based on the physician's failure to inform the patient of the risks of *not* consenting to a recommended Pap smear.[22] The Pap smear probably would have led to discovery of the patient's cancer in time to begin treatment that would have extended her life. The California informed consent rule also requires the primary physician to disclose the risks of not consulting a specialist.[23]

Proving Causation

The most difficult element for the patient to prove in an informed consent case is often causation. The patient must show a link between the inadequate informed consent and the injury by proving that he or she would not have consented if the risk that occurred had been disclosed. The courts have developed two standards for this proof. Some jurisdictions apply an objective standard, determining what a reasonable person in the patient's

---

[19]Korman v. Mallin, 858 P.2d 1145 (Alaska 1993).

[20]Johnson ex rel. Adler v. Kokemoor, 545 N.W.2d 495 (Wis. 1996).

[21]Wecker v. Amend, 918 P.2d 658 (Kan. Ct. App. 1996).

[22]Truman v. Thomas, 611 P.2d 902 (Cal. 1980).

[23]Moore v. Preventive Medicine Med. Group, Inc., 223 Cal. Rptr. 859 (Ct. App. 1986).

position would have decided if informed of the risk.[24] Other courts apply a subjective standard, determining whether the patient involved in the lawsuit would have refused to consent to the procedure if informed of the risk.[25] Either of these standards provides substantial protection for the conscientious health care provider who discloses the major risks, and whose patient suffers from a more remote risk. For example, in a Massachusetts case, a court held that a physician was not liable for failure to obtain informed consent where the risk he failed to disclose was remote.[26] The physician did not advise a pregnant patient whose membranes had ruptured that waiting for labor to proceed naturally posed a risk of streptococcus pneumonia for the infant, who died five days after birth. The court ruled in favor of the physician, ruling that because the risk of infection was negligible, disclosure would not have been material to the patient's decision to allow labor to proceed naturally.

Medical Experimentation and Research

Innovative treatments trigger special consent requirements, beyond properly informing the patient of risks and benefits. Federal, state, and local laws on human experimentation and the protection of human research subjects impose strict requirements for obtaining patient consent. These laws contain specific safeguards for research subjects and guidelines for informed consent, establishing detailed standards for documentation and record retention. The requirements vary depending on the legal status of the experimental treatment, agreements between the health care provider or research sponsor and government authorities, and health care facility policies and procedures. Thus, medical record requirements should be carefully examined whenever a patient undergoes an experimental treatment or takes part in a clinical study.

Exceptions to the Informed Consent Requirement

The courts have recognized four situations in which consent is required, but informed consent (i.e., adequate disclosure) is not necessarily required: emergencies, the therapeutic privilege, patient waiver, and treatment of criminal suspects or patients in custody.

---

[24]Canterbury v. Spence, 464 F.2d 772 (D.C. Cir.), *cert. denied*, 409 U.S. 1064 (1972).

[25]Feeley v. Baer, 295 A.2d 676 (R.I. 1972).

[26]Wilkinson v. Vesey, 679 N.E.2d 180 (Mass. 1997).

Emergencies

In some circumstances, the patient is competent and able to consent to treatment, but the health care provider does not have time to provide full disclosure of all possible treatment alternatives before initiating care. This situation does not meet the strict parameters of the emergency doctrine, discussed earlier, in which the patient is incapacitated and consent is presumed. For example, in a New Mexico case, a patient suffered from a snake bite that required immediate treatment.[27] The court recognized that even when there is time to secure consent, certain emergency situations may allow only an abbreviated disclosure of information as to the required treatment. Hospitals (the setting where such emergencies are most likely to be presented) should insist that staff engage in consultation with patients as time and circumstances permit. Findings supporting the existence of an emergency should be noted on the patient's record, with particular emphasis on the nature of the threat, immediacy, and magnitude. The initialing of such notations by consultant physicians is advisable. At the least, the physicians' names should be recorded.

Therapeutic Privilege

Many courts recognize an exception to the informed consent doctrine, called therapeutic privilege, that permits a physician to withhold information when disclosure of information poses a significant threat of detriment to the patient. Courts have carefully limited the therapeutic privilege by making it inapplicable when the physician fears only that the information might lead the patient to forgo needed therapy. Instead, physicians should rely on this privilege only when they can document that a patient's anxiety is significantly above the norm. In a federal appeals case, the court ruled that when the therapeutic privilege applies, the information must be disclosed to a relative.[28]

Statutes and regulations may also set the parameters of the therapeutic privilege.[29] In California skilled nursing facilities, for example, a physician may choose not to inform a patient of the risks of treatment if objec-

---

[27]Crouch v. Most, 432 P.2d 250 (N.M. 1967).

[28]Lester v. Aetna Cas. & Sur. Co., 240 F.2d 676 (5th Cir.), *cert. denied*, 354 U.S. 923 (1957); *but see* Nishi v. Hartwell , 473 P.2d 116 (Haw. 1970) (duty to make full disclosure arises from the physician-patient relationship and is owed only to the patient).

[29]*See, e.g.*, DEL. CODE ANN. tit. 18, § 6852(b)(3).

tive facts documented in the patient's record demonstrate that the disclosure would so seriously upset the patient that the patient would not have been able to rationally weigh the risks of refusing the recommended treatment. Unless inappropriate, the physician must obtain informed consent from the patient's representative.[30]

Patient Waiver

Some cases have indicated that a patient can waive the right to be informed before giving consent.[31] State laws and regulations may also narrowly define the circumstances where waiver is appropriate, such as requiring the patient to initiate the waiver, requiring the substituted consent of a representative, or allowing waiver only where risks are minimal. In New York, for example, a law states that it is a defense to a suit for failure to obtain informed consent that the patient assured the medical practitioner that he would undergo the treatment regardless of the risk, or told the practitioner that he did not want to be informed.[32] A physician should not suggest a waiver but instead should encourage reluctant patients to be informed. If the patient persists, the waiver should be documented in the patient's medical records and carefully witnessed. The documentation should describe the patient's waiver and the physician's effort properly to inform the patient.

Treatment of Criminal Suspects and Prisoners

In some instances, health care providers are asked by law enforcement officers to perform procedures on unconsenting patients. A health care provider might be asked to conduct a medical examination that will result in the discovery of criminal evidence (such as a test for alcohol or drugs in a suspect's blood) or to treat a prisoner against his wishes for venereal disease, drug addiction, or mental illness. In some states, health care providers are protected by state laws that grant them immunity when acting on the request of a police officer.[33] State laws may specifically address what procedures may be performed in the absence of prisoner consent.

---

[30]CAL. CODE REGS. tit. 22, § 72528.

[31]See, e.g., Putensen v. Clay Adams, Inc., 12 Cal. App. 3d 1062 (Ct. App. 1970).

[32]N.Y. PUB. HEALTH LAW § 2085-d.

[33]See, e.g., N.Y. VEH. & TRAF. LAW § 1194.

For example, Florida law authorizes the treatment of prisoners for venereal disease,[34] Maryland law allows prisoners to be enrolled in drug treatment programs,[35] Tennessee law authorizes complete physical examinations of prisoners, including blood tests,[36] and Iowa code implies consent (which may be withdrawn) by drivers to be tested for blood alcohol.[37]

There have been several cases addressing the appropriateness of procedures ordered by police officers or courts, such as pumping of a suspect's stomach to recover drugs,[38] blood tests performed despite patient refusal,[39] and bullet removal from a suspect's body.[40] However, those cases involve the constitutional rights of the patient, not the liability of the health care provider. Health care providers who are requested to perform examinations or administer treatment to a prisoner without consent should consider whether a state law, regulation, or court order authorizes the medical intervention. The provider should not rely on the police officer's assurance that the procedure is permitted by law, and should document the source of the authority to treat in the medical record.

WHO CAN GIVE CONSENT

The person who makes the consent decision must be legally and actually competent to make the decision and must be informed, unless one of the exceptions applies. Competent adults and some mature or emancipated minors make decisions regarding their own care. Someone else must make the decisions for incompetent adults and other minors.

Competent Adults

The age of majority is established by the legislature of each state. In most states, legal majority is now 18 years of age. In some states, a person can be considered an adult before the statutory age of majority by taking certain actions, such as by getting married or serving in the armed forces.

---

[34]FLA. STAT. ANN. § 384.32.

[35]MD. CODE ANN. Art. 27, § 700F.

[36]TENN. CODE ANN. § 41-4-138.

[37]IOWA CODE ANN. § 321J.6.

[38]Rochin v. California, 342 U.S. 165 (1952).

[39]Schmerber v. California, 384 U.S. 757 (1966).

[40]Winston v. Lee, 470 U.S. 753 (1985).

An adult is competent if (1) a court has not declared the person incompetent and (2) the person generally is capable of understanding the consequences of alternatives, weighing the alternatives by the degree to which they promote his or her desires, and choosing and acting accordingly. There is a strong legal presumption of competence. For example, in one case a court found a woman competent to refuse a breast biopsy even though she had been committed to a mental institution with a diagnosis of chronic schizophrenia and two of her three reasons for refusal were delusional.[41] In another case, a court found a woman competent to refuse the amputation of her gangrenous leg even though her train of thought sometimes wandered, her conception of time was distorted, and she was confused on some matters.[42] The fact that her decision was medically irrational and would lead to her death did not demonstrate incompetence. The court believed she understood the alternatives and the consequences of her decision.

Competence is not necessarily determined by psychiatrists. A practical assessment of competence should be made by the health care provider who obtains the consent or accepts the refusal. When it is difficult to assess competence, consultation with a specialist should be considered. If the provider suspects an underlying condition that affects brain function, the consultant should be a psychiatrist or other appropriate specialist. These assessments should be documented in the medical record.

Refusal of Consent

Competent adults have the right and capacity not only to consent to medical treatment but also to refuse such treatment. This refusal must be honored regardless of the basis on which it is grounded.

Some patients refuse treatment on religious grounds. The religious beliefs of Jehovah's Witnesses, for example, prohibit them from receiving blood transfusions. The majority of courts have ruled that such patients have the right to refuse blood transfusions even if such refusal will lead to their death.[43] Terminally ill competent adult patients constitute another category of those who may refuse consent to treatment. Documentation of

---

[41]In re Yetter, Pa. D. & C. 2d, 169 (Pa. C. Pl., Northampton County, 1973).

[42]Lane v. Candura, 376 N.E.2d 1232 (Mass. App. Ct. 1978).

[43]See, e.g., In re Melideo, 390 N.Y.S.2d 523 (1976); In re Brown, 478 So. 2d 1033 (Miss. 1985).

their wishes in the medical record is addressed in detail in Chapter 8, DOCUMENTATION AND DISCLOSURE: SPECIAL AREAS OF CONCERN.

In these sensitive situations, hospitals and physicians should seek the advice of legal counsel if the patient's refusal is a serious threat to health, as long as the delay involved in seeking that guidance would not further endanger the patient's life. Health care providers should exercise extreme caution when administering treatment to an unconsenting patient in the absence of a court order or other clear authority.

Incompetent Adults

If a patient is not competent to give informed consent or informed refusal, the patient's guardian or, if no guardian exists, the representative of the incompetent adult patient makes consent decisions on the patient's behalf. Representatives of patients have a narrower range of permissible choices regarding that person than they would have concerning their own care. In addition, the known wishes of the patient should be considered in reaching decisions about treatment.

When a court rules that a person is incompetent, it designates an individual to be the incompetent person's guardian. The guardian has the legal authority to make most of the decisions regarding the incompetent person's care.

Because some patients who actually are incompetent never have been determined to be incompetent by a court, they have no legal guardians. When decisions must be made concerning their care, it is common practice to seek a decision from the next of kin or others who have assumed supervision of the patient. In many states, statutes[44] or court decisions[45] support that practice.

If the incompetence is temporary, the medical procedure should be postponed until the patient is competent and capable of making the decision, unless the postponement presents a substantial risk to the patient's life or health; in this case, consent will be implied from the emergency.

Certain procedures, such as sterilization and organ donation, require special consideration. Traditionally, neither the courts nor a guardian can authorize involuntary sterilization of incompetent minors or adults with-

---

[44]*See, e.g.*, MISS. CODE ANN. §§ 41-41-3 & 41-41-5.
[45]*See, e.g.*, Farber v. Olkon, 254 P.2d 520 (Cal. 1953).

out specific statutory authority.[46] However, several state courts have held that courts have inherent authority to order the sterilization of incompetents.[47] Health care providers should not perform sterilization procedures on incompetents without appropriate legislative authority, case law authority, or a court order.

As for organ transplants involving incompetents as donors, the courts generally examine the situation to establish whether the procedure is in the best interest of the incompetent person. In some cases, courts have concluded that operations, such as kidney transplants, are not in the patient's best interest.[48] Other courts, however, have been willing to find indirect benefit to the incompetent sufficient to support consent to the procedure. Some courts have upheld the right of a guardian to authorize kidney donations because of the close relationship between the donor and the proposed recipient, the emotional injury to the donor if the recipient were to die, and the reasonable motivations of the patient and the patient's parent or guardian.[49]

Minors

Parental or guardian consent should be obtained before treatment is given to a minor unless (1) the patient requires emergency treatment, (2) a statute grants the minor the right to consent, or (3) a court or other legal authority orders treatment.

Emergency Care

As with adults, consent for treatment of a minor is implied in medical emergencies when an immediate threat to the patient's life or health exists. Most states have statutes addressing this issue. If the health care provider believes that the patient's parents would refuse consent to emergency treatment, and if time permits, the provider should seek court authorization for treatment or notify the appropriate government agency responsible for seeking court authorization. If the patient requires

---

[46]*See, e.g.*, Hudson v. Hudson, 373 So. 2d 310 (Ala. 1979).

[47]*See, e.g.*, In re C.D.M., 627 P.2d 607 (Alaska 1981); In re Grady, 426 A.2d 467 (N.J. 1981).

[48]*See, e.g.*, In re Guardianship of Pescinski, 226 N.W.2d 180 (Wis. 1975); Curran v. Bosze, 566 N.E.2d 1319 (Ill. 1991).

[49]*See, e.g.*, Strunk v. Strunk, 445 S.W.2d 145 (Ky. 1969); Hart v. Brown, 289 A.2d 386 (Conn. Super. Ct. 1972).

immediate treatment, the provider in most cases should treat the minor, even if the parents object. Health care administrators should establish policies for responding to these situations.

Emancipated Minors

Emancipated minors may consent to their own medical care. Minors are considered emancipated when they are married or otherwise no longer subject to parental control or regulation and are not supported by their parents. The specific factors necessary to establish emancipation usually are established by statute and vary from state to state. Some states require that the parent and child agree on the emancipation, so that a minor cannot become emancipated in those states simply by running away from home. In some states, emancipation is established by the courts, and no statutory definition of emancipation exists. Because the doctrine of emancipation is unsettled in many states, health care providers should try to obtain the consent of a parent in addition to that of the minor, or consider the existence of another basis upon which to treat a minor without parental or guardian consent (such as an emergency). A well-written policy established with the advice of legal counsel will help guide practitioners confronted with this issue.

Mature Minors

Mature minors may consent to some medical care under common law and constitutional principles and under the statutes of some states. Many states have statutes that authorize older minors to consent to any medical treatment. In other states, the age limits and scope of treatments to which a minor may consent vary. Many states have special laws concerning minors' consent to treatment for venereal or other communicable diseases and substance abuse without regard to age.

Most courts reject chronological age as the sole factor in determining maturity, and tend to balance a number of factors.[50] In one case, the Illinois Supreme Court ruled that a mature minor has the right to refuse life-sustaining medical treatment if state interests in preserving life, protecting third-party interests, preventing suicide, and maintaining the ethical integrity of the medical profession do not outweigh this right.[51] A 17-year-

---

[50]*See, e.g.,* Cardwell v. Bechtol, 724 S.W.2d 739 (Tenn. 1987).

[51]In re E.G., No. 66089 (Ill. 1989).

old patient needed blood transfusions to treat leukemia, but both she and her mother refused consent on religious grounds. The court held that the mature minor had the right to refuse medical treatment.

Consent requirements for minors seeking abortions are largely regulated by state law. The law varies from state to state, and currently is in a condition of flux. State statutes usually provide that a minor can avoid the necessity of parental consent by proving to a court that she is a mature minor capable of making such a decision on her own.

Generally, when treating a minor, a health care provider should urge the minor to involve his or her parents in making consent decisions. When a mature minor refuses to permit parental involvement, the health care provider can give the necessary care without substantial risk based on the minor's consent alone, unless there is likelihood of harm to the minor or others that can be avoided only through parental involvement. When the likelihood of such harm arises, parents usually should be involved, unless state law forbids notifying them.

Parental or Guardian Consent

Either parent can give legally effective consent for treatment of a minor child, except when the parents are legally separated or divorced. When the parents are legally separated or divorced, usually only the consent of the custodial parent must be obtained unless there is an agreement between the parents that both must consent to treatment. This often is specified in state statutes. The provider should rely upon the parent or parents to provide information concerning who has authority to consent to the minor's care. If a provider knows or suspects that one parent objects, the provider should use caution and seek the advice of its legal counsel.

RESPONSIBILITY FOR OBTAINING CONSENT

It is the physician's responsibility to provide the necessary information to the patient concerning the patient's condition and proposed treatment and to obtain informed consent before proceeding with diagnostic and therapeutic procedures. Other independent practitioners who order procedures have a similar responsibility concerning those procedures. The hospital, facility, or other health care setting where care is rendered generally is not liable for the failure of the physician or other independent practitioner to obtain informed consent unless the practitioner is an employee or otherwise acting on behalf of the corporate entity.[52] Some states have codified this principle in their statutes. For example, Ohio law states: "No hospital, home health agency, or provider of a hospice care program shall be held liable for a physician's failure to obtain an informed consent from his patient prior to a surgical or medical procedure or course of procedures, unless the physician is an employee of the hospital, home health agency, or provider of a hospice care program."[53]

The courts have ruled overwhelmingly that hospitals do not have an affirmative obligation to monitor the content of disclosures given by non-employed health care practitioners to patients being treated within the hospital's facilities to ensure that consent is informed.[54] This reasoning also applies to other types of health care facilities and organizations. However, there are circumstances that may lead to consent-related liability for these entities:

- The physician that failed to obtain informed consent is an employee of the facility. Liability of an employee may be "imputed" or attributed to the employer based on the reasoning that employers are responsible for supervising their employees.
- The facility knew or should have known that a physician did not comply with informed consent requirements but failed to intervene. In this case, a court may hold that the facility negligently breached its own duty to provide quality care to the patient.
- The facility's procedures for requiring, documenting, or verifying consent did not comply with the standards of the medical community, or the facility did not comply with its own policies, procedures, or usual practices with regard to a particular patient. As in the previous example, under these circumstances, the facility may be liable for breaching its direct duty to protect patients.

Another issue that may arise is which provider has the duty to disclose when there is more than one provider involved in rendering care. Courts

---

[52]*See, e.g.*, Fiorentino v. Wenger, 227 N.E.2d 296 (N.Y. 1967).

[53]Ohio Rev. Code Ann. § 2317.54.

[54]*See, e.g.*, Petriello v. Kalman, 576 A.2d 474 (Conn. 1990); Pauscher v. Iowa Methodist Med. Ctr., 408 N.W.2d 355 (Iowa 1987); Kershaw v. Reichert, 445 N.W.2d 16 (N.D. 1989). *But see* Magana v. Elie, 439 N.E.2d 1319 (Ill. App. Ct. 1982), in which an Illinois appeals court ruled that a hospital may have a duty to its patients to ensure that independent medical staff physicians inform them of the risks of and alternatives to surgery.

have held that if a primary treating physician remains active in the patient's treatment, that physician must obtain informed consent.[55] Responsibility for disclosure also may depend on whether the primary treating physician has asked for a consultation with another physician or whether the patient has been referred to a second physician. To avoid confusion, health care administrators should make certain that medical staff bylaws or policies clearly allocate the responsibility of obtaining informed consent.

The role of nonphysician health care practitioners (such as nurses and physician assistants) in the consent process varies among care settings. A typical approach to delineating the role of nonphysician employees in hospitals is to limit their role to (1) screening for completion of a consent form to ascertain that the hospital has documented the patient's consent in accordance with established hospital policy and (2) informing the responsible physician when the patient has concerns or questions about the consent form, seems to be confused about the proposed treatment, or has withdrawn or retracted consent. If the physician does not respond appropriately, hospital employees should notify medical staff and hospital officials so they may determine whether intervention is necessary.

Other health care entities permit nonphysician providers to obtain the required signature of the patient on the consent form once the physician has informed the patient of proposed procedures and obtained the patient's verbal authority to proceed with treatment. In some practices or facilities, nonphysicians may provide some or all of the information necessary for the patient to give an informed consent. Although these approaches can provide the patient with the information he or she needs for an informed consent, involving nonphysicians in the consent process could negatively affect the physician-patient relationship by reducing the opportunity for adequate communication. Involving nonphysicians also could shift the liability for inadequacies of consent from the (typically independent) physician to the nonphysician's employer. To avoid those adverse consequences, some health care entities prohibit nonphysicians from obtaining consent. State law should be considered in detail when developing a policy on who may participate in the consent process, as statutes and court decisions often outline who is or may be responsible for

---

[55]*See, e.g.*, Jones v. Philadelphia College of Osteopathic Med., 813 F. Supp. 1125 (E.D. Pa. 1993); Ritter v. Delaney, 790 S.W.2d 29 (Tex. Ct. App. 1990); Jacobs v. Painter, 530 A.2d 231 (Me. 1987).

obtaining informed consent. In Maine, for example, regulations specifically permit certified registered nurse anesthetists to verify consent.[56]

DOCUMENTATION

Consent is not merely a form, despite common belief to the contrary. The patient and everyone involved with providing health care should understand that obtaining the patient's consent means obtaining the patient's authorization for diagnosis and treatment. Once the patient has authorized the proposed care, it is important to document that authorization in the patient's medical record. Many commentators agree that the best way to document informed consent is to obtain the signature of the patient or the patient's representative on an appropriate form. Other experts recommend that the physician write a detailed note in the medical record reflecting the discussion of consent with the patient or the patient's representative. This approach is recommended out of concern that courts will view a consent form as all the information given to the patient and not believe the physician's testimony that additional information was provided. Some forms used today, however, may be more detailed than a practitioner's note in the medical record. A combination of a signed form and medical record notation is another method for documenting consent.

A typical consent policy outlines the circumstances under which a signed consent form is required. The types of procedures that may trigger a signed consent requirement include:

- major or minor invasive surgery
- procedures that involve more than a slight risk of harm
- forms of radiological therapy
- electroconvulsive therapy
- experimental procedures
- HIV tests
- sterilization
- abortion
- organ donation
- other procedures for which consent forms are required by statute or regulation

---

[56]CODE ME. R. § 02-380-008-1.

In developing or applying a policy on the use of consent forms, health care administrators should be aware that the actual process of providing information to the person giving consent and of determining the person's decision is more important than the consent form. The form is only evidence of the consent process and is not a substitute for the consent process. A senior administrator or medical staff officer should be responsible for determining that actual consent exists even when a consent form has been lost or inadvertently not signed before treatment, or when other circumstances make it difficult to obtain the necessary signature. In all cases, the information on a consent form must be consistent with the information given the patient by the physician. If the physician provides information different from that on the standard consent form, the doctor should revise the form before the patient signs it.

TYPES OF CONSENT FORMS

Once the decision has been made to use a consent form, rather than making a detailed note in the medical record, the type of form must be selected. There are two basic approaches to consent forms: the short consent form (also called a general or battery consent form) and the long consent form (also called a detailed or special consent form). These approaches to consent documentation are described below.

A third approach is not advisable, but should be noted. In the past, many hospitals asked patients being admitted for care to sign a consent form authorizing any procedure their physician wished to perform. These forms are known as blanket consents or admission consents. Courts have ruled that blanket consent forms are not evidence of consent to major procedures because the procedure is not specified on the form. Because admission consent forms may serve as valid evidence of consent to minor procedures and noninvasive treatments with insignificant risk of harm, some attorneys recommend their continued use. However, most believe that these admission forms provide no more protection than the implied consent that is inferred from admission and submission to minor procedures.

Short Consent Forms

The short consent form provides space for the name and description of the specific procedure and states that (1) the person signing has been told about the medical condition, consequences, risks, and alternative treatments and (2) all the person's questions have been answered to his or her satisfaction. The short form does not list the particular risks and benefits that were described to the patient. This type of consent form usually will defeat a claim of battery if the proper person signs the form and the procedures described in the form are the ones performed on the patient. Following the procedures for the use of the form also provides support for the health care provider's position that the person who signed was informed adequately. However, it is possible that the person who signed the short consent form could convince a court that he or she did not give informed consent, because he or she did not receive information as to consequences, risks, and alternatives to the treatment. When the short form is used, testimony of the health care providers who participated in the informed consent process, rather than the form itself, will serve as the most important evidence of informed consent. For this reason, practitioners who use the short form are well advised to make detailed notes in the patient's medical record regarding the risks and benefits that were discussed in the informed consent process.

Long Consent Forms

Some health care organizations use forms that include a detailed description of the patient's medical condition, proposed procedure, consequences, risks, and alternatives to treatment. These detailed forms may be mandated by statute, such as in the case of federally funded sterilizations and research involving human subjects. When a long form is used, it is much more difficult for the patient to prove that the information in the form was not disclosed, since it bears the patient's signature. The health care provider may hand-write the risks, benefits, alternatives, and other pertinent information on the long form, or the form may be preprinted. A preprinted detailed form for a particular procedure should be updated to reflect changes in the risks, benefits, and alternatives to the procedure so that the form does not become obsolete. Because the preprinted long form contains a full description of risks and benefits, there is a danger health care providers may come to rely on the form as an inadequate substitute for the consent process, rather than explaining the information carefully to each patient and ascertaining that the patient understands. Consent policies and procedures, as well as staff education, should be used to guard against this possibility.

Challenges to Consent Forms

As stated earlier, although consent forms are strong evidence of informed consent, they are not conclusive. The person challenging the adequacy of the consent process will have an opportunity to convince the court that informed consent was not actually obtained. For example, the person who signed the form may prove he or she was not competent as a result of the effects of medication. Thus, it is important that the explanation of a procedure's risks, benefits, and alternatives be given and the signature be obtained at a time when the consenting party is capable of understanding the decision being made. Consent forms may be challenged on the basis that the wording was too technical or that the form was written in a language the patient could not understand. Although persons are presumed to have read and understood documents they have signed, courts will not apply this presumption in the face of such challenges.

As a result, it is important that forms are understood by the person signing them. If the person has difficulty understanding English, someone, preferably a health care organization employee capable of understanding the technical information, should translate the form. It is advisable to have consent forms in the primary languages used by a substantial portion of the patients served by the health care organization or practice. However, it is usually sufficient to have the form translated orally and have the translator certify that the form and discussion of the procedure have been translated orally for the person signing the form. If a patient refuses to sign a consent form but is willing to give oral consent after receiving an adequate explanation of the procedures, the fact of oral consent and the reason for the patient's refusal to sign should be documented on the consent form, along with the witnessed signature of the person obtaining the verbal consent.

A consent form also may be challenged on the ground that the signature was not voluntary. Because the person signing would have to prove that there had been some threat or undue inducement to prove that the signature was coerced, it is difficult to prove coercion. However, if a physician misrepresents the probability of death or injury involved in refusing to undergo the proposed procedure, the patient or the patient's representative might be successful in showing coercion and thereby invalidate the patient's prior consent.

Withdrawal of Consent

Unless specified by statute, there is no absolute limit on the period of validity of a consent or the documentation of that consent by a signature on a consent form. If the patient's condition or the available treatments change significantly, the earlier consent no longer is valid, and a new consent should be obtained.

Whenever a patient refuses to consent to or withdraws consent for treatment, the patient's physician should be notified, and written acknowledgment of the refusal or withdrawal should be obtained from the patient after the physician has discussed the implications of the refusal or withdrawal with the patient. These steps generally will protect the health care provider and organization from liability. If the patient refuses to sign a form releasing the health care organization and providers from responsibility for the consequences of refusal or withdrawal of consent, these facts should be documented thoroughly in the medical record.

Because a claim that consent was withdrawn becomes more credible as time passes, it may be advisable to obtain informed consent for patients with ongoing treatment periodically. For example, some hospitals obtain a new consent each time the patient is admitted. The consent may be obtained in a physician's office before the admission, provided that the time between the consent and the admission is not too long. Some policies require consent forms to be signed no more than 30 days before the procedure; others require new consents periodically, especially in outpatient treatment settings. Carefully prepared policy should establish guidelines governing the validity and expiration of patient consent.

Impact of Statutes

When developing forms, health care administrators must consider state statutes. In some states, statutes provide that if the consent form contains certain information and is signed by the appropriate person, it creates a presumption of informed consent. For example, in Iowa a written consent is presumed to be an informed consent if it describes the nature and purpose of the procedure consented to, including specific risks listed in the statute such as death, brain damage, and quadriplegia, as well as an acknowledgment that the patient's questions have been answered satisfactorily.[57] Such statutes indicate how the courts will treat forms containing only the information specified in the statute. Although it is not a violation of these statutes to use a form that contains different language than that outlined in the statute, health care organizations should be sure that a de-

---

[57]Iowa Code § 147.137.

cision to use forms that do not meet the statutory requirements is based on careful consideration of the risks. In any case, organizations should not adopt such forms without the advice of their legal counsel.

6

Access to Medical Record Information

Chapter Objectives

- Explain the general rule regarding ownership of medical record information.
- Give examples of state laws that protect the confidentiality of medical record information.
- Describe the types of medical record information protected by federal law.
- Summarize the rights of patients and third parties to access medical record information, including sensitive information such as alcohol and drug abuse patient records and psychiatric records.
- Give examples of laws governing the release of patient information for medical research purposes.
- Describe the authority allowing health care providers to charge record duplication fees.
- Summarize the laws or accreditation standards governing the use of medical records in utilization review and quality assurance activities.

INTRODUCTION

This chapter discusses medical record confidentiality requirements and the general legal principles governing access to patient health care information. Health care organizations and providers must be aware of the various federal and state laws governing the confidentiality of medical record information. A variety of access issues can arise in a health care setting, including access to medical records by or on behalf of the patient, access to the medical records of minors, and staff access to medical record information. Patient records containing sensitive health information, such as psychiatric records, may have stricter confidentiality and release requirements. Health care organizations should also be aware of the law regarding disclosures for medical research. To comply with all of these laws, each health care organization must devise an effective record-security procedure that protects and preserves both the physical medical record and the patient's general interest in confidentiality. Utilization review laws and standards issued by voluntary accreditation organizations may also govern how health care organizations and providers may grant access to medical record information. Health care organizations and providers should consult the law in their jurisdiction to fully understand their obligation to keep patient information confidential and the circumstances in which medical record information may be disclosed.

Health care organizations and practitioners may be held liable for improperly disclosing patient information. In addition to facing statutory penalties, health care facilities, organizations, and providers may be liable under common law theories, including defamation, invasion of privacy, and breach of physician-patient privilege. (These common law theories are discussed in Chapter 11.)

OWNERSHIP OF THE MEDICAL RECORD

As a general rule, the health care facility or the provider owns the medical records subject to the patient's interest in the information it contains. The basic rule of record ownership is established by statute in many states.[1] Many state statutes provide that medical records are the property of the organization or provider that maintains or possesses the records. For example, the South Carolina statute states that the "[p]hysician is the owner of

---

[1]*See, e.g.*, TENN. CODE ANN. § 68-11-304(a)(1); MISS. CODE ANN. § 41-9-65.

medical records in his possession that were made in treating a patient and of records transferred to him concerning prior treatment of the patient."[2]

Many states with specific rules on record ownership include these provisions in their state hospital-licensing regulations. A typical regulation provides that medical records are the property of the hospital and shall not be removed from its premises except for court purposes.[3]

While the health care organization owns the physical medical record, the patient has an interest in information contained in the record. State legislation frequently subjects the health care organization's right of ownership to the patient's right of access to the information contained in the medical record. In Louisiana, for example, the statute provides that although the medical records are the property and business records of the health care provider, a patient has the right to obtain a copy of the record.[4] Thus, the patient has an ownership interest in the information contained in the medical record. At least one state, New Hampshire, explicitly recognizes the patient's interest in the medical information contained in the medical record.[5] Courts have recognized that a patient has the right to access health information, such as a copy of medical records or an interpretation of an X-ray, even though the patient might not have a right to possess original medical records or an X-ray negative.[6]

In the absence of statutory or regulatory authority, a few courts have held that a medical record is hospital property in which the patient has a limited property interest. In an Oklahoma case,[7] for instance, a patient's health insurer sought access to the hospital records for the purpose of settling an insurance claim where the patient had authorized disclosure. The court recognized that the "records maintained by [the hospital] pertaining to care and treatment of patients and to expenses incurred by patients . . . [were] the property of the hospital." However, the court did grant access to the insurer because the patient in this case had authorized disclosure.[8]

---

[2]S.C. CODE ANN. § 44-115-20; *see also* VA. CODE ANN. § 32.1-127.1:03.

[3]*See, e.g.*, 902 KY. ADMIN. REGS. 20:016(11)(c); OR. ADMIN. R. 333-505-050(12); 28 PA. CODE § 115.28; TENN. CODE ANN. § 68-11-304(a)(1).

[4]LA. REV. STAT. ANN. § 40:1299.96.

[5]N.H. REV. STAT. ANN. § 332-I:1.

[6]*See* Cannell v. Medical & Surgical Clinic, 315 N.E.2d 278 (3d Dist. 1974), McGarry v. J.A. Mercier Co., 262 N.W. 296 (Mich. 1935).

[7]Pyramid Life Ins. Co. v. Masonic Hosp. Ass'n of Payne County, 191 F. Supp. 51 (W.D. Okla. 1961).

[8]Pyramid Life Ins. Co. v. Masonic Hosp. Ass'n of Payne County, 191 F. Supp. 51 (W.D. Okla. 1961). *See also* Wallace v. University Hosps., 164 N.E.2d 917, 918 (Ohio C.P. 1959), *modified and aff'd*, 170 N.E.2d 261 (Ohio Ct. App. 1960)

While a patient may have a statutory interest in information contained in the medical record, there is no independent constitutional right to such information. In a New York case,[9] a former mental patient writing a book about her experiences was denied access to her medical records by her treating hospitals. At trial, the patient argued that the hospitals had violated her federal constitutional rights. The district court ruled that the hospitals' withholding of information did not violate any of the patient's rights, including her right to information as a corollary to her right of free speech, her right of privacy, her freedom from unreasonable searches and seizures of property, or deprivation of her property without due process of law. In affirming the district court opinion, the court of appeals refused to recognize that psychiatric patients have a constitutionally protected property interest in the direct and unrestricted access to their records.

A health maintenance organization (HMO), managed care organization (MCO), or other third-party administrator owns the medical records, even if the health plan sponsor is a self-insured employer. An employer might try to obtain access to confidential patient information by claiming ownership of the medical records. However, even if the third-party administrator is an agent of the employer, not every material used by the third-party administrator belongs to the employer. Most relationships between a third-party administrator and an employer are that of independent contractor. In that case, ownership interests are set by state law. No law in any state provides that information obtained or maintained while providing health care services to a self-insured employer is the property of the employer. Just as courts have determined that providers, not the patients who hire them, own the medical records, a court likely would find that a third-party administrator owns its records. Accordingly, confidential patient information can only be released in accordance with federal and state confidentiality laws.[10]

When questions of medical records ownership arise, the attorney for the health care organization or provider should be aware that, although the institution owns every medical record, patients generally have a right to review their records. When a patient seeks access to records, the health care organization or provider through its legal counsel should consult state and

---

[9]Gotkin v. Miller, 379 F. Supp. 859 (E.D.N.Y. 1974), aff'd, 514 F.2d 125 (2d Cir. 1975). The rules governing access to the medical records of mental health patients are more restrictive than those for other types of medical treatment in many jurisdictions.

[10]G. Bogossian, MCO's Protection of Confidential Information (Paper presented at National Health Lawyers Association Health Law Update and Annual Meeting, June 5-7, 1996)

federal statutes governing hospital licensure, mental health patients, and specific programs such as alcoholism and drug abuse treatment centers, along with any licensing regulations applicable to their facility and any special programs. In addition, all relevant court decisions must be reviewed before questions regarding a specific case can be answered.

CONFIDENTIALITY REQUIREMENTS

The obligation of health care organizations and providers to keep medical records confidential is governed by a patchwork of federal and state law. Federal law protects a very limited amount of health information. Most states have statutory requirements protecting the confidentiality of medical record information, although these statutory protections often vary between states and within a state, depending on who holds the information.

State Law

Statutory provisions concerning health information often are scattered throughout a state's code. For example, confidentiality requirements can be found in a state's medical records act, hospital licensing act, medical practice act, HMO act, or statutes dealing with human immunodeficiency virus (HIV). Often, these statutes protect only certain information—such as hospital medical records or physician's records. Some states might not impose confidentiality requirements on all entities that hold patient information. A state might require a physician to keep a patient's medical record confidential but not impose a similar requirement on an insurer even though the insurer has the same information. Another complication occurs because protection of health information can vary from state to state, leading to situations where information is protected in one state but not in another. The lack of uniform standards and variation in the law among the states can cause difficulty where interstate health care transactions, telemedicine, and ERISA health plans are common.[11]

---

[11]For a survey of law in this area, *see* L. Gostin, Z. Lazzarini, & K. Flaherty, Legislative Survey of State Confidentiality Laws, with Special Emphasis on HIV and Immunization, Final Report (Presented to the U.S. Centers for Disease Control and Prevention, the Council of State and Territorial Epidemiologists, and The Task Force for Child Survival and Development—Carter Presidential Center, Georgetown University Law Center, July, 1996).

Most states require physicians to keep their medical records confidential. Some states extend this confidentiality requirement to other licensed health care providers.[12] In California, a health care provider may not disclose medical information regarding a patient without the patient's authorization.[13] Similarly, Maryland requires health care providers to keep the patient medical record confidential.[14] Prior written consent is often needed before the physician can release the medical records.[15] Redisclosure by the individual or entity receiving the patient information commonly is not permitted unless the patient signs a new authorization.[16] Finally, most states do allow disclosure without authorization under a limited set of circumstances, such as for diagnosis or treatment purposes, quality control or peer review, or research purposes without patient identification information.[17]

As with physicians, most states require health care institutions to keep their medical records confidential. Many states locate these requirements in a licensing and regulation act. For example, Florida's hospital and licensing act provides that patient records are confidential and explains that the records may not be released without the patient's consent except under a narrow set of circumstances.[18] The Illinois Nursing Home Care Act provides that a resident's records are confidential.[19] Illinois law governing long-term care facilities states that all information contained in a resident's record is confidential and the facility must obtain written consent of the resident or a guardian prior to releasing the records.[20] Under certain circumstances, however, facilities may be able to release medical records without the consent of the patient. Florida allows hospitals to release patient records to licensed facility personnel and attending physicians for use in treating the patient; to facility personnel for administrative, risk

---

[12]*See, e.g.,* California, where the confidentiality requirement extends to medical doctors, doctors of osteopathy, chiropractors, and anyone else licensed or certified under the state's Business and Professions Code. CAL. CIV. CODE § 56.05(d).

[13]CAL. CIV. CODE § 56.10.

[14]MD. CODE ANN., HEALTH-GEN. § 4-302.

[15]*See, e.g.,* CAL. CIV. CODE § 56.11.

[16]*See, e.g.,* MD. CODE ANN., HEALTH-GEN. § 4-302(d).

[17]*See, e.g.,* CAL. CIV. CODE § 56.10(c).

[18]FLA. STAT. ANN. § 395.3025(4).

[19]210 ILL. COMP. STAT. 45/2-206.

[20]ILL. ADM. CODE tit. 77 § 390.1630.

management, and quality assurance activities; to Florida's public health agency for the purpose of health care cost containment; and if subpoenaed in any civil or criminal action.[21]

Insurers and MCOs increasingly require patient information before making utilization review or reimbursement decisions. Some states have enacted statutory provisions requiring HMOs or other insurers to keep patient information confidential. A statute in Colorado concerning HMOs provides that any data or information pertaining to the diagnosis, treatment, or health of any enrollee is confidential and may be disclosed under very limited circumstances or upon the consent of the individual.[22] Texas is another state where the state's HMO Act requires HMOs to keep patient information confidential.[23] In New York, utilization review agents are required to keep patient information confidential.[24]

Several states have adopted the National Association of Insurance Commissioners Insurance Information and Privacy Protection Model Act (NAIC Model Act) or similar legislation.[25] The NAIC Model Act requires "insurance institutions, agents, and insurance support organizations" to keep health information confidential.[26] Health information may not be disclosed without the authorization of the individual. The NAIC Model Act, however, allows disclosures without authorization in the following situations. The insurer can disclose health information under limited circumstances, including:

- with the written authorization of the individual;
- to persons performing business, professional, or insurance functions for the insurer, subject to an agreement that the individual not redisclose the information;
- to prevent or detect criminal activity or fraud;

---

[21]FLA. STAT. ANN. § 395.3025(4).

[22]COL. REV. STAT. § 10-16-423.

[23]TEX. INS. CODE ANN. § 20A.25.

[24]N.Y. INS. LAW § 4905.

[25]National Association of Insurance Commissioners, Insurance Information and Privacy Protection Model Act, Model #670-1. States that have adopted this Model Act include Arizona, California, Connecticut, Georgia, Illinois, Kansas, Massachusetts, Minnesota, Montana, Nevada, New Jersey, North Carolina, Oregon, and Virginia.

[26]National Association of Insurance Commissioners, Insurance Information and Privacy Protection Model Act, Model #670-1.

- to a provider or institution to verify coverage or audit the provider or institution;
- to insurance regulators, law enforcement agencies, and other government agencies; in response to court orders;
- to conduct actuarial or research studies;
- to an entity buying, selling, or merging with the insurer subject to the entity's agreement not to redisclose the information;
- to the group policyholder for reporting claims experience or for conducting an audit of the insurer; and
- to peer review organizations.[27]

Employers that self-insure may have access to their employees' patient health care information. However, very few states have enacted legislation protecting the confidentiality of patient information held by the patient's employer. One state that has passed legislation protecting this information is California. California law provides that employers who receive medical information are required to develop procedures to ensure the confidentiality of this information. The statute also states that the health care information may be used only for administering and maintaining employee benefit plans.[28]

Some states have enacted patient rights legislation that covers the confidentiality of medical information. For example, New Jersey's Patient Bill of Rights Act specifies that all patients admitted to a hospital licensed in the state are entitled to privacy and confidentiality of all records.[29] Illinois has a patient rights statute that protects a variety of health information. The Illinois Patient Rights Act directs physicians, health care providers, health services corporations, and insurance companies not to disclose the nature or details of services provided to patients. The Act has several exceptions to this directive. Disclosure may be made to the patient; to the party making treatment decisions if the patient is not capable of making them; to parties directly involved with providing treatment or processing payment for that treatment; to parties responsible for peer review, utilization review, and quality assurance; and to those parties where disclosure is authorized or required under the law.[30]

---

[27]National Association of Insurance Commissioners, Insurance Information and Privacy Protection Model Act, Model #670-1.

[28]CAL. CIV. CODE § 56.20.

[29]N.J. STAT. ANN. § 26:2H-12.8(g).

[30]410 ILL. COMP. STAT. 50/3.

Some states have adopted comprehensive health information statutes. The states of Montana and Washington have adopted the Uniform Health Care Information Act (UHCIA).[31] The UHCIA forbids a health care provider, an individual who assists a health care provider in the delivery of health care, or an agent or employee of a health care provider from disclosing health care information without the patient's written authorization. However, the UHCIA has some exceptions to this general rule, allowing disclosure in several situations, including to an individual providing health care to the patient, to an individual needing this information for quality assurance or peer review purposes, and to immediate family members of the patient or any other individual known to have a close personal relationship with the patient if the disclosure is made in accordance with good medical or professional practice and the patient has not instructed the provider otherwise.

State Open Records Laws

Many states have freedom of information laws granting public access to records maintained by state agencies.[32] In some states, the statute is called the "public records" or "open records" law. Like the federal Freedom of Information Act (FOIA), these typically contain exceptions for medical records where disclosure would constitute an unwarranted invasion of personal privacy.[33] A few states simply exempt all hospital or medical records from the public records law[34] or include them in a list of public records available only upon court order and in other limited circumstances.[35] Most case law arising under the state acts deals with determining whether a private interest in confidentiality outweighs the public interest in disclosure.

In *Child Protection Group v. Cline*,[36] for example, a West Virginia court outlined five factors for determining whether release of personal information under the state freedom of information act would constitute an "un-

---

[31]MONT. CODE ANN. §§ 50-16-501 through 50-16-553; WASH. REV. CODE §§ 70.02.005 through 70.02.904.

[32]*See, e.g.*, ALA. CODE § 36-12-40; FLA. STAT. ANN. § 119.01; MD. CODE ANN., STATE GOV'T § 10-611.

[33]*See, e.g.*, 20 ILL. COMP. STAT. 2215/4-3.

[34]*See, e.g.*, LA. REV. STAT. ANN. § 44:7; MISS. CODE ANN. § 41-9-68.

[35]*See, e.g.*, IOWA CODE ANN. § 22.7.

[36]Child Protection Group v. Cline, 350 S.E.2d 541 (W. Va. 1986).

reasonable" invasion of privacy: (1) whether disclosure would result in a substantial invasion of privacy and, if so, how serious the potential consequences would be; (2) whether the extent or value of the public interest and the purpose or object of individuals seeking the information justify disclosure; (3) whether the information was available from other sources; (4) whether the information was given with an expectation of confidentiality; and (5) whether it is possible to mold relief to limit the invasion of privacy.[37] After examining these issues, the court in this case authorized release of a bus driver's psychiatric records to parents of schoolchildren after the driver acted in a manner raising serious questions about his ability to operate the bus safely.

Whether specific documents are the kind covered by an exception to a state public records law sometimes is unclear. In *Head v. Colloton*,[38] for instance, a state hospital objected to an attempt to access its bone marrow transplant registry under the Iowa Public Records Act, arguing that the registry was protected from disclosure under the statutory exemption to the Act for "hospital and medical records of the condition, diagnosis, care, or treatment of a patient or former patient, including outpatient." Although the court concluded that only hospital records relating to patient care and treatment are exempt from disclosure under the law, it concluded that the bone marrow records related to a patient and therefore were not accessible.

Federal Law

A small amount of health information is protected by federal law. Sources of federal protection of medical record information include the Constitution, the Privacy Act, the Freedom of Information Act, and the Medicare Act.

Constitution

The constitutional right to privacy provides very limited protection for patient health information. The Supreme Court noted that in some situations the duty to avoid disclosing confidential medical record information has its roots in the Constitution.[39] Thus, an absolute privacy interest in

---

[37]Child Protection Group v. Cline, 350 S.E.2d 541 (W. Va. 1986).

[38]Head v. Colloton, 331 N.W.2d 870 (Iowa 1983).

[39]Whalen v. Roe, 429 U.S. 589 (1977).

confidential medical records information does not exist. Constitutional claims are further limited by the requirement that any violation of the right to privacy must be caused by state action. However, at least one state, California, has created a right of privacy that applies to an invasion of privacy by a private party.[40]

Privacy Act

The Privacy Act of 1974,[41] designed to give private citizens some control over information collected by the federal government, restricts the type of information that a federal agency lawfully may collect concerning an individual citizen or legal alien and limits the uses of such information. Under the Privacy Act, an agency may maintain only information that is relevant and necessary to its authorized purpose.[42] An agency may not disclose any information about a private individual through any means of communication to any person or other agency except as authorized in writing by the person or under certain conditions described in the Act.[43]

The Privacy Act also requires each federal agency to allow individuals to gain access to their records or any information pertaining to them and copy any or all of the information.[44] Individuals also may make requests to amend or modify their records, and the agency must either make the changes or provide an explanation for declining to do so.[45] In certain cases, the head of the agency must review the decision to deny a requested change.[46]

The Privacy Act allows an agency to disclose information about an individual without that person's consent only in certain circumstances. Disclosures may be made: to officers and employees of the agency who need the information to perform their duties; under the Freedom of Information Act; for certain statistical and law enforcement purposes; to Congress, the Comptroller General, or the National Archives and Records Administration; pursuant to a valid court order; or where a person shows compelling

---

[40]CAL. CONST. art. 1, § 1.
[41]5 U.S.C. § 552a.
[42]5 U.S.C. § 552a(e)(1).
[43]5 U.S.C. § 552a(b).
[44]5 U.S.C. § 552a(d)(1).
[45]5 U.S.C. § 552a(d)(2).
[46]5 U.S.C. § 552a(d)(3).

circumstances affecting the health or safety of the individual to whom the information relates.[47]

The Privacy Act provides civil remedies for individuals aggrieved by an agency's failure to comply with the law.[48] An injured individual may bring suit against the agency in federal court and, possibly, enjoin the agency from continuing its action and recover reasonable attorney fees and court costs. The Act provides for criminal fines against an officer or employee of an agency for certain willful violations of the statute.[49]

It is important to emphasize that the Privacy Act applies only to federal agencies and to government contractors. Hospitals operated by the federal government, therefore, are bound by the Act's requirements with respect to the disclosure of the medical records of their patients. In addition, medical records maintained in a records system operated under a contract with a federal government agency are subject to the Privacy Act.[50] MCOs that provide health insurance to government employees and MCOs with Medicare contracts are also covered by the Act.[51] Private or state-owned hospitals and MCOs that do not contract with the federal government generally are not subject to civil or criminal liability under the Act for their unlawful disclosure of patient information, or for any unlawful disclosure by a federal agency to which the hospital properly reports. The fact that a hospital or other health care facility receives federal funding or is subject to federal regulation does not automatically subject it to the Act.[52]

Freedom of Information Act

The Freedom of Information Act (FOIA),[53] enacted in 1966, provides public access to information on the operations and decisions of federal administrative agencies. A hospital does not become a federal agency by receiving federal funds, so FOIA applies to few hospitals outside of the Veterans Administration and Defense Department hospital systems. The law provides that specific categories of information are available to the

---

[47] 5 U.S.C. § 552a(b).
[48] 5 U.S.C. § 552a(g)(1).
[49] 5 U.S.C. § 552a(i)(1).
[50] 5 U.S.C. § 552a(m)(1).
[51] 42 C.F.R. § 417.486(c).
[52] St. Michael's Convalescent Hosp. v. California, 643 F.2d 1369 (9th Cir. 1981).
[53] 5 U.S.C. § 552.

public unless one of the nine specific exceptions to the general rule of disclosure applies. Medical records may be exempt from FOIA under specific circumstances.

The FOIA requires each federal agency to make certain information available for public inspection and copying, including final opinions, concurring and dissenting opinions, and orders made in the adjudication of cases;[54] statements of policy and interpretations adopted by the agency and not published in the *Federal Register*;[55] and administrative staff manuals and instructions to staff that affect a member of the public.[56] Each agency must make the information available unless the materials are published promptly and copies offered for sale.[57]

All other records, except those specifically excluded under the FOIA, must be made available promptly to any person upon request if he or she reasonably describes such records and complies with the agency's published rules covering the time, place, and fee for inspecting and copying.[58] Each agency also is required to maintain and make available a current index for public inspection and copying. The index must provide identifying information as to matters covered by the FOIA.[59] However, an agency may delete identifying details when it makes available an opinion, statement of policy, interpretation, or staff manual or instruction to prevent a clearly unwarranted invasion of an individual's personal privacy. In each case, justification for the deletion must be explained fully in writing.[60]

Nine specific exceptions to the general FOIA disclosure are provided.[61] One of these exceptions, known as "Exception Six," covers "personnel and medical files and similar files, the disclosure of which would constitute a clearly unwarranted invasion of personal privacy.[62]

To qualify for protection from FOIA disclosure, medical records information must satisfy the three elements described in Exception Six:

---

[54] 5 U.S.C. § 552(a)(2)(A).

[55] 5 U.S.C. § 552(a)(2)(B).

[56] 5 U.S.C. § 552(a)(2)(C).

[57] 5 U.S.C. § 552(a)(2).

[58] 5 U.S.C. § 552(a)(3).

[59] 5 U.S.C. § 552(a)(2).

[60] 5 U.S.C. § 552(a)(2).

[61] 5 U.S.C. § 552(b).

[62] 5 U.S.C. § 552(b)(6).

1. The information must be contained in a personnel, medical, or similar file.
2. Disclosure of the information must constitute an invasion of privacy.
3. The invasion clearly is unwarranted.[63]

An agency seeking to withhold information has the burden of showing that the requested material satisfies each and every element of Exception Six.[64]

In determining whether the information sought falls within this exception, the relevant consideration is whether the privacy interests associated with the information are similar to interests that generally arise from personnel or medical information, and not whether the data are recorded in a manner similar to a personnel or medical file.[65] A file is considered similar to personnel and medical files if it contains intimate details of an individual's life, family relations, personal health, religious and philosophical beliefs, and other matters that, if revealed, would prove personally embarrassing to a person of normal sensibilities. Whether file materials are similar turns on whether the facts that would be revealed would infringe on some privacy interest as highly personal or as intimate in nature as that at stake in personnel and medical records.

Once a court determines that requested information is the type of material covered by Exception Six, it must address whether disclosure of such information would constitute an invasion of privacy. Several courts have emphasized that Exception Six was intended to prevent public disclosure of intimate details about an individual's life, such as marital status, legitimacy of children, identity of fathers of children, medical conditions, welfare payments, alcohol consumption, family fights, and reputation.[66] On

---

[63]Sims v. C.I.A., 642 F.2d 562 (D.C. Ct. App. 1980), rev'd and aff'd on other grounds, 471 U.S. 159 (1985); see also Citizens for Envtl. Quality Inc. v. United States Dep't of Agric., 602 F. Supp. 534, 537 (D.D.C. 1984), where the court characterized its analysis under Exception Six as a two-step inquiry to determine: first, whether information sought is contained in personnel, medical, or similar files and, second, whether release would constitute a clearly unwarranted invasion of personal privacy.

[64]Sims v. C.I.A., 642 F.2d 562, 566 (D.C. Ct. App. 1980), rev'd and aff'd on other grounds, 471 U.S. 159 (1985).

[65]Harbolt v. Department of State, 616 F.2d 772, 774 (5th Cir. 1980), cert. denied, 449 U.S. 856 (1980).

[66]Sims v. C.I.A., 642 F.2d 562, 574 (D.C. Ct. App. 1980), rev'd and aff'd on other grounds, 471 U.S. 159 (1985), quoting Rural Hous. Alliance v. United States Dep't of Agric., 498 F.2d 73, 77 (D.C. Cir. 1974).

the other hand, information connected with commercial matters, business judgments, or professional relationships is not covered by the exception.[67]

If a court concludes that the release of information would constitute an invasion of personal privacy as contemplated by Exception Six, it must balance the personal interest in preventing disclosure against the public interest in obtaining access to the information.[68] In this regard, courts have interpreted the language "clearly unwarranted invasion of personal privacy" as an expression of a congressional policy that favors disclosure and an instruction to tilt the balance in favor of disclosure.[69] An agency seeking to prevent the release of information under Exception Six, therefore, must make a detailed and factual showing of the likely consequences of disclosure in individual cases.[70] The possibility of embarrassing an agency or speculation about the identity of an individual that would result from disclosure will not outweigh the public interest.[71]

An agency is required to provide reasonably segregable nonexempt portions of an otherwise exempt record to any person requesting such record.[72] Federal agencies that maintain medical records or have obtained medical records legitimately are required, both by the Privacy Act and by this exception to the FOIA, to withhold disclosure of such records unless a court, in balancing individual and public interests in the information, orders disclosure or unless such records are requested by Congress.

Although original medical records maintained by a federal agency are exempt from disclosure under Exception Six, disclosure may be required under the FOIA of any information taken from these records in connection with government-funded medical research and incorporated into re-

---

[67]Sims v. C.I.A., 642 F.2d 562, 574 (D.C. Ct. App. 1980), *rev'd and aff'd on other grounds,* 471 U.S. 159 (1985), citing Board of Trade of Chicago v. Commodity Futures Trading Comm'n, 627 F.2d 392, 399-400 (D.C. Cir. 1980).

[68]Sims v. C.I.A., 642 F.2d 562, 573 (D.C. Ct. App. 1980), *rev'd and aff'd on other grounds,* 471 U.S. 159 (1985).

[69]Sims v. C.I.A., 642 F.2d 562, 575 (D.C. Ct. App. 1980), *rev'd and aff'd on other grounds,* 471 U.S. 159 (1985); Citizens for Envtl. Quality Inc. v. United States Dep't of Agric., 602 F. Supp. 534, 538 (D.D.C. 1984).

[70]Sims v. C.I.A., 642 F.2d 562, 575 (D.C. Ct. App. 1980), *rev'd and aff'd on other grounds,* 471 U.S. 159 (1985).

[71]Sims v. C.I.A., 642 F.2d 562, 573 n. 139 (D.C. Ct. App. 1980), *rev'd and aff'd on other grounds,* 471 U.S. 159 (1985); Citizens for Envtl. Quality Inc. v. United States Dep't of Agric., 602 F. Supp. 534, 538 (D.D.C. 1984).

[72]5 U.S.C. § 552(b).

search reports to a sponsoring agency. Determining whether the data belong to the researchers or to the agency is crucial in resolving a request for access under these circumstances because only the agency is subject to FOIA.

The U.S. Supreme Court has ruled[73] that "written data generated, owned, and possessed by a private controlled organization receiving federal study grants are not 'agency records' within the meaning of the [Freedom of Information] Act when copies of those data have not been obtained by a federal agency subject to the FOIA. Federal participation in the generation of the data by means of a grant from the Department of Health, Education, and Welfare (HEW) does not make the private organization a federal 'agency' within the terms of the Act."[74] The Court held that the grantee's data would become agency records if it could be shown that the agency directly controlled the day-to-day activities of the grantee.[75]

Health care organizations and hospitals receiving federal funds for medical research can minimize the risk of disclosure of research data under FOIA, therefore, by limiting the agency's supervision of studies conducted by staff. The health care organization or hospital also should obtain the agency's acknowledgment that the data are confidential and will not be disclosed except as required by law.

Medicare Conditions of Participation

The Medicare Conditions of Participation require institutions participating in the Medicare and Medicaid programs to keep medical records confidential. The Conditions of Participation apply to a number of institutions participating in federal health care programs, including hospitals, long-term care facilities, home health agencies, substance abuse agencies, and hospices.[76]

---

[73]Forsham v. Harris, 445 U.S. 169 (1980).

[74]Forsham v. Harris, 445 U.S. 169, 171 (1980).

[75]Forsham v. Harris, 445 U.S. 169, 180 (1980).

[76]*See, e.g.*, Conditions of Participation for Hospitals, 42 C.F.R. § 482.24(b)(3).

Accreditation Organizations

Hospitals, HMOs, and health care organizations that seek accreditation from private authorities will be required to meet standards concerning medical records confidentiality. The Joint Commission on Accreditation of Healthcare Organizations (Joint Commission), which accredits various entities including hospitals, home health agencies, and managed care organizations, has standards regarding the management of information. For example, entities accredited under the Joint Commission's health care network standards are required to develop a process to protect the confidentiality of medical record information.[77] The National Committee for Quality Assurance (NCQA), which accredits managed care entities, also has standards concerning medical record confidentiality. Physician organizations that seek accreditation from the NCQA are required to have policies and procedures that protect the confidentiality of medical records.[78] (Refer to "Record Security" later in this chapter for further discussion of standards issued by accreditation agencies.)

ACCESS TO MEDICAL RECORD INFORMATION

The medical record is a confidential document and access to it generally should be limited to the patient or an authorized representative, the attending physician, and other staff members possessing legitimate interests in the record relating to the patient's care. Usually, a parent must authorize disclosure of a minor's medical record. However, in some situations the minor might be able to authorize disclosure of medical record information. Certain types of health information, such as psychiatric records, records of alcohol and drug abuse treatment, and genetic testing information are particularly sensitive. Special laws may govern access to these medical records, usually imposing stricter requirements for confidentiality. Health care administrators involved with the release of medical information must understand all of these rules and exceptions.

---

[77]Joint Commission, 1996-97 Comprehensive Accreditation Manual for Health Care Networks, Standard IM 2.

[78]National Committee for Quality Assurance, Standards for the Certification of Physician Organizations, Standard MR 1 (1997).

Access by or on Behalf of the Patient

The patient or the patient's representative has the right in most jurisdictions to authorize disclosure of confidential patient information. Most state laws expressly allow a patient or authorized representative to examine and copy the patient's medical records.[79] The person seeking access typically must make a written request and pay reasonable clerical costs before the records become available.[80] The health care organization or provider usually is responsible only for making the records available at reasonable times and places. Connecticut law states that upon written request, a provider must furnish patients with copies of their health records at a cost of no more than 45 cents per page plus postage and the cost of X-ray materials.[81] South Carolina's Physicians' Patient Records Act provides that a patient has the right to receive a copy of his or her medical records.[82] In California, facilities must provide for patient inspection of records within five working days of the request and provide copies within 15 working days and upon payment of fees.[83] Georgia also requires hospitals to provide records access to patients upon receipt of a written request,[84] but allows the institutions to require payment of the copying and mailing costs before releasing the records.[85]

Depending upon the state, patients may be able to review their medical records while they are still in the hospital. Many statutes allow patients to review their records upon request during the course of hospitalization.[86] Other statutes grant patients an unrestricted right of access to their medical records only after discharge from the hospital.[87] Florida has similar legislation, providing that a licensed facility, upon receiving a written request after discharge of the patient, must furnish a patient or patient representative a true and correct copy of the record.[88]

---

[79]*See, e.g.*, MD. CODE ANN., INS. § 4-403; WIS. STAT. ANN. § 146.82.

[80]*See, e.g.*, N.H. REV. STAT. ANN. § 332-I; MONT. CODE ANN. §§ 50-16-526 & 50-16-541.

[81]CONN. GEN. STAT. § 20-7c(b).

[82]S.C. CODE ANN. § 44-115-30.

[83]CAL. HEALTH & SAFETY CODE § 123110.

[84]GA. CODE ANN. §§ 31-33-2 & 31-33-3.

[85]Cotton v. Med-Cor Health Info. Solutions, Inc., 472 S.E.2d 92 (Ga. App. Ct. 1996), *cert. denied*, No. S96C1434 (Ga. Oct. 4, 1996) (unpublished); GA. CODE ANN. § 31-33-3.

[86]*See, e.g.*, MINN. STAT. § 144.335(2).

[87]*See, e.g.*, 735 ILL. COMP. STAT. ANN. 5/8-2001.

[88]FLA. STAT. ANN. § 395.3025(1).

In addition to meeting its legal obligations, a hospital may have some practical reasons for allowing a patient to examine the records during hospitalization. Hospitals should consider whether refusal to permit such an inspection will create unnecessary problems for the institution and its staff. An inpatient who is denied access to a chart may become hostile and more difficult to treat. Moreover, the patient may be more likely to file a claim against the hospital if treatment ends in a poor result.

Therefore, unless the attending physician has a reasonable basis for believing that disclosure of the medical record will harm the patient, the hospital should allow the individual to review the record. In some instances, a record review coordinated by the patient's attending physician will enhance the patient's understanding of actions taken by the physician, thereby promoting better hospital-patient relations and decreasing the likelihood of any claims being filed against the facility. If inpatients are allowed to examine their records, however, the hospital should employ its customary record security procedures. (Record security is discussed later in this chapter.)

Many statutes allow the health care organization or provider to refuse to grant the patient's request for disclosure where the individual seeks access to psychiatric information, where release of psychiatric information would be detrimental to the patient's mental health,[89] or where release of any medical information would adversely affect the general health of the person.[90] In some instances, the psychiatric patient can obtain at least a summary of the records following termination of the treatment program.[91] In New York, the provider may deny access to a patient's records where the requested information can reasonably be expected to cause substantial and identifiable harm to the subject or others that outweighs the right to access.[92] In most states where a patient lawfully can be denied access to records, however, the health care organization may be required to deliver copies of the record to the patient's representative or attorney.[93]

---

[89]*See, e.g.*, CAL. HEALTH & SAFETY CODE § 13115(b); COLO REV. STAT. § 25-1-801.

[90]*See, e.g.*, HAW. REV. STAT. § 622-57; ME. REV. STAT. ANN. tit. 22, § 1711; MINN. STAT. § 144.335(2)(c).

[91]*See, e.g.*, COLO. REV. STAT. § 25-1-801(1)(a).

[92]N.Y. PUB. HEALTH LAW § 18(3)(a).

[93]*See, e.g.*, HAW. REV. STAT. § 622-57; ME. REV. STAT. ANN. tit. 22, § 1711; MINN. STAT. § 144.335(2)(c) (provider may withhold information from patient and may supply the information to appropriate third party); OKLA. STAT. ANN. tit. 76, § 19.

Several states' statutes contain special provisions concerning a patient's access to particular portions of the record, such as X-rays;[94] others have separate rules governing access by a minor patient;[95] and still others allow a provider to prepare a summary of the record for inspection and copying rather than permit the patient access to the entire record.[96]

Some statutes and regulations providing access to records by patients prescribe a time limit for a response. For example, New York requires the provider to respond to a request to review records within ten days after receiving the request.[97] California law requires the hospital to provide for inspection of records within five working days after receiving a request and to provide copies of the record within 15 days.[98] Illinois allows 60 days to respond.[99] Minnesota law states that a provider must furnish copies of a medical record to a patient "promptly" after receiving the request.[100] As the laws in each state vary with respect to the time allowed for a response, every health care organization and provider must check requirements in its own area. Where the laws are silent on the matter, a health care organization or provider should develop a policy for providing copies of patient records as soon as possible after the institution reasonably can locate the record and prepare a copy for the patient.

In the absence of statute or regulation, courts in some jurisdictions have recognized a common law duty to allow a patient limited access to records.[101] In *Cannell v. Medical and Surgical Clinic*, for instance, the court found that the fiduciary qualities of the physician-patient relationship require the provider to disclose medical data to the patient or agent upon request, and that the patient need not engage in legal proceedings to attain higher status in order to receive such information.[102] Other courts have held that, although a hospital may have a common law duty to disclose all or part of a patient's record, there is no obligation to do so free of

---

[94]*See, e.g.*, CAL. HEALTH & SAFETY CODE §§ 123110(c) through (e).

[95]*See, e.g.*, CAL. HEALTH & SAFETY CODE § 123115; N.Y. PUB. HEALTH LAW § 18(2)(c).

[96]*See, e.g.*, CAL. HEALTH & SAFETY CODE § 123130; MINN. STAT. § 144.335(2)(b).

[97]N.Y. PUB. HEALTH LAW § 18(2)(a).

[98]CAL. HEALTH & SAFETY CODE § 123110(b).

[99]735 ILL. COMP. STAT. ANN. 5/8-2001.

[100]MINN. STAT. § 144.335(2)(b).

[101]*See, e.g.*, Hutchins v. Texas Rehabilitation Comm'n, 544 S.W.2d 802 (Tex. Ct. App. 1976); In re Weiss, 147 N.Y.S.2d 455 (Sup. Ct. 1955).

[102]Cannell v. Medical & Surgical Clinic, 315 N.E.2d 278 (Ill. Ct. App. 1974); *see also* Emmett v. Eastern Dispensary & Cas. Hosp., 396 F.2d 931 (D.C. Cir. 1967); Parkson v. Central DuPage Hosp., 435 N.E.2d 140 (Ill. Ct. App. 1982).

charge.[103] However, because the vast majority of states now grant statutory recognition to a patient's right of access, courts are less likely to become involved in enunciating legal precedent on this issue.

MCOs also have an obligation to disclose medical record information to the patient unless the MCO can determine that such access would be harmful to the patient. The NAIC Privacy Protection Model Act requires MCOs that are insurers to give enrollees access to information about themselves, as well as the chance to correct or object to the accuracy of the information.[104] Under ERISA, plan participants and their authorized representatives have the right to review documents used to support claim denials.[105] These documents include medical records used to justify the denial.[106] Finally, an MCO that is an ERISA plan fiduciary may have to provide plan participants access to health care information held by the MCO. The reasoning discussed above concerning the fiduciary qualities of the physician-patient relationship can also be applied to the MCO-participant relationship.[107]

Copies of health care records and other medical information should never be disclosed to any third party in the absence of a medical records release authorization signed by the patient. Third-party payers usually require the patient to sign a consent form for release of patient records as a condition of the patient's payment contract. A health care organization or provider should request a copy of this release from the third-party payer before releasing a copy of the patient's medical information to the third-party payer.

Before a health care organization provides access to a third party with the patient's authorization, it may take reasonable precautions to verify the authority of the person seeking the information. Some state statutes specifically authorize hospitals to take these measures.[108] Courts also have recognized a hospital's right to verify the validity of a patient's authorization. In one case, a state appeals court held that a hospital records clerk properly refused to release certain files on the basis of a signed authoriza-

---

[103]Rabens v. Jackson Park Hosp. Found., 351 N.E.2d 276, 279 (Ill. Ct. App. 1976).

[104]National Association of Insurance Commissioners, Insurance Information and Privacy Protection Model Act, Model #670-1, § 8.

[105]29 C.F.R. § 2560.503-1(g).

[106]Groves v. Modified Retirement Plan, 803 F.2d 109 (3d Cir. 1986).

[107] G. Bogossian, MCO's Protection of Confidential Information (Paper presented at National Health Lawyers Association Health Law Update and Annual Meeting, June 5-7, 1996).

[108]*See, e.g.,* CAL. HEALTH & SAFETY CODE § 123110(d).

tion form containing alterations that were unacceptable under hospital records policy.[109] On the other hand, a hospital will be liable for unreasonably restricting access to medical records as tantamount to refusal to release the records.[110]

Determining who is the patient's representative for purposes of accessing records also can generate difficulties. In *Emmett v. Eastern Dispensary and Casualty Hospital*,[111] for instance, the son of a deceased patient requested to see his father's medical record in order to bring a wrongful death action against the hospital. However, the hospital refused to release the records because the son was not the father's administrator and, therefore, not the father's legal representative. The court ruled that, while the decedent's proper legal representative is the only person authorized to bring a suit for wrongful death, the purpose of a suit is to benefit the spouse and next of kin. Therefore, the court concluded, the hospital's duty of disclosure to the patient extended to the patient's son, his only surviving relative and next of kin.

Records of Minors

Generally, a health care organization or provider may disclose the medical record of a minor patient only with authorization from one of the parents of that individual. Parents typically are allowed access to such records on behalf of a minor patient. If a guardian has been appointed to act in the child's behalf, only the guardian may access the patient's records and authorize release of information to others.

A number of state statutes governing access to medical records include specific directions about disclosing the records of a minor. For example, Minnesota defines the term "patient" to include a parent or guardian of a minor and then directs each hospital to provide copies of the record to the "patient" upon request.[112] The California statute has separate provisions dealing with access to a minor's records and disclosure of such records to third parties.[113] The provision on access provides that any adult patient, any minor patient authorized by law to consent to treatment, and any pa-

---

[109]Thurman v. Crawford, 652 S.W.2d 240, 242 (Mo. Ct. App. 1983).

[110]Thurman v. Crawford, 652 S.W.2d 240, 242 (Mo. Ct. App. 1983).

[111]Emmett v. Eastern Dispensary & Cas. Hosp., 396 F.2d 931 (D.C. Cir. 1967).

[112]MINN. STAT. § 144.335(1)(a).

[113]CAL. HEALTH & SAFETY CODE § 123110(a); *see also* N.Y. PUB. HEALTH LAW § 17 (release of medical records), and N.Y. PUB. HEALTH LAW § 18 (access to patient information).

tient representative shall be entitled to inspect patient records upon written notice and payment of reasonable fees. However, a minor patient shall be entitled to inspect only records pertaining to health care of the type for which the minor may lawfully consent.

Notwithstanding the general right of access granted to a minor's representative under California law, a representative may not access the minor's records if the minor has a right of inspection under the general rule of patient access by virtue of his or her authority to consent to the type of medical treatment described in the record.[114] In addition, a health care provider may deny access to a minor's representative if it determines that access would have a detrimental effect on the provider's professional relationship with the minor.[115] The California statute defines "representative" as a parent or guardian of a minor who is a patient or former patient.[116]

A minor patient may authorize release of medical information to third parties if the information was obtained during the course of providing health care services to which the minor lawfully could consent under other provisions of the law.[117] In all other cases, the minor's legal representative must consent.[118]

The New York law on access to a minor's record is similar to California's; however, New York allows the provider to deny access where release of information would have a detrimental effect on an infant's relationship with parents or guardian.[119] Further, a minor patient's records involving abortion or venereal disease never can be released to the parent or guardian.[120] In all other cases, the parent or guardian can authorize release to third parties.

The statutes of many states simply are not clear on the question of parental or guardian access to a minor's records. Most statutes permit ac-

---

[114]CAL. HEALTH & SAFETY CODE § 123115(a)(2).

[115]CAL. HEALTH & SAFETY CODE § 123115(a)(2). *See* In re Daniel C.H., 269 Cal. Rptr. 624 (Ct. App. 1990), in which the court applied this provision to deny a parent access to a minor child's psychotherapy records. The parent contended that he was entitled to access the child's confidential communications because, as a parent, he has the right to receive information concerning the medical condition of his child. The court ruled, however, that access would cause substantial harm to the child, who might refuse to be open with the therapist out of fear of disclosure to the parent.

[116]CAL. HEALTH & SAFETY CODE §§ 123105(c) through (e).

[117]CAL. CIV. CODE § 56.11(c)(1).

[118]CAL. CIV. CODE § 56.11(c)(2).

[119]N.Y. PUB. HEALTH LAW § 18(2)(c).

[120]N.Y. PUB. HEALTH LAW § 17.

cess with the consent of the patient,[121] or the patient or his authorized representative.[122] In those states, health care organizations and providers should follow the general rule and obtain the authorization of the minor's parent before disclosing the patient's records to third parties. However, when the minor has the authority under state law to consent to medical treatment, the minor must give his or her consent to disclose this information, even to the minor's parents or legal guardians.

In this regard, health care organizations and providers must examine carefully the definitions of terms such as "patient" and "representative" in the statute because not all states define those terms in the same way. Moreover, the same state may provide one definition under the provisions on direct access and another definition for disclosure to third parties.

Most importantly, a health care organization or provider treating or planning to treat a young person must double-check the legal age for giving consent to the particular treatment involved. While a "minor" in most states is a person under 18 years of age,[123] many jurisdictions create exceptions for certain types of medical treatment. For example, in California, a 12-year-old may consent to mental health treatment if the child presents a serious danger to self or others, or has been the victim of alleged incest or child abuse,[124] and an emancipated minor of any age lawfully can consent to any hospital, medical, or surgical care.[125] In Illinois, a 17-year-old can consent to a blood donation.[126]

Access by Staff

Hospitals and health care organizations generally allow certain staff members to access medical records without patient consent for certain authorized purposes. Staff members must access medical records for patient care reasons, as well as for certain administrative purposes such as auditing, filing, billing, replying to inquiries, and defending against lawsuits. At the same time, health care entities are responsible for safeguarding

---

[121]*See, e.g.,* COLO. REV. STAT. § 25-1-801(1)(a); FLA. STAT. ANN. § 395.3025(1); HAW. REV. STAT. § 622-57.

[122]*See, e.g.,* ME. REV. STAT. ANN. tit. 22, § 1711; TENN. CODE ANN. § 68-11-304(a)(1).

[123]*See, e.g.,* CAL. FAM. CODE § 6500.

[124]CAL. FAM. CODE § 6924(B)(b).

[125]CAL. FAM. CODE § 7002 & 7050.

[126]210 Ill. COMP. STAT. ANN. 15/1.

each record and its content against unauthorized access or use.[127] Guidelines addressing this generally are found in hospital or medical staff bylaws, policies and procedures, and, less frequently, in state statutes or regulations.

State law and standards promulgated by accreditation agencies such as the Joint Commission permit disclosure of confidential patient information under certain conditions. Several state statutes permit the release of confidential patient information to qualified personnel for the purpose of conducting scientific research, audits, program evaluations, official surveys, education, and quality control activities, without patient authorization.[128] In addition, the Joint Commission says that clinical and administrative data can be aggregated and analyzed to support decisions, track trends over time, make comparisons within the organization and among organizations, and improve performance.[129]

Some state statutes provide that hospital or health care organization staff members can have access to patient records. In most states, hospital licensing regulations permit access to patient records by "authorized" personnel or persons granted access by hospital policy for purposes related to the patient's care.[130] The hospital then is made responsible for ensuring that only authorized persons review the records.[131] Some states, such as Rhode Island, permit qualified personnel and health care providers within the system to have access to medical records for the purpose of coordinating care.[132] State law may also permit release of patient information for administrative reasons, such as for billing purposes.[133] Finally, the confi-

---

[127]JOINT COMMISSION, 1997 ACCREDITATION MANUAL FOR PREFERRED PROVIDER ORGANIZATIONS, Standard IM.2; NATIONAL COMMITTEE FOR QUALITY ASSURANCE, STANDARDS FOR THE CERTIFICATION OF PHYSICIAN ORGANIZATIONS, Standard PO 2 (1997); JOINT COMMISSION, 1996-97 COMPREHENSIVE ACCREDITATION MANUAL FOR HEALTH CARE NETWORKS, Standard IM.2.3; JOINT COMMISSION, 1997 HOSPITAL ACCREDITATION MANUAL, Standard IM. 2.3.

[128]*See, e.g.*, R.I. GEN. LAWS § 5-37.3-4(b)(3); CAL. CIV. CODE § 56.10.

[129]JOINT COMMISSION, 1997 HOSPITAL ACCREDITATION MANUAL, Standard IM.8 through IM 8.1.12; JOINT COMMISSION, 1997 ACCREDITATION MANUAL FOR PREFERRED PROVIDER ORGANIZATIONS, Standard IM.4 through IM 4.3.

[130]*See, e.g.*, CAL. CIV. CODE § 56.10(c)(1); FLA. STAT. ANN. § 395.3025(4)(a); WIS. STAT. ANN. § 146.82(2).

[131]*See, e.g.*, 902 KY. ADMIN. REGS. 20:016 (11)(C)(1); MO. CODE REGS. ANN. tit. 19, § 30-20.021(D)(7).

[132]R.I. GEN. LAWS § 5-37.3-4(b)(5).

[133]*See, e.g.*, WIS. STAT. ANN. §§ 146.82(2) & (3).

dentiality statutes in many states expressly permit access to patient records by health care providers and others for purposes of providing diagnosis or treatment, and during medical emergencies.[134]

Access to certain patients' records is expressly governed by some state and federal laws. For example, there are special federal statutes and regulations on access to certain alcohol or drug abuse treatment records (discussed later in this chapter). These provide for the general confidentiality of drug and alcohol patients' records with an exception for disclosure to persons in connection with their duties to provide diagnosis, treatment, or referral for treatment of abuse.[135] There also is a statutory exception to confidentiality for release of patient record information during a bona fide medical emergency.[136]

Some states also address alcohol and drug abuse patient records. These laws typically provide an exception to the general ban on disclosure of such records for the exchange of information relating to the patient's treatment among qualified personnel involved in the treatment.[137] Other states incorporate the federal alcohol and drug abuse regulations directly into their own laws.[138]

Some states have special laws on staff access to records of mental health patients[139] and AIDS patients.[140] Not all staff members have access to those types of records. Again, the laws vary from state to state, and health care organizations should consult the particular rules applicable to them.

Accreditation organizations such as the Joint Commission and the National Committee for Quality Assurance require health care and physician organizations to be especially careful about maintaining the confidentiality of sensitive information.[141] In the Joint Commission's Management of

---

[134]*See, e.g.,* CAL. CIV. CODE § 56.10(c)(1); FLA. STAT. ANN. § 395.3025(4)(a) R.I. GEN LAWS § 5-37.3-4(b)(1).

[135]42 C.F.R. § 2.12(c)(3).

[136]42 U.S.C. § 290dd-2(b)(2)(A); 38 U.S.C. § 7332(b)(2)(A).

[137]*See, e.g.,* WIS. STAT. ANN. § 51.30(4).

[138]*See, e.g.,* MD. CODE ANN., HEALTH-GEN. § 8-601(c).

[139]WASH. REV. CODE ANN. § 71.05.390.

[140]*See, e.g.,* HAW. REV. STAT. § 325-101; WIS. STAT. ANN. § 146.82.

[141]*See* JOINT COMMISSION, 1997 HOSPITAL ACCREDITATION MANUAL, Intent of Standard IM.2 through IM.2.3; JOINT COMMISSION, 1997 ACCREDITATION MANUAL FOR PREFERRED PROVIDER ORGANIZATIONS, Intent of Standard IM.2; JOINT COMMISSION, 1996-97 COMPREHENSIVE ACCREDITATION MANUAL FOR HEALTHCARE NETWORKS, Standard IM.2 through IM.2.3.

Information Standards, the Joint Commission recognizes that some data are more sensitive and require a higher level of confidentiality.[142]

Health care organizations should carefully develop policies and procedures for staff members to follow to obtain access to medical records. The Joint Commission suggests that the organization begin by determining the levels of confidentiality necessary for different types of information, such as a high level of confidentiality for sensitive health care information. The organization should next decide who has access to what information. Health care organizations should consider allowing access on a need-to-know basis. Access may differ depending upon the staff member's job title, responsibilities, and function. For example, physicians do not need to access information on all patients; their access should be limited to the patients that they are treating. Certain parts of the medical record may be very sensitive and require extra protection of the patient's privacy. A health care organization might choose to store sensitive portions of the medical record, such as psychiatric records, in a separate location.[143] (See also the discussion of Record Security later in this chapter.)

Psychiatric Records

In some states, the rules on access to the medical records of mental health patients differ from those applicable to medical records generally. In past years, mental health patients were denied access to their medical records even where non–mental health patients in the same jurisdiction had such a right. It was widely believed that authorizing psychiatric patients to review their records would be injurious to their health.

Mental health patients in some states have the same right to inspect their records as do other patients, although only a few laws expressly grant such individuals a right to access their records.[144] In other states, the laws provide that records of psychiatric patients or institutionalized persons are confidential and shall be disclosed only as provided by the statute. In New Jersey, for example, the statute governing psychiatric patients makes confidential all records that directly or indirectly identify an

---

[142]JOINT COMMISSION, 1995 MANAGEMENT OF INFORMATION STANDARDS, pp 40-41. The Management of Information Standards, which currently are being phased in, are directed to hospitals and health care networks.

[143]JOINT COMMISSION, 1995 MANAGEMENT OF INFORMATION STANDARDS, pp 40-45.

[144]*See, e.g.*, HAW. REV. STAT. § 334E-2(a)(15); 740 ILL. COMP. STAT. ANN. 110/4(a).

individual who is receiving or has received mental health services, except if the person or legal guardian consents.[145] Such a provision, granting the patient a statutory right to records confidentiality, can be construed to create a corresponding implied right of access for the patient. A federal trial court has ruled that this provision allows patients confined in mental institutions to obtain access to all of their records maintained by the state, even if their guardians do not consent to disclosure, unless the state can challenge the patients' capacity to give informed consent.[146]

A Florida federal trial court has ruled that a state statute excluding individuals with psychiatric conditions from accessing their medical records violates the Americans with Disabilities Act (ADA). A Florida statute provides discharged patients a legal right of access to their medical records, but excludes individuals with mental or emotional conditions from this right of access.[147] An organization advocating on behalf of individuals with mental disabilities sued the state of Florida, alleging that Florida's medical records access statute violates the ADA by excluding patients with mental disabilities from all other individuals who have a right of access to their medical records and imposing additional burdens on individuals with mental disabilities who want access to their treatment records. A Florida federal trial court has ruled that this statute violated the ADA, concluding that the state of Florida cannot impose an extra burden on patients seeking access to their medical records because they received mental health treatment.[148]

Even where a patient has a clear right to review the records, state legislation frequently imposes limits on the exercise of that right. For example, the New York Mental Hygiene Law establishes the confidentiality of clinical records and authorizes the patient to make a written request to review the files.[149] The facility maintaining the records must inform the patient's treating physician upon receipt of the request. The facility must permit the patient to inspect the records or provide copies unless the treating practitioner determines that the requested review could "reasonably be expected to cause substantial and identifiable harm to the patient."[150] If review is denied, the patient has a right to obtain review of that decision without

---

[145]N.J. STAT. ANN. § 30:4-24.3.

[146]Bonnie S. v. Altman, 683 F. Supp. 100 (D.N.J. 1988).

[147]FLA. STAT. ANN. § 395.3025.

[148]Doe v. Stincer, No. 96-2191-CIV-MORENO (S.D. Fla. Dec. 2, 1997).

[149]N.Y. MENTAL HYG. LAW § 33.16(b)1.

[150]N.Y. MENTAL HYG. LAW § 33.16(c)(1).

cost by the appropriate records committee.[151] The patient also has a right to judicial review of an adverse determination by the committee.[152]

State legislation in some jurisdictions allows mental health patients to petition a court to seal the records of treatment. Under New York legislation, for example, patients must demonstrate by competent medical evidence that they are not currently suffering from mental illness, that they have not received inpatient services for treatment of mental illness for a period of three years, and that the interests of both the petitioners and society would be served best by sealing the records.[153] One court has ruled that society has an interest in sealing mental health records to remove the barriers that would prevent a former psychiatric patient from participating fully in society without fear of stigma or discrimination.[154] In the absence of a statutory right to expunge mental health records, some courts have authorized such action for records that result from an illegal commitment or illegal involuntary examination proceeding involving falsehood or perjury.[155]

If a state does not have specific legislation governing access to psychiatric records, access falls under the general rules of confidentiality effective in the jurisdiction. Typically, only a person authorized by a competent patient can obtain access to that patient's records, including those relating to psychiatric treatment. If a patient is incompetent, the duly authorized legal guardian may access the records in the same manner as a competent patient.[156] However, the health care organization or provider should request to see the appropriate authorization before permitting access to a person who claims to be acting on behalf of an incompetent patient. A guardian who has been appointed for a specific purpose does not necessarily have the authority to review an incompetent patient's records.[157]

---

[151]N.Y. MENTAL HYG. LAW § 33.16(c)(4).

[152]N.Y. MENTAL HYG. LAW § 33.16(c)(5); *see also* Davis v. Henderson, 549 N.Y.S.2d 241 (App. Div. 1989) where the court remitted the petitioner's claim for judicial review that a psychiatric facility had denied his request to review his records but had failed to inform him of his right to committee review. The court ordered the case returned to the facility for further proceedings under the New York Mental Hygiene Law.

[153]N.Y. MENTAL HYG. LAW § 33.14(a)(1) & (b).

[154]Smith v. Butler Hosp., 544 N.Y.S.2d 711 (Sup. Ct. 1989).

[155]Johnston v. State, 466 So. 2d 413 (Fla. Dist. Ct. App. 1985) *citing* Wolfe v. Beal, 384 A.2d 1187 (Pa. 1978).

[156]*See, e.g.*, Gaertner v. State, 187 N.W.2d 429 (Mich. 1971).

[157]*See, e.g.*, In re Patarino, 142 N.Y.S.2d 891 (Ct. Cl. 1955).

Similarly, where an incompetent patient has a guardian assigned by a court to act in the person's best interests, the health care organization or provider should be careful not to release the records to other persons associated with the patient. In one case, for example,[158] the mother of an involuntarily committed minor requested access to records pertaining to her daughter's treatment, but the child's court-appointed guardian objected. The mother alleged but could not prove that decisions made by the hospital were not in the best interests of her daughter. The court denied the mother's request, emphasizing that one purpose of appointing a guardian is to protect the minor from parental efforts to terminate treatment for reasons unrelated to the best interests of the child.[159]

Alcohol and Drug Abuse Patient Records

Provisions in the Public Health Service Act[160] address access to the records of drug or alcohol abuse patients. Under these provisions, records of the "identity, diagnosis, prognosis, or treatment" of any patient maintained in connection with the performance of any educational, training, treatment, rehabilitative, or research program concerning drug or alcohol abuse may not be disclosed except for certain purposes and under certain circumstances.[161] Any person or program that releases information in violation of the Act is subject to criminal fines.[162]

The Secretary of the Department of Health and Human Services (HHS) has promulgated regulations on access to records of alcohol and drug abuse patients covered by the Act.[163] The regulations, like the statutes,

---

[158]In re J.C.G., 366 A.2d 733 (N.J. Hudson County Ct. 1976).

[159]Cases involving a guardian purportedly acting on behalf of a mental health patient should be distinguished, however, from those involving an "interested person" who may have independent rights under state law to participate in mental health proceedings affecting a patient. *See, e.g.*, In re Wollan, 390 N.W.2d 839 (Minn. Ct. App. 1986), where the court granted records access to the sister of a mentally ill and dangerous patient as an "interested person" entitled to notification of any change in the patient's status and the right to request review of the change of status under Minnesota law. *See also* In re New York News, 503 N.Y.S.2d 714 (1986), where the court granted a newspaper access to sealed mental health records as a party "properly interested" in such records under applicable New York law.

[160]Originally enacted as Drug Abuse Prevention, Treatment, and Rehabilitation Act. *See generally* 21 U.S.C. §§ 1101 through 1800 and the Comprehensive Alcohol Abuse and Alcoholism Prevention, Treatment, and Rehabilitation Program Act, 42 U.S.C. §§ 4541 through 4594.

[161]42 U.S.C. § 290dd-2(a).

[162]42 U.S.C. § 290dd-2(f).

[163]The regulations are codified at 42 C.F.R. §§ 2.1 through 2.67.

generally prohibit disclosure of certain types of information about an alcohol or drug abuse patient except as specifically authorized.[164]

Virtually every alcohol and/or drug abuse treatment center is subject to the statute and regulations. Under the regulations, any facility operating a "program" that is "federally assisted" falls within the scope of this legislation.[165] "Federal assistance" is defined broadly to include any program that receives a state or municipal grant if the state or local government in turn has received any unrestricted grants or funds from the federal government.[166] If contributions to a program are deductible under federal income tax law, the program is regarded as a recipient of federal financial assistance. Few programs are totally privately funded, receive no tax deductions for contributions, and/or are neither licensed nor regulated by the federal government. Accordingly, almost every drug or alcohol abuse program is governed by this legislation.[167]

"Program" refers to an individual, partnership, corporation, governmental agency, or other legal entity holding itself out, in whole or part, as providing, and does provide, alcohol or drug abuse diagnosis, treatment, or referral for treatment. For a general medical care facility or any part of it to qualify as a "program," it must have an identified unit that provides such services, or medical personnel whose primary function is to provide such services and who are identified as providers of such services.[168] The terms "diagnosis," "treatment," "alcohol abuse," and "drug abuse" are defined specifically in the regulations.[169]

The provisions for the release of information apply only if an individual is a "patient" under the law. The regulations define "patient" as any individual who has requested or received a diagnosis or treatment for alcohol

---

[164]42 C.F.R. §§ 2.12(a) & 2.13(a).

[165]42 C.F.R. § 2.12(a)(1)(ii).

[166]However, if a state receives federal money earmarked for certain purposes not including an alcohol or drug abuse treatment program, a facility receiving state funds is not subject to the federal laws governing alcohol and drug abuse patient records. *See* Listion v. Shelby County, No. 93007-3 R.D. (Tenn. Ct. App. Oct. 23, 1987) (unpublished).

[167]Whenever a person or program seeks to invoke the protection of the federal statute and regulations in order to assure the confidentiality of patient records, that person or program bears the burden of demonstrating the applicability of the federal laws. *See* Samaritan Health Serv. v. City of Glendale, 714 P.2d 887 (Ariz. Ct. App. 1986), where the facility claiming protection under 42 U.S.C. § 290ee-3 failed to show that it operated a program subject to the law; *see also* State v. Gullekson, 383 N.W.2d 338 (Minn. Ct. App. 1986).

[168]42 C.F.R. § 2.11.

[169]42 C.F.R. § 2.11.

or drug abuse at a federally assisted program.[170] One court ruled that a person who enters a hospital emergency room for immediate treatment of conditions arising from a drug overdose is a "patient" under the regulations because that individual clearly "applied for treatment or diagnosis of drug abuse."[171] Further, the court ruled, the emergency room qualified as a "program" because it provides diagnoses, treatment, and referrals and because many drug users enter the hospital through the emergency room as the first step to further drug treatment.

An alcohol or drug abuse treatment program under this legislation may not disclose any information, recorded or not, that would identify a patient as an alcohol or drug abuser either directly, by reference to other publicly available information, or through verification by another person.[172] This blanket prohibition clearly covers a broad range of information about a patient, including nonwritten information and indirect indications of a patient's identity.[173]

Health care organizations subject to these rules must be wary of implicit disclosure of confidential information. If a general care hospital or other health care organization fails to disclose information about a drug or alcohol abuse patient that it routinely discloses about other patients, it could be liable for implicitly admitting that the patient was being treated for drug or alcohol abuse. Hospitals and health care organizations therefore should delete such patients from their registers unless the individuals consent to having their presence acknowledged. Although that practice will protect the patients' identity as required by the alcohol and drug abuse regulations, it can create other problems. For example, hospitals that maintain patient registers at their switchboards and information desks may encounter difficulties. Health care organizations must devise methods for identifying drug or alcohol abuse patients that do not allow its personnel to release information inadvertently.

The medical records of alcohol and drug abuse patients may be disclosed with their consent under certain circumstances. The regulations provide a list of elements required for lawful consent, along with a sample

---

[170]42 C.F.R. § 2.11.

[171]United States v. Eide, 875 F.2d 1429, 1435 (9th Cir. 1989).

[172]42 C.F.R. § 2.12(a)(1)(i).

[173]*But see* State v. Brown, 376 N.W.2d 451 (Minn. Ct. App. 1985), where the court held that personal observations made to police officers by a counselor at a drug treatment center relating to a patient's parole for drug-related offenses were not "records" under the regulations, even if reduced to writing by the counselor.

consent form.[174] In general, the consent must be in writing, signed by the patient or authorized signatory, and must describe the kind of information to be disclosed and the purpose for disclosure. The person releasing the medical records must notify the recipient of the fact that the recipient in turn is bound by the regulations and prohibited from further disclosure.[175] A facility releasing information in accordance with this provision should document its notice to the recipient in writing; a routine form letter sent to each recipient of alcohol and drug abuse patient records would facilitate meeting this requirement.

Under the regulations, minors may consent to the release of their drug and alcohol abuse records if, under state law, they may consent to the treatment.[176] The regulations do not address directly the circumstances under which a minor may consent to such treatment, but instead expressly defer to state law on the issue. Consequently, a minor's ability to consent to the release of treatment records covered by the federal law will vary from state to state. Where state law mandates parental consent to alcohol and drug abuse treatment for a minor, the federal regulations require parental consent to any disclosure of information relating to such treatment.[177] Federal regulations also specifically authorize disclosure to parents or guardians of facts relevant to reducing a substantial threat to a minor's life or physical well-being where the individual lacks capacity to make a rational decision about whether to release the records.[178] The regulations also contain a special provision on release of information by incompetent patients.[179]

Disclosure without consent is permitted under limited circumstances. For example, disclosure to medical personnel may be made in a medical emergency posing an immediate threat to health.[180] A program proceeding under this provision must enter the following information directly into the patient's record:

- the name of the medical personnel to whom disclosure was made and their affiliation with any health care facility

---

[174]42 C.F.R. §§ 2.31(a) & (b).

[175]42 C.F.R. § 2.32.

[176]42 C.F.R. § 2.14(b).

[177]42 C.F.R. § 2.14(c).

[178]42 C.F.R. § 2.14(d).

[179]42 C.F.R. § 2.15.

[180]42 C.F.R. § 2.51(a).

- the name of the individual making the disclosure
- the date and time of the disclosure
- the nature of the emergency[181]

Another important exception to the general ban on disclosure without the patient's consent applies to communications between persons who need the information to perform duties arising out of diagnosis, treatment, or referral for treatment of alcohol or drug abuse. However, such exchanges of information are permitted only if they occur within a program or between a program and an entity that has direct administrative control over the program.[182] The ban on disclosure does not apply to communications between a program and a "qualified service organization,"[183] defined as including companies providing data processing, bill collecting, lab work, legal work, and other services to the program.[184] On the other hand, the ban on disclosure expressly is extended to third-party payers; entities with direct administrative control over programs receiving information from the program related to diagnosis, treatment, or referral; and persons receiving information from a covered program with the patient's consent as provided under the regulations.[185] This provision could apply to MCOs that, for example, receive protected information related to payment of benefits even though the MCO does not maintain actual treatment records.

Disclosure without consent may be made for audit and evaluation[186] or for research purposes.[187] The regulations provide for additional measures in these situations to protect patient information and identification. The regulations allow certain disclosures of information to the Food and Drug Administration (FDA) where a tainted drug may threaten the health of an individual under the FDA's jurisdiction.[188] Other exceptions are made for disclosures to law enforcement officials relating to a patient's commission of or threat to commit a crime on program premises or against program

---

[181] 42 C.F.R. § 2.51(c).
[182] 42 C.F.R. § 2.12(c)(3).
[183] 42 C.F.R. § 2.12(c) (4).
[184] 42 C.F.R. § 2.11.
[185] 42 C.F.R. § 2.12(d) (2).
[186] 42 C.F.R. § 2.53.
[187] 42 C.F.R. § 2.52.
[188] 42 C.F.R. § 2.51(b).

personnel[189] and for reporting suspected child abuse and neglect under state law.[190]

Disclosure without consent also may be made in response to a court order. A person with a legally recognized interest in disclosure of records covered by the federal provisions may apply for a court order to use the records for noncriminal purposes.[191] In general, the statute provides that an order for disclosure may issue only for good cause.[192] For "good cause" to exist, the evidence must demonstrate that the information is not available through other means or would not be effective, and that the public interest and need for disclosure outweigh the potential injury to the patient, the physician-patient relationship, and the treatment services.[193]

If the records are to be used in a criminal investigation or prosecution of a patient, different criteria govern their release. These criteria relate to the seriousness of the underlying crime; the value of information in the records to the investigation or prosecution; the unavailability or ineffectiveness of other ways to obtain the information; the public interest and need for disclosure versus the potential injury to the patient, physician-patient relationship, and the ability of the program to provide services to others; and the availability of independent counsel for the person holding the records.[194]

Many of the programs subject to the federal laws on alcohol and drug abuse patient records also are governed by state law, including state rules on confidentiality and state mandatory reporting laws. The operation of both sets of rules may create conflicts for the program.

The federal regulations provide that the statutes authorizing them do not preempt state law.[195] They instruct that if disclosure permitted by the federal regulations is prohibited under state law, federal law should not be interpreted to authorize a violation of the state law. On the other hand, the regulations provide that state law may not authorize or compel any disclosure prohibited by the federal regulations. In other words, if the federal law permits disclosure prohibited by state law, the disclosure is not to be

---

[189]42 C.F.R. § 2.12(c)(5).

[190]42 C.F.R. § 2.12(c)(6).

[191]42 C.F.R. § 2.64.

[192]42 U.S.C. § 290dd-2(b)(2)(C); *see also* 42 C.F.R. § 2.64.

[193]42 C.F.R. § 2.64(d).

[194]42 C.F.R. § 2.65(d).

[195]42 C.F.R. § 2.20.

made; and if federal law prohibits disclosure, disclosure should not be made, regardless of the state law governing the issue. Nevertheless, a program subject to both sets of rules must be careful to release only the particular information required by state law. Any release of information beyond that required by state law constitutes a breach of the federal regulations.

Several states have enacted their own provisions for access and disclosure of alcohol and drug abuse patient records.[196] These statutes typically impose a general ban on disclosure of records by covered programs except as provided in the law. Exceptions to confidentiality generally are created for disclosures relating to financial and compliance audits and program evaluations, between qualified personnel involved in the patient's treatment, and to qualified persons responding to a medical emergency. Alcohol and drug abuse treatment programs in each state must be aware of the particular state laws applicable to them in addition to the federal laws governing their patient records.

Genetic Information

The advent of the Human Genome Project (HGP) in 1990 has raised many legal issues. The goal of the HGP is to map the location of genes in the human genome. Researchers have already successfully identified the genes responsible for diseases such as Huntington's disease, amyotrophic lateral sclerosis (Lou Gehrig's disease), and cystic fibrosis. The HGP is also identifying genes associated with diseases caused by environmental and social influences as well as by hereditary factors, such as breast and colon cancer, diabetes, and hypertension.

Breaching the confidentiality of genetic information can make an individual vulnerable to discrimination by insurance companies or employers. In addition, the offspring of these individuals can be susceptible to the same form of discrimination because they too might have inherited genes making it more likely that they will develop a particular disease. Recognizing the sensitivity of genetic information, the Ninth Circuit has stated that genetic information is entitled to the highest expectation of privacy.[197]

---

[196]*See, e.g.*, CAL. HEALTH & SAFETY CODE § 11977; MD. CODE ANN., HEALTH-GEN. § 8-601(c); WIS. STAT. ANN. § 51.30(4).

[197]Bloodsaw v. Lawrence Berkeley Laboratory, No. 96-16526 (9th Cir. Feb. 3, 1998).

In response to concerns about genetic privacy, many states have passed legislation regulating access to genetic information. For example, Georgia's statute provides that genetic test information is confidential and privileged. In addition, an insurer that possesses genetic information may not release the information to any third party without the written consent of the individual tested.[198] In Missouri, genetic test information cannot be released before fully informing the individual of the scope of information that will be released, as well as the risks, benefits, and purposes of disclosure and the identity of those to whom the information will be released.[199] Colorado's genetic privacy law applies to health insurers, HMOs, nonprofit hospitals, and medical-surgical and health service corporations.[200] Under the statute, information derived from genetic testing is confidential and privileged. It may not be released for purposes other than diagnosis, treatment, and therapy without the written consent of the patient. Any entity that receives genetic test information may not use or keep the information for any nontherapeutic purpose, or for a purpose connected with the provision of health, group disability, or long-term care insurance coverage.[201]

DISCLOSURES FOR MEDICAL RESEARCH

Many medical research projects involve the use of patients' medical records. These records are important for determining responses to specific types of therapy, tracking relationships involving population characteristics and incidence of illness, or obtaining statistical information important for developing more efficient treatments. Several states have adopted specific provisions allowing disclosure of patient information for research purposes.[202]

The California research provision is found in its records confidentiality statute.[203] Other states have independent medical research statutes allowing providers to release patient information for research purposes.[204]

---

[198]GA. CODE ANN. § 33-54-3. *See also* LA. REV. STAT. ANN. § 40:1299.6.

[199]MO. REV. STAT. § 191.317.

[200]COLO. REV. STAT. § 10-3-1104.7.

[201]*See also*, MD. CODE ANN., INS. § 223.1.

[202]*See, e.g.*, CAL. CIV. CODE § 56.10(c)(7); FLA. STAT. ANN. § 405.01.

[203]CAL CIV. CODE § 56.10.

[204]*See, e.g.*, FLA. STAT. ANN. §§ 405.01 through 405.03.

When responding to requests for patient data for research, a health care provider must consult the provision effective in its state, if one exists. The statutes vary in terms of who can release information, what information can be released, and to whom and for what purposes it may be released.

Some states have special rules for access to certain types of records for research purposes. In addition to its general rule on research, for example, California has a special provision governing access to records of patients with developmental disabilities.[205] The District of Columbia and Iowa have special statutes addressing researcher access to mental health records.[206]

Federal regulations also cover research involving human subjects and the release of patient information for research purposes where HHS conducts or funds the study in whole or part or by grant, contract, cooperative agreement, or fellowship.[207] Hospitals that are federal grantees or contractors conducting experimental medical research on human subjects are required to establish an Institutional Review Board (IRB) to evaluate proposed research protocols.[208] The IRB is responsible for determining whether the research would be beneficial to society and whether adequate safeguards are available to protect the human subjects at risk.[209] The facility engaged in research must give assurances that the medical research projects will be subject to continuing review by the IRB.[210]

Health care organizations permitting their staffs to conduct medical research studies must establish an IRB to evaluate the risks posed to the patient by disclosure of medical records information and the potential benefits of the research. The IRB must reconcile the health care organization's duty to protect the confidentiality of patients' records with its interest in conducting medical research projects and the corresponding public interest in advancing medical science. Often, the best way to achieve both goals is for the health care organization to impose controls and limitations on staff access to medical records for authorized continuing research. Some health care organizations inform patients on admission or at their first appointment that their records may be made available to approved in-

---

[205]Cal. Welf. & Inst. Code § 4514(e).

[206]D.C. Code Ann. § 6-2025; Iowa Code § 229.25.

[207]45 C.F.R. §§ 46.101 through 46.124.

[208]45 C.F.R. § 46.103.

[209]45 C.F.R. § 46.111.

[210]45 C.F.R. § 46.103(b).

vestigators. This practice informs potential subjects that their records may be used in a research project undertaken by someone who is not a member of the staff but whose project is approved by the IRB or medical committee of the hospital.

A health care organization should try to obtain written authorization by the patient for access to medical records; however, it often is impractical to obtain patient consent for retrospective studies. Therefore, in the absence of such consent, the IRB must implement safeguards consistent with applicable federal regulations and state law for medical investigators seeking access to the past medical records of discharged patients.

The federal regulations on medical research generally require informed consent when studies involve a human being. The regulations provide that certain information must be presented to prospective subjects under circumstances allowing them sufficient opportunity to consider whether to participate in the study. One of the items that must be disclosed is a statement describing the extent to which the confidentiality of records identifying the person will be maintained.[211]

The federal regulations governing alcohol and drug abuse patient records also allow release of information from alcohol and drug treatment records without consent for certain research activities.[212] The director of an alcohol or drug treatment program covered by the rules must determine that the recipient of patient-identifying information is qualified to conduct research and has research protocols protecting the information and preventing unauthorized redisclosure of the material. The researcher must provide a satisfactory written statement that three or more individuals independent of the research project have reviewed the protocol and determined that patients' rights and welfare are protected adequately and that the risks of disclosing patient-identifying information are outweighed by the potential benefits of the research.[213]

The federal regulations governing research contain special rules for studies involving the fetus, pregnant women, or in vitro fertilization,[214] biomedical and behavioral research projects involving prisoners,[215] and

---

[211]45 C.F.R. § 46.116(a)(5).

[212]42 C.F.R. § 2.52.

[213]42 C.F.R. § 2.52(a)(3).

[214]45 C.F.R. §§ 46.201 through 46.211.

[215]45 C.F.R. §§ 46.301 through 46.306.

studies involving children as the research subjects.[216] State laws may impose special requirements on certain types of research.[217]

Even after a health care organization properly releases patient data to an authorized researcher whose final project omits any patient identifiers, problems still arise over access to identifying material by third parties. The general rule is that no academic privilege exists to protect research from discovery by third parties in litigation and the fact that researchers promise confidentiality to research participants does not confer absolute immunity.[218]

In one case, for example, a drug company sought production of research documents maintained by a university relating to a certain type of cancer in women.[219] The company served a subpoena for the documents on the university as part of its defense against a products liability suit filed by several women who alleged that their cervical and uterine cancer had been caused by in vitro exposure to the manufacturer's drug diethylstilbestrol (DES). Researchers at the university had compiled the only centralized repository of data on genital tract cancer in the country. The data, which included the medical records and follow-up information on many women with the disease, had been delivered voluntarily to the researchers by medical practitioners across the country relying on the researchers' written promises of confidentiality. The court weighed the hardship to the university researchers and the registry that disclosure would cause compared with the hardship to the drug company if it were denied access to the information. The court held that, because the public holds a vital interest in promoting research, the registry enjoys a qualified privilege against unnecessary disclosure, but that the privilege was not absolute. The court ruled that in this case, access to the registry was "absolutely essential" for the company to analyze its accuracy and methodology in preparing a proper defense at trial. It thus concluded that, while the company had no right to all materials in the registry as it originally had requested, not all of the data in the registry were protected from discovery.

In the absence of state regulations establishing standards for disclosing patients' medical records for biomedical or epidemiological research pur-

---

[216]45 C.F.R. §§ 46.401 through 46.409.

[217]See, e.g., CAL. WELF. & INST. CODE § 4514(e) (persons with developmental disabilities).

[218]See, e.g., Snyder v. American Motors Corp., 115 F.R.D. 211, 213 (D. Ariz. 1987).

[219]Deitchman v. Squibb & Sons, Inc., 740 F.2d 556 (7th Cir. 1984). See also Anker v. G.D. Searle & Co., 126 F.R.D. 515 (D.N.C. 1989).

poses without patient consent, the IRB or research committee should require the medical researchers to satisfy the following safeguards before authorizing disclosure of confidential records to them:

- The information must be treated as confidential.
- The information must be communicated only to qualified investigators pursuing an approved research program designed for the benefit of the health of the community.
- Adequate safeguards to protect the record or information from unauthorized disclosure must be established.
- The results of the investigation must be presented in a way that prevents identification of individual subjects.[220]

Absent statutory law, health care organizations should prohibit access to medical records by investigators whose medical studies do not include these minimum safeguards as determined by the IRB or another appropriate committee.

RECORD DUPLICATION AND FEES

Although health care organizations and providers have a duty to permit patients and their representatives to inspect and copy their medical records, health care organizations and providers are not obligated to do so at no cost. The authority to charge duplication fees and the amounts of those fees result from either specific statutory provisions or case law.

In some states, a health care organization or provider may impose a reasonable charge for copying records as a matter of statute. While some of the statutory or regulatory provisions on fees enunciate a "reasonable" standard to determine the amount, many other states have stipulated specific maximum amounts that may be charged for these services. For example, in Louisiana, a provider may require payment of a reasonable copying charge before releasing a patient's medical record. The amount may not exceed $1 per page for the first 25 pages, 50¢ for pages 26 through 500, and 25¢ per page thereafter. Hospitals may charge a maximum handling charge of $10, other health care providers may charge a maximum handling charge of $5, and all providers may charge actual postage.[221]

[220] L. Walters et al., "The Use of Medical Records for Research at Georgetown University," IRB, *Review of Human Subjects Research* (March 1981): 1.

[221] LA. REV. STAT. ANN. § 40:1299.96(A)(2)(b).

In the absence of a statute, courts have applied similar rules to a hospital's right to charge fees for accessing a medical record. For example, a court in Mississippi held that a hospital obligated to disclose record information to the patient could charge a fee for reproducing that information.[222] In an Illinois case,[223] a court held that the hospital properly refused to reproduce and release voluminous patient records when it received only a form request and offer to pay for "reasonable access." The court ruled that the hospital properly could allow the person making the request to review the full record and indicate what parts he was willing to pay to have copied.

Whether the authority to charge an access fee derives from legislation or case law, the price a provider charges for reproducing any portion of a patient's medical record should be based on the actual or reasonable cost to remove the record from the record library and duplicate the portions requested.[224] A health care organization should not make a profit from a patient's request for copies of his or her records. A Michigan appeals court declared, in determining whether a hospital's copying charges were reasonable, that the charge billed to paying requesters could not include any amount subsidizing the expense of photocopying for nonpaying parties who received free copies of records under hospital policy.[225] In a California case, an appeals court decided that a health care provider may not decline to release a patient's medical records because the patient has refused to sign a lien for payment of the fees owed the provider.[226] In setting copying charges, health care organizations and providers should consider checking the charges of local courts and their libraries because it will be difficult for courts to find comparable charges unreasonable.

In responding to patient requests for photocopying records, a health care organization may contract with a third party to perform the work. Whenever the health care organization makes such an arrangement, it must ensure confidentiality of the records in its contract with the party providing the copying services. In an Illinois case, an appeals court ruled that hospitals that send patient medical records to photocopy shops to be reproduced when patients ask for copies of their records are not violating

---

[222]Young v. Madison Gen. Hosp., 337 So. 2d 931 (Miss. 1976).

[223]Rabens v. Jackson Park Hosp. Found., 351 N.E.2d 276 (Ill. App. Ct. 1976).

[224]See Casillo v. St. John's Episcopal Hosp., 580 N.Y.S.2d 992 (Sup. Ct. 1992).

[225]Graham v. Thompson, 421 N.W.2d 694 (Mich. Ct. App. 1988).

[226]Person v. Farmers Ins. Group of Cos., 52 Cal. App. 4th 813 (Ct. App. 1997).

state law regarding confidentiality.[227] Under Illinois law a hospital can use independent contractors, agents, or employees in providing patients access to their records, the court held. Finally, the court refused to find that ministerial duties, like photocopying, breach a patient's right to confidentiality, as long as the photocopying is done in a reasonable manner. (For more about liability for improper disclosures of medical record information, see Chapter 11.)

Alternatively, patients might choose to rent a portable photocopy machine and copy the records themselves. Patients choosing that option must reimburse the health care organization for retrieving the file and for time spent by a health care organization employee supervising the copying.[228] A patient does not have the right to unsupervised off-premises inspection and copying of records.[229] When responding to the patient's request to access and copy records, the health care organization has the obligation to make the records available at a reasonable time and place.[230] Those arrangements must be made within the time prescribed by law or within a reasonable time after the health care organization receives the request for information.

RECORD SECURITY

It is essential that each health care organization and health care delivery site establish an effective procedure for safeguarding medical records. Record security is critical to protecting patient confidentiality and preventing intentional alteration or falsification of records by employees or others. Unfortunately, some providers have learned through experience that, given the opportunity, patients occasionally will remove important sections or alter significant information in their records simply to improve their chances of bringing a successful negligence action against the facility. Other organizations or individuals also have strong interests in the in-

---

[227]Clay v. Little Co. of Mary Hosp., 660 N.E.2d 123 (Ill. App. Ct. 1995). The relevant part of Illinois law provides as follows: "Examination of records. Every…hospital shall…permit the patient, his or her physician or authorized attorney to examine the hospital records…kept in connection with the treatment of such patient, and permit copies of such records to be made by him or her or his or her physician or authorized attorney…" 735 ILL. COMP. STAT. 5/8-2001.

[228]McDonald v. State Univ., 514 N.Y.S.2d 789 (App. Div. 1987); Paterna v. Zandieh, 515 N.Y.S.2d 54 (App. Div. 1987); *see also* Hayes v. County of Nassau, 512 N.Y.S.2d 134 (App. Div. 1987).

[229]Paterna v. Zandieh, 515 N.Y.S.2d 54 (App. Div. 1987).

[230]*See, e.g.,* N.Y. PUB. HEALTH LAW § 18(2)(f).

formation in certain medical records, and these people may go to great lengths to discover that information.[231]

To protect medical records from abuse, health care organizations and delivery sites should adopt the following security measures as a minimum:

- Medical records should be stored in secure, restricted-access locations.
- Competent medical records or risk management personnel should review every record before it is examined by the patient or patient representative. The reviewer should notify a designated individual if the record is incomplete or otherwise defective, or if it reveals a problem that could give rise to negligence liability by the facility or its staff.
- An original medical record should never be removed from the premises unless required by legal process, or pursuant to a defined procedure that permits patients going to another facility for testing to take their medical records with them, or permits medical records to be sent out for photocopying. Patients should be permitted to take their records only if the patient is returning to the facility the same day, and provided that the patient is accompanied by a responsible employee.
- Anyone who is not an authorized employee or staff member should not be allowed to examine a medical record without supervision. That includes a patient and/or a patient representative. Where a patient or other person is properly authorized to review a record under the principles of law discussed above, the facility should provide accommodations for record inspection in its medical records department or in another location under proper surveillance.

Security for computerized medical records raises special concerns, which are discussed in Chapter 13.

PRO RECORDKEEPING

The Tax Equity and Fiscal Responsibility Act of 1982[232] repealed the Professional Standards Review Organization (PSRO) program and replaced it with a similar one, the Peer Review Organization (PRO) program. Under the revised statute, a PRO, or "utilization and quality control peer

---

[231]*See, e.g.*, People v. Home Ins. Co., 591 P.2d 1036 (Colo. 1979), where agents of an insurance company obtained confidential information about two hospitalized insurance claimants by hiring an investigator to telephone an unnamed source at the hospital.

[232]42 U.S.C. §§ 1320c through 1320c-12.

review organization," means an entity composed of a substantial number of licensed doctors of medicine and osteopathy in the area representative of practicing physicians, or an entity with a sufficient number of such doctors available under arrangement to assure adequate peer review of services provided by the various specialties and subspecialties.[233]

At least one member of the PRO's governing body must be an individual representing consumers.[234] A PRO must be able to perform the required review functions efficiently and effectively, and must measure the pattern of quality of care provided in the area against objective criteria that define acceptable and adequate practice.[235]

PROs are charged with a number of functions. Most importantly, they must review some or all of the professional activities conducted by physicians and providers who receive federal reimbursement under Medicare. In conducting these reviews, PROs must determine (1) whether services and items were reasonable and medically necessary; (2) whether the quality of services met professionally recognized standards; and (3) whether inpatient services could have been provided more economically on an outpatient basis or in an inpatient health care facility of a different type.[236] The statute also requires PROs to conduct certain other reviews, including readmissions occurring within 31 days of discharge[237] and some or all ambulatory surgical procedures.[238]

In carrying out its functions, a PRO must collect and maintain records of relevant information, and permit access to such records and use of the collected information as required by the Secretary of HHS, subject to the statutory provisions prohibiting disclosure of certain PRO information.[239] Under the PRO regulations,[240] the Health Care Financing Administration (HCFA) or any person, organization, or agency authorized by HHS or federal statute to monitor a PRO will have access to, and may obtain copies of, medical records of Medicare patients maintained by institutions or health care practitioners.[241] The statute and regulations address access and

---

[233] 42 U.S.C. §§ 1320c-1(1)(A) & (B).

[234] 42 U.S.C. § 1320c-1(3).

[235] 42 U.S.C. § 1320c-1(2).

[236] 42 U.S.C. §§ 1320c-3(a)(1)(A) through (C).

[237] 42 U.S.C. § 1320c-3(a)(13).

[238] 42 U.S.C. § 1320c-3(d).

[239] 42 U.S.C. § 1320c-3(a)(9)(A).

[240] 42 C.F.R. §§ 462.1 through 476.143.

[241] 42 C.F.R. § 476.131.

disclosure of medical records and PRO information in other contexts considered below.

PRO Access to Individual Patient Records

The Act grants PROs broad authority to access patient records and other information. First, it provides that each PRO shall examine the pertinent records of any practitioner or provider of health care services subject to its review[242] and may require the institution or practitioner to provide copies of records or information to the PRO.[243] Second, a PRO is authorized to access and require copies of Medicare records or information held by intermediaries or carriers if the PRO determines that such material is necessary to carry out its review functions.[244] Third, a PRO has the right to all information collected by institutions or other entities for PRO purposes.[245] Finally, all information collected or generated by institutions or practitioners to carry out quality review studies must be disclosed to the PRO.[246] The regulations add that a PRO may have access to records of non-Medicare patients in accordance with its quality review responsibilities under the Act if authorized by the institution or practitioner.[247] Clearly, PROs have authority to review and copy confidential patient medical records and related information collected by physicians, facilities, intermediaries, and carriers.

Third Party Access to Information Collected by a PRO

The statute provides that, in general, any data or information acquired by a PRO in the exercise of its duties and functions shall be held in confidence and not disclosed except as specifically authorized under the law.[248] A PRO may disclose information to the extent necessary to carry out the purposes of the statute.[249] It also may release information for purposes specifically authorized by statute, including to assist with investigations

---

[242] 42 U.S.C. § 1320c-3(a)(7)(C).
[243] 42 C.F.R. § 476.111(a).
[244] 42 C.F.R. § 476.112.
[245] 42 C.F.R. § 476.113(a).
[246] 42 C.F.R. § 476.113(b).
[247] 42 C.F.R. § 476.111(c).
[248] 42 U.S.C. § 1320c-9(a).
[249] 42 U.S.C. § 1320c-9(a)(1).

into cases and/or patterns of fraud or abuse; with matters where a risk to the public health is presented; with issues involving state licensing, certification, or accreditation; and with health planning.[250] A PRO may disclose information as authorized by the Secretary of HHS to assure adequate protection of the rights and interests of patients, practitioners, or providers of health care.[251]

PROs are required to provide reasonable physical security measures to prevent unauthorized access to the information and to ensure the integrity of the data.[252] The PRO must instruct its officers and employees and employees of health care institutions participating in its activities of their responsibility to maintain confidentiality. No individual participating in the PRO review process on a regular basis shall have authorized access to confidential PRO information unless that person has been properly trained and has signed a statement indicating an awareness of the legal penalties for unauthorized disclosure.[253] PRO information may be stored in a shared health data system unless such storage would prevent the PRO from complying with the regulations.[254] PRO information may not be disclosed by the shared health data system unless the source of the information consents or the PRO requests disclosure as permitted by the regulations.[255]

The regulatory provisions governing disclosure of PRO information distinguish "confidential" from "nonconfidential." "Confidential information" is defined as:

- information that explicitly or implicitly identifies an individual patient, practitioner, or reviewer[256]
- sanction reports and recommendations
- quality review studies that identify patients, practitioners, or institutions
- PRO deliberations[257]

---

[250] 42 U.S.C. §§ 1320c-9(a)(3) & 1320-9(b).

[251] 42 U.S.C. § 1320c-9(a)(2).

[252] 42 C.F.R. § 476.115(a).

[253] 42 C.F.R. § 476.115(d).

[254] 42 C.F.R. §§ 476.143(a) & (b).

[255] 42 C.F.R. § 476.143(c).

[256] *See* General Care Corp. v. Mid-South Found. for Med. Care, 778 F. Supp. 405 (W.D. Tenn. 1991), where a federal district court in Tennessee, interpreting this provision, granted a hospital a permanent injunction to prevent a PRO from disclosing information relating to its investigation of care rendered to a patient at a hospital.

[257] 42 C.F.R. § 476.101(b).

The phrase "implicitly identifies" is defined to mean "data so unique or numbers so small that identification of an individual patient, practitioner, or reviewer would be obvious."[258] Nonconfidential information is not defined by the regulations, but the term presumably refers to information falling outside the definition of "confidential information."

A PRO is required to disclose nonconfidential information to any person upon request. Such information may relate to the norms, criteria, and standards used for initial screening of cases and other review activities; routine reports submitted by the PRO to HCFA to the extent they do not contain confidential information; and quality review studies from which the identification of patients, practitioners, and institutions has been deleted.[259] A PRO also must disclose to state or federal health planning agencies all aggregate statistical information that does not implicitly or explicitly identify individual patients, practitioners, or reviewers.[260] In addition to these mandatory disclosures, a PRO may disclose any of the above nonconfidential information to any person, agency, or organization on its own initiative.[261]

The regulations generally require a PRO that intends to disclose nonconfidential information to give 30-day advance notice to any institution identified in the material and to provide a copy to the institution. The institution may submit written comments to the PRO that must be included with the information disclosed or forwarded separately.[262] Where the PRO plans to disclose "confidential information," it also must give advance notice. If the request for information comes from a patient or patient representative, the PRO must provide the notice to the practitioner who treated the patient.[263] On the other hand, if the request comes from an investigative or licensing agency, the PRO must: (1) notify the practitioner or institution, (2) provide the practitioner or institution with a copy of the requested information, and (3) include comments submitted by the practitioner or institution in the disclosure to the agency.[264]

---

[258] 42 C.F.R. § 476.101(b).
[259] 42 C.F.R. § 476.120(a).
[260] 42 C.F.R. § 476.120(b).
[261] 42 C.F.R. § 476.121.
[262] 42 C.F.R. § 476.105(a).
[263] 42 C.F.R. § 476.105(b)(1).
[264] 42 C.F.R. § 476.105(b)(2).

There are three exceptions to the general requirement that a PRO give advance notice to a practitioner or institution before confidential information is disclosed:

1. If a PRO determines that the requested information is necessary to protect against an imminent danger to individuals or the public health, notice of the disclosure may be sent to the practitioner or institution at the same time the disclosure is made, rather than 30 days in advance.[265]

2. If the disclosure is made during a fraud and abuse investigation conducted by the Office of the Inspector General (OIG) or the General Accounting Office (GAO), no notice is required.[266]

3. If the disclosure is made during a fraud and abuse investigation conducted by any other state or federal agency, no notice is required if the agency specifies in writing that the information is related to a potentially prosecutable criminal offense.[267]

All disclosures of confidential information by a PRO must be accompanied by a written statement informing the recipient that the information may not be further disclosed except as provided by the regulations.[268]

Records held by a PRO that identify patients are not subject to subpoena or discovery in a civil action, including an administrative, judicial, or arbitration proceeding.[269] However, this last restriction does not apply to HHS, OIG, or GAO, or to administrative subpoenas issued during the course of HHS program audits and investigations, or during administrative hearings held under the Social Security Act.[270]

There is no access or disclosure of PRO information beyond that described in the statute and regulations.[271] That provision is designed to avoid the litigation experienced under the former PSRO law where attempts to characterize PSROs as federal agencies under FOIA led to conflicting court decisions.[272]

---

[265]42 C.F.R. § 476.106(a).

[266]42 C.F.R. § 476.106(b)(1).

[267]42 C.F.R. § 476.106(b)(2).

[268]42 C.F.R. § 476.104(a)(2).

[269]42 C.F.R. § 476.138(a)(3).

[270]42 C.F.R. § 476.138(b)(1).

[271]42 C.F.R. § 476.138(b)(2).

[272]*See, e.g.*, Public Citizen Health Research Group v. Department of Health, Educ. & Welfare, 668 F.2d 537 (D.C. Cir. 1981).

Patient Access to PRO Information

Generally, a PRO must disclose patient-identifying information in its possession to that individual or his or her representative upon written request, provided that all other patient and practitioner identifiers have been removed.[273] First, however, the PRO must discuss the appropriateness of disclosure with the patient's attending practitioner. If the practitioner states that the released information could harm the patient, the PRO must disclose the material to the patient's representative rather than directly to the patient.[274] If the patient is mentally, physically, or legally unable to designate a representative, the PRO must disclose the information to a person responsible for the patient as determined by the PRO in accordance with the regulations.[275] The PRO must disclose patient information directly to the patient unless knowledge could be harmful.[276]

UTILIZATION REVIEW AND QUALITY ASSURANCE

In addition to their uses in medical research, patients' records play a critical role in each health care organization's effort to improve the quality of health care services and to increase the efficiency with which they are provided. Patients' records are a primary source of data for such utilization review and other quality assurance activities. Health care providers and health law practitioners must be aware of the statutes, regulations, and judicial opinions in their jurisdictions that affect the ability to use medical records for these purposes.

Two types of review processes occur in hospitals. The first type is the federal PRO system, part of the Medicare program governed by federal statute and regulation.[277] Hospitals seeking federal reimbursement for Medicare services must contract with a PRO as a condition of participation in the program.[278] PROs have authority to review patient records in carrying out their responsibilities to assess the reasonableness and adequacy of medical care.[279] PRO access and disclosure of patient records is discussed in detail earlier in this chapter.

---

[273]42 C.F.R. § 476.132(a)(1).

[274]42 C.F.R. §§ 476.132(a)(2) & (c)(2).

[275]42 C.F.R. § 476.132(c)(3).

[276]42 C.F.R. § 476.132(c)(1).

[277]*See generally* 42 C.F.R. §§ 476.101 through 476.143.

[278]42 C.F.R. § 476.102.

[279]42 C.F.R. §§ 476.111 & 476.112.

The second type of review is hospital utilization review and quality assurance. These two review programs are conducted by hospital staff members and consist of in-house monitoring of both the quality and cost of providing services. The basic requirements for these review programs are set forth in the standards of accreditation adopted by the Joint Commission and in various state laws.

Quality assurance and utilization review programs also are an important aspect of managed health care. State laws usually condition issuance of an HMO or MCO certificate of authority on the submission and approval of a quality assurance program. Statutes and regulations mandating quality assurance activities vary in terms of level of detail.[280] State laws also vary widely on utilization review. Many laws, however, indicate that the HMO must have procedures for developing, compiling, evaluating, and reporting statistics relating to the cost of its operations, the pattern of utilization of its services, and the availability and accessibility of its services.[281]

Accreditation organizations have standards related to quality assurance and utilization review. The Joint Commission standards applicable to hospitals, PPOs, and health care networks are located in the chapters on "Leadership" and on "Improving Organizational Performance."[282] The standards in those chapters concentrate on the monitoring, evaluation, and comparison of various data in order to identify and correct problems. In its Standards for the Certification of Physician Organizations, the NCQA has developed standards for quality management and improvement as well as utilization management.[283] Like the Joint Commission standards, the NCQA standards stress collecting and analyzing data in order to monitor service and improve performance.

Although utilization management and quality assurance rely on many data sources, the most valuable sources clearly are patients' medical records. Many states have enacted laws protecting the confidentiality of medical records used in utilization management and quality assurance

---

[280]*See, e.g.,* IDAHO CODE § 41-3905(6)(a); MD. CODE ANN., HEALTH-GEN. §§ 19-705.1(d), (e), & (f).

[281]*See, e.g.,* GA. CODE ANN. § 3-21-3(b)(3).

[282]JOINT COMMISSION, 1997 HOSPITAL ACCREDITATION STANDARDS, Standards LD.1 through LD4.5 and PI.1 through PI.5.1; JOINT COMMISSION, 1997 ACCREDITATION MANUAL FOR PREFERRED PROVIDER ORGANIZATIONS, Standards LD.1 through LD.5.1 and PI.1 through PI.4.1; JOINT COMMISSION, 1996-97 COMPREHENSIVE ACCREDITATION MANUAL FOR HEALTH CARE NETWORKS, Standards LD.1 through LD.6 and PI.1 through PI.5.1.

[283]NATIONAL COMMITTEE FOR QUALITY ASSURANCE, STANDARDS FOR THE CERTIFICATION OF PHYSICIAN ORGANIZATIONS, QI Standards 1 through 13; UM Standards 1 through 9 (1997).

functions. For example, some states require entities applying for a utilization review organization (URO) license to submit information about the URO's policies for protecting the confidentiality of medical records.[284] In addition, many state laws require UROs to protect the confidentiality of medical information.[285] An Illinois statute provides that all information used in the course of internal quality control or in other ways designed to improve patient care is strictly confidential. However, a claim of confidentiality may not be used to deny a physician access to any information used to make a decision in any HMO proceeding concerning the physician's services or the physician's staff privileges.[286]

Many states have enacted statutes authorizing disclosure of patient records to staff quality control, peer review, and medical review committees. Some of these statutes provide that a health care practitioner *may* release confidential patient information to a peer review committee.[287] On the other hand, the Nebraska law states that a provider is *obligated* to give a review committee information it requests.[288] Other statutes indicate that physicians or other health care practitioners who provide information to a review committee are immune from liability if their actions were taken in good faith.[289] Each type of statute permits review committees access to confidential patient information as is relevant and necessary to carry out their functions.

Some states without statutes specifically granting record access to quality control committees may have case law that permits disclosures. In a Missouri appeals court case, for example, a staff physician sought to prevent the disclosure of his patients' records to a hospital committee that was investigating his qualifications and competency.[290] Missouri had a physician-patient privilege statute that decreed that a physician was incompetent to testify as to any information received during a professional consultation with a patient. The physician argued that the privilege should prevent the use of patient records in a competency determination because

---

[284]*See, e.g.,* MD. CODE ANN., HEALTH-GEN § 19-1305(a)(4); R.I. GEN. LAWS § 23-17.12-4.

[285]*See, e.g.,* LA. REV. STAT. ANN. § 40:2731; ALA. CODE § 27-3A-5(a)(7); MINN. STAT. § 62M.08.

[286]735 ILL. COMP. STAT. 5/8-2101.

[287]*See, e.g.,* ALASKA STAT. § 18.23.010(b); CAL. CIV. CODE § 56.10(c)(4).

[288]NEB. REV. STAT. § 71-2047.

[289]*See, e.g.,* CONN. GEN. STAT. ANN. § 19a-17b; DEL. CODE ANN. tit. 24, § 1768; FLA. STAT. ANN. § 766.101(3)(a).

[290]Klinge v. Lutheran Med. Ctr., 518 S.W.2d 157, 161 (Mo. Ct. App. 1975).

that would constitute a type of testimony at what basically was a hearing. The court reviewed the privilege's history and noted that no state ever had treated the privilege as an absolute prohibition against a physician's disclosure. After balancing the parties' opposing interests, the court concluded the privilege was inapplicable because "[t]he public's interest in the disclosure of the information to the internal staff of the hospital and in assuring proper medical and hospital care outweigh[ed] the patient's interest in concealment."[291]

If a third party asks to review records for utilization management and quality assurance purposes, the health care organization will need to evaluate each request individually to determine if the patient has given permission for the release of his or her health information. The health care organization will need to review a copy of the agreement that the patient signed when the patient enrolled in the health plan to determine if it authorizes representatives of the plan to access medical records. If the patient has not provided such an authorization, the patient's medical records should not be released before obtaining the patient's written authorization.

State quality assurance and utilization management laws vary from state to state. Health care administrators and health law practitioners therefore should consult the statutes, regulations, and case law in their jurisdictions before authorizing the use of patients' medical records for quality assurance and utilization review.

---

[291]Klinge v. Lutheran Med. Ctr., 518 S.W.2d 157, 166 (Mo. Ct. App. 1975).

7

Reporting and Disclosure Requirements

Chapter Objectives

- Give examples of mandatory reporting laws.
- Discuss the persons or facilities subject to the reporting requirement under mandatory disclosure laws.
- Give examples of information that must be included in a child abuse report and adult abuse report.
- Summarize the requirements of communicable disease reporting laws.
- Discuss whether mandatory reporting laws apply to managed care organizations.

INTRODUCTION

Many state laws and some federal laws allow the disclosure of confidential medical record information without the patient's consent. Certain disclosures, such as child abuse reports, are mandatory; others are permissive. Some laws require hospitals and other facilities to make reports; other laws place the responsibility on the individual health care professional to perform this function. Certain laws may also permit or require managed care organizations (MCOs) to disclose confidential medical record information.

Disclosure of medical record information under statutory or regulatory requirements does not subject a health care organization or practitioner to civil liability, even if the disclosure is made against the patient's express wishes. Health care organizations and providers must be aware of the special disclosure rules applicable in their jurisdictions because the rules often vary among states.

Health care organizations choosing to participate in cancer or other registries should seek the creation of statutory or regulatory authority for release of medical record information to such registries. If legislative action is impractical, participating organizations should exercise care in drafting agreements with registries. Such contracts should contain safeguards against improper disclosure of confidential information by the registry and should include indemnification of the health care organization for claims that may result from release of data to the registry or from improper disclosure by the registry.

Child Abuse

Laws in most jurisdictions require hospitals and practitioners to report cases of actual or suspected child abuse. The exact list of persons and facilities subject to the reporting requirement varies among the states, and persons working in various health care institutions should check their state's particular child abuse law. It is important that health care organizations and practitioners understand who in their facility must report, when reports are due, and what information must be presented in a child abuse report. While most statutes protect persons required to report from civil liability, voluntary reports or release of extra information not required or permitted by law do not have similar protections.

To comply with child abuse reporting requirements, health care organizations must first determine whether a patient is a "child" under the relevant statute. A "child" for abuse reporting purposes is not necessarily synonymous with "minor" under state law. Definitions of these terms vary in different state laws. In Massachusetts, for example, child abuse reports must be filed for all persons under 18 years of age who satisfy other criteria for reporting.[1] In New York, an "abused child" may be older than 18 in some cases.[2]

---

[1] MASS. GEN. LAWS ch. 119, § 51A.
[2] N.Y. SOC. SERV. LAW § 412.

The exact list of persons and facilities subject to the reporting requirement varies among the states, and persons working in various health care
institutions should check their state's particular child abuse law. Some
states have broad mandatory requirements that all "persons" with certain
knowledge of child abuse make a report.[3] This type of statute imposes
obligations on all personnel, not only on practitioners who treat victims of
child abuse. Most statutes require reporting by practitioners and others
who know or have "reason" to suspect or believe that a child they know or
observe in their official or professional capacity is abused or neglected.[4]

Other states impose mandatory reporting obligations on specific categories of people, including designated health care professionals. Practitioners and other health care workers subject to mandatory reporting may
be listed directly in the child abuse reporting provisions[5] and/or may be
cross-referenced to the state health care professional licensing statute.
Most child abuse reporting requirements are mandatory for health practitioners; at least one state, Mississippi, has a permissive child abuse reporting law.[6]

In some states, the list creates a fixed group of professionals subject to
reporting;[7] in other states, the list is merely illustrative, stating that all individuals who provide health care services, including those listed, must
report.[8] In a few states, persons involved with hospital admissions have an
explicit duty to report, along with practitioners.[9]

Only certain conditions diagnosed in children are reportable, and the
child abuse statute in each state includes definitions of conditions that
trigger the duty to report. Some statutes define an "abused and neglected"
child as a single term.[10] Others distinguish "abuse" from "neglect."[11] Still

---

[3]*See, e.g.*, 23 PA. CONS. STAT. § 631; N.J. STAT. ANN. § 9:6-8.10.

[4]*See, e.g.*, FLA. STAT. ANN. § 415.504(1); MD. CODE ANN., FAM. LAW § 5-704; N.Y. SOC. SERV. LAW
§ 413.

[5]*See, e.g.*, HAW. REV. STAT. § 350-1.1(a); MD. CODE ANN., FAM. LAW §§ 5-701(h) & 5-704(a); N.Y.
SOC. SERV. LAW § 413.

[6]MISS. CODE ANN. § 93-21-25.

[7]*See, e.g.*, N.Y. SOC. SERV. LAW § 413.

[8]*See, e.g.*, FLA. STAT. ANN. §§ 415.504(1)(a) & (b); HAW. REV. STAT. § 350-1.1(a); TENN. CODE ANN.
§ 37-1-403(a).

[9]*See, e.g.*, FLA. STAT. ANN. § 415.504(1).

[10]*See, e.g.*, FLA. STAT. ANN. § 415.503(1); HAW. REV. STAT. § 350-1.

[11]*See, e.g.*, LA. REV. STAT. ANN. § 603; D.C. CODE ANN. § 6-2131; *see also* New York law, which defines "abused child" and "maltreated child" separately. N.Y. SOC. SERV. LAW § 412.

others provide definitions of other related terms such as "sexual abuse."[12] Some states refer to abuse by the child's parent or other person responsible for the child's welfare.[13] A few statutes apply to child abuse or neglect of a child caused by "any" person.[14]

The definitions in every state generally include both physical and mental harm or threats of harm caused by the acts or omissions of certain persons. Sexual abuse, unusual punishment, or unexplained physical injuries constitute signs of abuse under most laws.[15] Impairment of the child's ability to perform or function and other signs of emotional or psychological distress indicate potential abuse in many states.[16] Exploitation and abandonment are typical elements of child abuse, along with failure to provide adequate supervision, food, clothing, shelter, or health care.[17]

Most statutes require certain information to be included in a child abuse report. Typically, the name of the person making the report, the name and address of the child, the extent of the child's injuries, and the child's present whereabouts must be disclosed, along with other pertinent information relating to the cause of abuse and the identity of the individual(s) responsible.[18] Massachusetts requires the child's age and sex to be disclosed in addition to the child's parents' names and addresses.[19] In New York, persons making the reports must reveal their identities and any actions they have taken, including photographs or X-rays and removal or keeping of the child.[20]

Persons who comply with the reporting provisions generally are immune under the statute from any resulting civil or criminal liability.[21] Several courts have extended civil immunity to reports made in good faith but based on a negligent diagnosis.[22] California legislation that grants immu-

---

[12]*See, e.g.*, CAL. PENAL CODE § 11165.1.

[13]*See, e.g.*, FLA. STAT. ANN. § 415.503(1); HAW. REV. STAT. § 350-l; LA. REV. STAT. ANN. § 603.

[14]*See, e.g.*, ARIZ. REV. STAT. ANN. § 13-3620(A).

[15]*See, e.g.*, FLA. STAT. ANN. § 415.503; HAW. REV. STAT. § 350-1.

[16]*See, e.g.*, HAW. REV. STAT. § 350-1.

[17]*See, e.g.*, FLA. STAT. ANN. § 415.503; HAW. REV. STAT. § 350-1.

[18]*See, e.g.*, N.Y. SOC. SERV. LAW § 415; TENN. CODE ANN. § 37-1-403; WASH. REV. CODE ANN. § 26.44.040.

[19]MASS. ANN. LAWS ch. 119, § 51A.

[20]N.Y. SOC. SERV. LAW § 415.

[21]*See, e.g.*, FLA. STAT. ANN. § 415.511; HAW. REV. STAT. § 350-3.

[22]*See, e.g.*, Maples v. Siddiqui, 450 N.W.2d 529 (Iowa 1990).

nity to health care providers when they make mandated reports of child abuse also protects providers from liability when they make reports that are not required but merely are authorized under the law.[23] On the other hand, persons who fail to make required reports or who knowingly make false reports may be criminally liable.[24]

Most child abuse statutes stipulate that both the report and the identity of the individual who makes it are confidential.[25] Moreover, in most states, disclosures authorized by such laws do not violate the physician-patient privilege that otherwise would prevent the use of confidential medical information at trial or in other legal proceedings. (For a more extensive discussion of how physician-patient privilege operates in conjunction with child abuse reporting laws, see Chapter 8.)

Abuse of Adults and Injuries to Disabled Persons

Many states have enacted reporting requirements for cases of known or suspected abuse of senior citizens, institutionalized persons, nursing home residents, and persons suffering from physical or mental impairments.[26] Like the child abuse statutes discussed above, the laws on abuse of adults typically define terms such as "abuse" and "neglect" and require various health practitioners to report instances where they have a reasonable basis for believing such abuse or neglect has occurred. The statutes usually list the kinds of information to be included in a report, such as the identity of the person reporting, the name and address of the victim, the time and place of the incident of abuse, the name of the suspected wrongdoer, and other information concerning the victim's statements and persons with knowledge of the incident. A practitioner usually may make an initial incident report by telephone, then follow up with a written report within a certain time period.

Most jurisdictions have general reporting requirements. Some states also require reports based on particular diagnoses of institutionalized or disabled adults—for example, Maryland mandates general reports of

---

[23]See Ferraro v. Chadwick, 270 Cal. Rptr. 379 (Ct. App. 1990); rev. denied, No. 501657 (Cal. Aug. 15, 1990) (unpublished).

[24]See, e.g., HAW. REV. STAT. § 350-1.2; MASS. ANN. LAWS ch. 119, § 51A.

[25]See, e.g., FLA. STAT. ANN. § 415.51; HAW. REV. STAT. § 350-1.4; TENN. CODE ANN. § 37-1-612.

[26]See, e.g., CAL. WELF. & INST. CODE §§ 15600 through 15657.3; FLA. STAT. ANN. §§ 415.101 through 415.113; IOWA CODE §§ 235B.1 through 235B.20.

abuse suffered by developmentally disabled[27] or mentally impaired persons.[28]

The Minnesota Vulnerable Adult Act defines the terms "vulnerable adult," "abuse," and "neglect," and requires a mandated reporter to report known abuse or neglect, in instances where the professional has reasonable cause to believe maltreatment is occurring or has occurred, or who has knowledge that a vulnerable adult has sustained an unexplained physical injury.[29] The Minnesota Act extends immunity for reports made in good faith under the law, and imposes criminal liability on mandated reporters who intentionally fail to report and liability for damages on those who negligently fail to report.[30]

Controlled Drug Prescriptions and Abuse

Some states require physicians and others to identify patients obtaining prescriptions for certain controlled drugs and to report their names to the appropriate state or federal agency.[31] Other states require the provider to maintain records of such prescriptions for government inspection.[32]

Other states require physicians to report diagnoses of drug abuse. New Jersey requires health care practitioners to report the names of drug-dependent persons within 24 hours after determining that the person uses a controlled dangerous substance for purposes other than treatment of sickness or injury as prescribed and administered under the law.[33]

Occupational Diseases

A few states require physicians to report diseases or abnormal health conditions caused by or related to conditions in the workplace.[34] The re-

---

[27]MD. CODE ANN., HEALTH-GEN. § 7-1005.

[28]MD. CODE ANN., HEALTH-GEN. § 10-705.

[29]MINN. STAT. ANN. § 626.557.

[30]MINN. STAT. ANN. §§ 626.557(5) & (7).

[31]*See, e.g.*, CAL. HEALTH & SAFETY CODE § 11164; MASS. ANN. LAWS ch. 94C, § 24; N.Y. PUB. HEALTH LAW § 3333.

[32]*See, e.g.*, MASS. ANN. LAWS ch. 94C, § 9(d).

[33]N.J. STAT. ANN. § 24:21-39; *but see* Commonwealth v. Donoghue, 358 N.E.2d 465 (Mass. Ct. App. 1976), where a Massachusetts state court struck down its drug abuse reporting statute as unconstitutionally vague because practitioners could not define the term "chronic use" triggering such reports under the existing version of the law.

[34]*See, e.g.*, TEX. HEALTH & SAFETY CODE ANN. § 84.004.

ports are made to the state's department of public health and usually include the name, address, occupation, and illness of the patient, and the name and address of the patient's employer. The reports are confidential except for statistical purposes and in extreme medical emergencies.[35] The purpose of these statutes is to enable public health officials to investigate occupational diseases and to recommend methods for eliminating or preventing them.

Abortion

Several states require hospitals and practitioners to report abortions they perform, along with a variety of information about the patient, the procedure, and any resulting complications.[36] Some states impose independent reporting requirements on physicians who diagnose a woman as having complications from an abortion.[37] A few states require reports only for abortions performed on minors.[38] At least one court has upheld the requirement that physicians disclose the names and addresses of women receiving abortions as rationally related to a compelling state interest in maternal health and not an infringement upon the physician-patient relationship, the right to an abortion, or any personal right of privacy.[39]

Birth Defects and Other Conditions in Children

Many states require, or at least permit, health practitioners and others to report diagnoses of various birth defects and children's conditions to the state department of health.[40] Reportable conditions include congenital and acquired malformations and disabilities,[41] Sudden Infant Death Syndrome,[42] sentinel birth defects,[43] Reye's syndrome,[44] diseases of the eyes of infants,[45] and abnormal spinal curvature.[46]

---

[35]Tex. Health & Safety Code Ann. § 84.006.

[36]See, e.g., Fla. Stat. Ann. § 390.002; Tex. Health & Safety Code Ann. § 245.011.

[37]See, e.g., 720 Ill. Comp. Stat. Ann. 510/10.1.

[38]See, e.g., Ala. Code § 26-21-8(c).

[39]See, e.g., Schulman v. New York City Health and Hosp. Corp., 342 N.E.2d 501 (1975).

[40]See, e.g., N.J. Rev. Stat. § 26:8-40.21; Wis. Stat. Ann. § 253.12.

[41]See, e.g., Ala. Code § 21-3-8; Fla. Stat. Ann. § 383.14.

[42]See, e.g., Cal. Health & Safety Code § 102865.

[43]See, e.g., Md. Code Ann., Health-Gen. § 18-206.

[44]See, e.g., Mass. Ann. Laws ch. 111, § 110B.

[45]See, e.g., Mass. Ann. Laws ch. 111, § 110.

[46]See, e.g., Tex. Health & Safety Code Ann. § 37.003.

Cancer

Many states require disclosure of information from the medical records of cancer patients to central state or regional tumor registries.[47] These registries usually contain demographic, diagnostic, and treatment information about patients who suffer from the same or similar diseases and are designed to provide raw data for studies concerning the incidence of a disease in the population; long-term prognosis of the disease; type, duration, and frequency of treatment rendered to patients with the disease; and other indicators of the health care industry's ability to manage the disease. Usually operated by statewide, tax-exempt organizations funded by federal grants, the registries rely to a large extent on the cooperation of individual hospital registries and obtain patient information directly from participating hospitals pursuant to agreements between the hospitals and the registry.

Death or Injury from Use of a Medical Device

The Safe Medical Devices Act,[48] a federal statute enacted in 1990, requires hospitals to report any death resulting from the use of a medical device to the Department of Health and Human Services (HHS) within ten days of discovery. The hospital must identify in the report the device's manufacturer, if known, and must notify the manufacturer when a device caused or contributed to a patient's serious illness or injury. If the hospital cannot determine the manufacturer, the report of the illness or injury must be sent to the Secretary of HHS. The Joint Commission on Accreditation of Healthcare Organizations (Joint Commission) also requires compliance with the Safe Medical Devices Act as one of its accreditation standards.[49]

Communicable Diseases

Communicable disease reporting laws require hospitals and practitioners to inform public health authorities of cases of infectious, venereal, or sexually transmitted diseases. These are among the oldest compulsory reporting statutes in many states. The statutes or regulations usually list the particular diseases that must be reported and direct practitioners to give

---

[47]*See, e.g.*, CAL. HEALTH & SAFETY CODE § 103885; FLA. STAT. ANN. § 385.202; HAW. REV. STAT. § 324-21.

[48] 21 U.S.C. § 360i.

[49]JOINT COMMISSION, 1997 HOSPITAL ACCREDITATION MANUAL, Standard EC.1.8.

local public health officials the patient's name, age, sex, address, and identifying information, as well as the details of the illness.[50] The health department may have authority to request patient records for purposes of conducting epidemiological investigations.[51] Hospitals should disclose only the information required by the statute.

The majority of states have enacted special laws governing reports of acquired immune deficiency syndrome (AIDS) and human immunodeficiency virus (HIV) cases. Many of the statutes require both AIDS and HIV to be reported; the information required in these reports varies from state to state. Providers should know what information should be released in their jurisdictions. (For a detailed discussion of access and disclosure issues involving AIDS and HIV patients' records, see Chapter 9.)

A few states have laws authorizing hospitals to disclose confidential information when emergency medical personnel come into contact with a patient suffering from a reportable condition.[52] The procedures for notifying the emergency personnel vary among the states, and hospitals should know the proper routine before releasing any information. Some states allow the hospital to directly notify the person at risk; others require the hospital to notify authorities at the state board of health, who then contact the emergency personnel. In either case, the hospital usually is precluded from revealing the name of the afflicted patient.

Misadministration of Radioactive Materials

Federal regulations require hospitals or practitioners using radioactive materials in the practice of nuclear medicine to obtain a federal license[53] and report any misadministration of radioactive materials to the Nuclear Regulatory Commission (NRC).[54] "Misadministration" is defined as the administration of a radiopharmaceutical or radiation other than the one intended, or to the wrong patient, or by route of administration other than that intended by the prescribing physician; as a diagnostic or therapy dosage of radiopharmaceutical that differs from the prescribed dosage by

---

[50]*See, e.g.,* ALA. CODE §§ 22-11A-1 through 22-11A-73; FLA. STAT. ANN. §§ 384.21 through 384.34; HAW. REV. STAT. §§ 325-2 & 325-3.

[51]*See, e.g.,* FLA. STAT. ANN. § 395.3025.

[52]*See, e.g.,* CAL. HEALTH & SAFETY CODE § 1797.188; FLA. STAT. ANN. § 395.1025.

[53]10 C.F.R. §§ 35.11 & 35.12.

[54]10 C.F.R. § 35.33.

certain amounts; or as a therapy radiation dose with certain errors causing a total treatment dose differing by more than 10 percent from the final prescribed total treatment dose.[55]

Death

All deaths must be reported so that authorities are informed in the event the deceased was the victim of a crime and so that accurate statistical records can be kept. Death certificates usually are signed by the physician pronouncing the death. Any suspicious or unusual deaths must be reviewed by state authorities to rule out criminal activity. Unnatural deaths usually are referred to the medical examiner for review. The medical examiner usually reviews cases involving suicides, deaths caused by criminal neglect, any type of violent death, or any type of death under suspicious or unusual circumstances. The medical examiner may conduct an investigation or perform an autopsy to determine the cause of death.

Gunshot and Knife Wounds

Most states require the reporting of certain types of wounds that ordinarily result from some type of criminal activity. Gunshot and knife wounds are always included. A state may, however, require the reporting of any wound apparently inflicted by a sharp instrument or that may have resulted from a criminal act. For example, New York requires the reporting of any wound inflicted by a sharp instrument that may result in the death of the patient.[56] Iowa requires reporting of wounds that appear to have resulted from criminal acts.[57]

State laws that require reporting may provide criminal prosecution or civil or administrative sanctions against the professional who fails to report the appropriate incident. Failure to report may be the basis of professional disciplinary action against the professional, as well. On the other hand, a professional making such a report required by law is usually given immunity from any type of civil liability for making the report.

---

[55]10 C.F.R. § 35.2.

[56]N.Y. PENAL LAW § 265.25.

[57]IOWA CODE ANN. § 147.122.

Other Health-Related Reporting Requirements

Hospitals and practitioners in the various states may be required or permitted to report other instances of health-related conditions and injuries to the appropriate state board of health. Examples of miscellaneous reporting laws include instances of veterans' exposure to Agent Orange or other causative agents,[58] diagnosis of brain injuries in patients,[59] burn injuries and wounds in cases of suspected arson,[60] cases of cerebral palsy,[61] identities of women who took diethylstilbestrol (DES) during pregnancy,[62] adverse reactions from investigational drug products,[63] environmentally related illnesses and injury,[64] and lead poisoning.[65]

Wisconsin requires reports by coroners and medical examiners concerning the results of mandatory blood tests performed on victims of snowmobile[66] and boating[67] accidents. That state allows a physician to report a patient's name and other information to the state department of transportation without the patient's consent when the physician believes the patient's physical or mental condition affects the person's ability to reasonably control a motor vehicle.[68]

Some states provide reimbursement for certain health services provided to qualified persons. Facilities wishing to participate in these programs typically are subject to reporting requirements as to the care provided. Programs may involve primary health care services,[69] maternal and infant care,[70] or other services funded by the state.

---

[58]IOWA CODE ANN. §§ 36.1 through 36.10; TEX. HEALTH & SAFETY CODE ANN. §§ 83.001 through 83.010.

[59]IOWA CODE § 135.22.

[60]LA. REV. STAT. ANN. § 14:403.4.

[61]MASS. ANN. LAWS ch. 111, § 111A.

[62]N.J. STAT. ANN. § 26:2-116.

[63]FLA. STAT. ANN. § 499.019.

[64]HAW. REV. STAT. §§ 321-311 through 321-317.

[65]CAL. HEALTH & SAFETY CODE §§ 124125 through 124160.

[66]WIS. STAT. ANN. §§ 350.15 & 350.155.

[67]WIS. STAT. ANN. § 30.67.

[68]WIS. STAT. ANN. § 146.82.

[69]See, e.g., TEX. HEALTH & SAFETY CODE ANN. §§ 31.001 through 31.017.

[70]See, e.g., TEX. HEALTH & SAFETY CODE ANN. §§ 32.001 through 32.021.

REQUIRED DISCLOSURE BY MANAGED CARE ORGANIZATIONS

While the duty of hospitals and health care providers to report child abuse and other medical conditions is fairly well-established, an MCO's duty to disclose this same information is not quite as clear. MCOs possess a large amount of patient and medical record information that they use for utilization review, quality assurance, or other evaluation processes. The same laws that require health care providers or hospitals to disclose confidential patient information may also permit or require MCOs to disclose this information. Although many of the statutes were written with health care providers or hospitals in mind, some of the statutes, particularly concerning mandatory reporting of abuse, are broad enough to include MCOs.

In some states, non-provider entities are subject to mandatory reporting requirements even though they do not directly deliver health care services to patients. In Maryland, for example, the definition of "health care provider" under the state's Medical Records Act includes HMOs and the agents, employees, officers, and directors of a health care professional or a health care facility.[71] Maryland requires a health care provider to disclose medical record information for the purposes of investigating suspected abuse or neglect of a child or an adult.[72] Accordingly, MCOs that lawfully come into contact with patient information through, for example, claims processing or utilization review tasks, have a duty to disclose patient information under certain circumstances and are protected from liability for good faith actions.[73] Similarly, Hawaii requires "[e]mployees or officers of any public or private agency or institution, or other individual, providing social, medical, hospital, or mental health services . . ." to report suspected child abuse.[74] Depending upon the structure of the MCO, employees or officers of the MCO may be required to make a report.

In many states, statutory language may be broad enough to encompass MCOs. Many reporting statutes require or allow "any" person to report suspected abuse or neglect. For example, Arizona law provides that any

---

[71] MD. CODE ANN., HEALTH GEN. § 4-301.

[72] MD. CODE ANN., HEALTH GEN. § 4-306.

[73] MD. CODE ANN., HEALTH GEN. § 5-708. *See* Edward J. Krill, "Required Disclosure of Medical Record Information-Applications to Managed Care" in ABA Forum on Health Law Monograph 3, Health Care Facility Records: Confidentiality, Computerization and Security (July 1995) 11–25.

[74] HAW. REV. STAT. § 350-1.1.

person other than one required to report may report suspected child abuse and will received immunity for making such a report.[75] Other states, such as Florida, require "any" person who has reasonable cause to suspect that a child is abused or neglected to make a report.[76] Statutes requiring or allowing "any" person to report suspected abuse can allow or require MCO employees to make such a report.

MCOs should carefully examine the laws in the states in which they operate to determine whether the statutes in these states are written broadly enough to require or allow disclosure of otherwise confidential patient information. Research may reveal that MCOs and their employees have a duty to disclose patient information. Although some states may permit but not require MCOs to disclose medical record information under certain circumstances, MCOs should determine whether they would be immune from liability for disclosing this information before developing a workplace policy concerning this issue.

---

[75] ARIZ. REV. STAT. § 13-3620.

[76] FLA. STAT. ANN. § 415.504; *see also* MD. CODE ANN., FAM. LAW § 5-705(d)(2).

8

Documentation and Disclosure: Special Areas of Concern

Chapter Objectives

- Discuss state statutes, accreditation standards, and the Emergency Medical Treatment and Active Labor Act (EMTALA) requirements pertaining to the content of emergency department records.
- Discuss documentation and disclosure concerns associated with celebrities, hostile patients, possible child abuse victims, and adoption records.
- Outline documentation requirements and related obligations placed on health care providers by the Patient Self-Determination Act (PSDA).
- Distinguish between advance directives, living wills, and durable powers of attorney for health care, and discuss statutory requirements for documentation.
- Explain how do-not-resuscitate (DNR) orders impact health care providers' decisions on patient treatment.
- Recommend documentation steps to protect health care providers from liability triggered by disagreements among professional staff.
- List purposes for which managed care organizations (MCOs) may legitimately request access to patient health care information and recommend procedures for ensuring authorized disclosure.

- Discuss the scope of law enforcement agencies' authority to obtain access to medical records.
- Discuss the use of search warrants to obtain medical records, and give examples of court-approved warrantless searches of health care facilities.
- Outline the differences between a subpoena and a court order, and recommend procedures for health care records managers to follow in responding to subpoenas.
- Discuss the increasing trend of fraud and abuse investigations and appropriate response strategies for health care providers.
- Outline statutory/regulatory requirements and recommended procedures related to the disposition of medical records upon change of ownership or closure.

INTRODUCTION

This chapter discusses a number of special problems involving documentation and disclosure of medical records that arise frequently in health care settings. Some of these problems are derived simply from the fact that health care organizations provide medical services for special categories of patients on a daily basis, and special documentation issues arise in dealing with these patients; these categories include patients in need of emergency care, celebrity patients, hostile patients, victims of child abuse, patients who refuse treatment, dying patients, and recently deceased persons (i.e., dead bodies that require authorization for autopsy). Special attention to documentation is also required, however, in situations that do not involve any of these patient categories; for example, careful documentation is particularly important where patient care has generated disagreements among professional staff as to the appropriate treatment or medication. As will be discussed in the first part of this chapter, individuals making medical record entries relating to any of these areas must be extraordinarily precise and objective in their notations.

Health care professionals, and particularly health care records managers, also regularly encounter special disclosure issues. These issues are commonly triggered by certain requests for medical records made by individuals other than the patient. Such requests include: managed care organizations requesting enrollees' record information for purposes of utilization review or quality improvement; adoptees or adoptive parents requesting health-related information about biological parents; state and federal investigators seeking relevant information in the course of law enforcement activities; and attorneys or agency officials on a quest for information that may bolster their positions in a pending legal or enforcement action. Some of the disclosure problems arising in these situations are discussed in the second part of this chapter, with a particular emphasis on the potentially competing interests that come into play in deciding whether disclosure is appropriate; other special problems involving access, however, are discussed in Chapter 6. In these situations, the health care organization is best prepared if it has developed, with the assistance of legal counsel, a workable and appropriate policy to provide its personnel and medical records practitioners with a consistent protocol.

The chapter concludes with a discussion of two additional areas of concern for health care records managers in today's rapidly changing health care environment: (1) medical records containing test results as reported from outside diagnostic and laboratory facilities and (2) record maintenance and retention under circumstances where a health care facility is either undergoing a change of ownership or permanently closing its doors. As more and more facilities contract with independent laboratories for particular services, and form alliances or other health care delivery networks to achieve more cost-effective and higher quality patient care, medical records practitioners must be aware of the health information management issues arising from these developments.

SPECIAL DOCUMENTATION CONCERNS

Emergency Department Records

Various state and federal regulations and laws discussed throughout this book govern medical records, including emergency department records.[1] Some state laws and regulations specify the information to be recorded; other states specify which broad areas of information concerning the patient's treatment must be included, or simply declare that the medical record shall be "adequate," "accurate," or "complete." State hospital licensure rules and regulations also may provide requirements and standards for the general maintenance, handling, signing, filing, and retention of medical records. (For a more detailed discussion of these laws, regulations, and standards, see Chapter 3.)

---

[1] Medicare regulations on the conditions of participation formerly specifically addressed emergency service or emergency department records, but now no longer differentiate between the two. 42 C.F.R. § 482.24.

In addition, some states specifically regulate the contents of emergency department records. Alaska requires that the emergency services record contain patient identification, the time and means of transportation to the facility, current condition, diagnosis, record of treatment provided, condition on discharge or transfer, and disposition, including instructions given for follow-up care and the name of the physician who saw the patient.[2] Arkansas specifies content requirements for emergency department records, and mandates that they must be completed immediately or, if the physician treats the patient by telephone orders, within 24 hours.[3] Indiana imposes the same content requirements for emergency and outpatient records,[4] while Maine specifies the requisite content of emergency department records in addition to requiring that all such records contain documentation of notification of appropriate authorities in suspected medicolegal cases.[5] In Oklahoma, regulations require that an emergency medical record contain documentation if a patient leaves against medical advice.[6]

The Joint Commission on Accreditation of Healthcare Organizations (Joint Commission) also has set up standards for emergency care records. The standards for accreditation of hospitals provide that in addition to the information required for all medical records,[7] emergency care records should contain:

- the time and means of arrival
- the patient's leaving against medical advice
- conclusions at the termination of treatment, including final disposition, patient's condition at the time of discharge, and any instructions for follow-up care[8]

---

[2]ALA. ADMIN. CODE tit. 7, § 12.870(f). *See also* WIS. ADMIN. CODE § 124.24 (emergency department record must contain patient identification, history of disease or injury, physical findings, lab or x-ray reports if any, diagnosis, record of treatment, disposition of case, authentication, and other appropriate notations, such as patient's arrival time, time of treatments, and time of patient discharge or transfer).

[3]ARK. REG. 0604.2.

[4]IND. ADMIN. CODE tit. 410, r. 15-1-9.

[5]CODE OF ME. R. § 10-144-112.

[6]OKLA. HOSP. STANDARDS, 310:667-19-11.

[7]JOINT COMMISSION ON ACCREDITATION OF HEALTHCARE ORGANIZATIONS, 1997 ACCREDITATION MANUAL FOR HOSPITALS, STANDARD IM 7.2.

[8]JOINT COMMISSION ON ACCREDITATION OF HEALTHCARE ORGANIZATIONS, 1997 ACCREDITATION MANUAL FOR HOSPITALS, STANDARD IM 7.5 through 7.5.2.

The Joint Commission also states that a copy of an emergency care record should be available to the practitioner or medical organization responsible for follow-up care.[9] Finally, in accordance with the Emergency Medical Treatment and Active Labor Act (EMTALA),[10] discussed next, the Joint Commission requires that a hospital's decision to refer, transfer, or discharge a patient to a different level of care or another health professional or setting be based on the patient's needs and the organization's capability to provide the care needed.[11]

The importance of establishing complete and accurate emergency care records increased significantly with the enactment of federal legislation designed to prevent the transfer of hospital patients for economic reasons. In 1985, Congress enacted EMTALA as part of the Consolidated Omnibus Reconciliation Act of 1986 (COBRA).[12] An amendment to the Medicare statute, COBRA's emergency care requirements apply to every hospital that participates in the Medicare program and that has an emergency room. COBRA, sometimes called the federal "antidumping" law, was enacted largely out of legislative concern that hospital emergency departments were turning away or transferring patients who could not pay for treatment but needed emergency medical care.

Because COBRA has detailed requirements, and because violations may lead to serious administrative consequences as well as liability (discussed later), hospital administrators should review their emergency department procedures for compliance with this important federal law. Under COBRA, any hospital with an emergency department must provide for an appropriate medical screening examination (MSE) to any individual who comes to the department and requests treatment for a medical condition. A hospital must use ancillary services routinely available to the emergency department when providing medical screening. A hospital cannot delay an MSE, further medical examination, or treatment to inquire about the individual's method of payment or insurance status.[13]

Although COBRA was enacted to prevent disparate treatment of patients without insurance, it also prohibits disparate emergency department

---

[9]JOINT COMMISSION ON ACCREDITATION OF HEALTHCARE ORGANIZATIONS, 1997 ACCREDITATION MANUAL FOR HOSPITALS, Standard IM 7.5.3.

[10]42 U.S.C. § 1395dd.

[11]JOINT COMMISSION ON ACCREDITATION OF HEALTHCARE ORGANIZATIONS, 1997 ACCREDITATION MANUAL FOR HOSPITALS, Standard CC.6.

[12]42 U.S.C. § 1395dd.

[13]42 U.S.C. § 1395dd(a) & (h).

treatment of patients enrolled in managed care plans. For example, a hospital would violate COBRA by sending a patient to an HMO for a full examination after a partial MSE at the hospital because the hospital is not providing the HMO patient with the same MSE provided to other patients.[14]

Although the emergency care provisions of COBRA contain no specific requirements for documentation of an MSE, a hospital should carefully document this type of patient care to defend against charges that it violated the law. Accordingly, the emergency department should create and retain a record of each MSE it conducts. If the MSE indicates that the individual does not have an emergency condition, the hospital will have satisfied its obligations under the law. For evidence purposes, however, emergency department records should demonstrate that the MSE was conducted and that such a conclusion was reached.

Proper documentation is particularly important if the individual refuses to consent to the MSE or refuses to undergo recommended treatment. The hospital is required to obtain, or attempt to obtain, the individual's written informed consent to refuse treatment. Similarly, if a hospital offers to transfer the individual and informs the person of the risks and benefits of the transfer, but the individual refuses to consent, the hospital will have fulfilled its obligations under the law. A hospital must take all reasonable steps to obtain written informed consent when an individual has refused an examination, treatment, or transfer.

Documentation on the stabilization of a patient's condition or on a transfer must be accurate and complete in order to prove that the hospital complied with its duties under COBRA. The documentation should indicate the status of the individual's condition and the treatment provided to achieve stabilization. In the event of a transfer, the record also should include a statement by medical personnel that within reasonable medical probability, no material deterioration of the patient's emergency medical condition will result from the transfer or will occur during the transfer process.[15] In addition, COBRA requires that specific records accompany

---

[14]Health care administrators should note that courts generally have ruled that managed care organizations, including HMOs, cannot be held responsible for COBRA violations. *See, e.g.*, Bangert v. Christian Health Servs., No. 92-613 (S.D. Ill. Dec. 17, 1992) (unpublished) (patient's right to sue for COBRA violations limited to claim brought against Medicare-participating hospital); Dearmas v. Av-Med., Inc., 814 F. Supp. 1103 (S.D. Fla. 1993) (HMOs not subject to liability for failing to satisfy COBRA requirements).

[15]42 C.F.R. § 489.24(b).

the patient to the receiving facility. The transferring hospital must send a copy of all medical records related to the emergency conditions that are available at the time of transfer, including observations of signs or symptoms, preliminary diagnosis, treatment provided, results of any tests, the informed consent to transfer or the physician's certification, and the name and address of any on-call physician who has refused or failed to appear within a reasonable time to provide necessary stabilizing treatment.[16] Health care administrators also should know that states have become increasingly involved in the problems of patient transfer, and thus in some jurisdictions appropriate documentation and the implementation of hospital policies regarding patient transfers is necessary to prove compliance with state antidumping laws.[17]

If the person conducting the MSE (e.g., a physician or other "qualified" individual) determines that the patient has an emergency medical condition or is in active labor, the hospital must stabilize the patient before discharge.[18] The hospital may transfer the patient only upon the signed certification of a physician that the benefits of the transfer outweigh the risks. If a physician is not physically present in the emergency department at the time of transfer, a "qualified medical person" may sign a certification after consultation with a physician, but the physician must subsequently countersign the certification.[19]

At least two federal appeals courts interpreting COBRA have examined whether a physician actually evaluated the risks and benefits of transfer. COBRA certification must be a true assessment, not merely a signature, according to one of the earliest cases to arise under the law. The Fifth Circuit ruled that a physician's failure to weigh the medical risks and benefits before transferring a severely hypertensive woman in active labor violated the law. Although the physician had signed the "Physician's Certificate Authorizing Transfer," the court concluded that he had not engaged in a

---

[16]42 C.F.R. § 489.24(d). COBRA also requires that hospitals with emergency departments adopt a policy to ensure that records of all patient transfers are maintained for at least five years.

[17]*See, e.g.*, Tex. Health & Safety Code Ann. § 241.027 (hospital licensing statute requiring that hospitals adopt procedures that ensure patient transfers are accomplished through hospital policies that result in medically appropriate transfers, and specifying the policies' content, including the steps physicians must take in making patient transfer determinations and in documenting transfers).

[18]*See, e.g.*, 42 C.F.R. § 489.24(a). The qualifications for who may perform an MSE are not outlined in federal regulations; rather, the relevant regulations only require that hospital bylaws or rules identify which individuals are qualified to perform screening examinations.

[19]42 C.F.R. § 489.24(d).

meaningful weighing of the risks and benefits.[20] The Ninth Circuit, on the other hand, has ruled that a hospital did not violate COBRA by failing to enumerate the risks and benefits of a patient's transfer on a form, if the hospital could show that a physician actually considered the medical risks and benefits. In refusing to impose COBRA liability, the court concluded that even though the hospital technically violated a recordkeeping provision, the purpose of the statute was satisfied in light of evidence demonstrating that the physician deliberated over the risks and benefits before signing the transfer certification form.[21]

COBRA's enforcement provisions impose a civil monetary penalty of up to $50,000 for each violation against hospitals that negligently violate the law, or up to $25,000 against those with fewer than 100 beds. Hospitals that fail to substantially meet the COBRA requirements are subject to suspension or termination of their Medicare provider agreements.[22] Although many hospitals have been fined, few have been terminated. Civil liability is another potential consequence of COBRA violations. An individual who suffers personal harm as a direct result of a hospital's violation of the law can sue the hospital for personal injury damages and equitable relief.[23]

Since COBRA was enacted, an estimated 700 hospitals have been subject to enforcement actions, and the agency imposed fines on more than 500 hospitals between 1986 and 1995. Penalties and settlements have ranged from $5,000 to $150,000.[24] Given the increase in enforcement activity in this area, hospital administrators are well advised to work with hospital legal counsel in reviewing hospital policy and procedures to ensure full compliance with all applicable federal and state statutes and reg-

---

[20]Burditt v. United States Dep't of Health & Human Servs., 934 F.2d 1362 (5th Cir. 1991).

[21]Vargas ex rel. Gallardo v. Del Puerto Hosp., 98 F.3d 1202 (9th Cir. 1996).

[22]42 U.S.C. § 1395dd(d)(1), 52 C.F.R. § 489.53.

[23]Although courts have consistently ruled that physicians cannot be found liable under COBRA, hospital administrators should know that state laws may provide for individual liability for COBRA violations, and that hospitals found liable may be able to recover from individuals who actually committed the violations. See McDougal v. Lafourche Hosp. Serv. Dist. No. 3, No. 92-2006 (E.D. La. May 25, 1993) (unpublished) (allowing hospital to recover damages from staff physician); but see Griffith v. Mt. Carmel Med. Ctr., 842 F. Supp. 1359 (D. Kan. 1994) (jury award cannot be apportioned between hospital and physician in COBRA suit).

[24]Eric Weissenstein, Modern HealthCare, Vol 26, No. 13 at 5 (Mar. 25, 1996); Stephen A. Frew, "Welcome to COBRA Online," Executive Summary, Version 2.1, available on the Internet at http://www.medlaw.com/handout.htm.

ulations pertaining to emergency department records and recordkeeping requirements.

Celebrity Patients

When patients who are subject to close scrutiny by news media are hospitalized for conditions that might be embarrassing for them, special care often must be taken to protect records confidentiality. While news media take an interest in patients who may have become newsworthy temporarily, they often use more aggressive tactics in obtaining information concerning celebrities. As a result, some hospitals have established special procedures for handling celebrity patient records; such procedures typically allow the patient to control the amount and type of information released unless otherwise required by law.

As an extra precaution against unauthorized disclosure, some hospitals omit the patient's name from the record or use a code name that corresponds to a master code maintained by the medical records director and hospital chief executive officer.[25] Also, the celebrity patient has the right to request an alias name, and upon receiving such a request, the hospital should assign the alias name upon admission of the patient, use that name throughout the patient's visit, and then make necessary corrections to the records after discharge. The hospital also may adopt a policy reserving its right to issue an alias to a patient if it considers this action to be in the best interest of the patient and the medical facility admitting the patient. Although assigning an alias may give added protection to the patient, it may conflict with state statutes and regulations, and therefore should be employed only with the advice of legal counsel.

Policies and procedures should be established to quickly assess the need for patient anonymity at admission and assign an alias if necessary. For example, the hospital should have policies that specify exactly who is authorized to assign patient anonymity, and who should be notified to ensure greater protection of that anonymity (e.g., security, public relations, and/or administration). Some hospitals place the medical records of celebrity patients in a special secure file accessible only to the medical records director and other designated persons. This approach may not provide the same degree of protection as the former method, but it is not

---

[25]Some health care institutions prefer using an alphanumeric code in place of the patient's real name, rather than assign a generic name (e.g., "John Doe"). One code format, for example, is a combination of the patient's initials and business office account number.

likely to violate record content requirements of state law. A spokesperson, preferably an individual experienced in health care public relations, should be designated to address any inquiries received from the media or any other authorities.[26] The hospital also should establish procedures to ensure that any information approved for release is consistent and accurate, and that any information regarding the patient's condition or presence in the facility is released only upon the patient's authorization. (For a more extensive discussion of media access to medical records, see "Invasion of Privacy," covered in Chapter 11.)

Health care records managers developing special procedures for handling the records of patients who request anonymity should consider a number of other steps for preventing unauthorized disclosure, including:

- Replacing the patient's name with an assigned code or alias on all bed boards, bulletin boards, and patient room signs.
- Restricting computer access to those users who need to know the patient's identity to perform their jobs, and employing mechanisms that will alert a security officer when a system user attempts to access information beyond his or her security clearance.
- Designating one individual to be responsible for controlling access to the restricted medical record in facilities with paper record systems.
- Providing employees, medical staff members, students, and volunteers with specific training about their responsibility to protect the confidentiality of medical records information, and requiring them to sign a nondisclosure agreement.
- Allowing access to the patient's record after the patient has been discharged only to those employees with a valid need to know (for example, those involved in the chart completion process).

Health care records managers and risk managers also should establish a system for performing periodic audits to ensure that policies in this area are being followed and are still effective.

---

[26]Health care administrators should consider advising designated spokespersons to follow established guidelines when releasing information about patients. *See, e.g.*, Society for Healthcare Strategy and Market Development, American Hospital Association, General Guide for the Release of Information on the Condition of Patients (Chicago, Ill. 1997).

Hostile Patients

Hostile patients present problems for everyone in a health care facility. Whether the hostility arises from the patient's condition, general nature, or the treatment received at the institution, the hostile individual often is more inclined to take legal action if a problem in treatment actually occurs. Moreover, hostile patients may be less inclined to remember all the facts of a treatment situation or to view them in a light favorable to the health care facility, and therefore physicians and other health care personnel should take greater care in documenting hostile patients' treatment.

No special rules of law apply to records of hostile patients, but health care practitioners should take a common-sense approach to documentation in such records. All relevant staff members should be trained to recognize the hostile patient, and should know that prudent handling of that patient's medical care must include the creation of a detailed medical record that leaves little ambiguity about the care that has been provided. Obviously, such staff members also should avoid making derogatory remarks about a hostile patient in the medical record; remarks of this nature contribute nothing to the ability of other practitioners to care for the patient, and instead generate the risk that these comments will be used by the litigious hostile patient as further proof of the practitioners' bad faith. A medical record should contain remarks concerning the patient's hostility only if such conduct is clinically relevant; in those cases, notations should be limited to concise descriptions in clinical terms.

Recording Indicators of Child Abuse

When the physician assesses a child to determine whether reasonable cause exists to believe the youngster is abused or neglected, careful notations must be made in the medical record. Specifically, a detailed and objective documentation and description of all pertinent physical findings should be noted clearly in the record. In addition, any tests performed or photographs taken to document the suspected abuse should be noted carefully. This information will be the basis upon which a determination of abuse is made, and thus attention to detail in recording the information is very important. The record should include a history of the injury, including details reported by the parent or guardian of how the injury allegedly happened, date and time of the injury, sequence of events, names of witnesses, interval between the injury and the time medical attention was sought, and identities of the interviewers. If the parents, guardians, and child are interviewed separately, the date, time, and place of each session should be documented. (For a more detailed discussion of disclosure issues in relation to records indicating child abuse, see "Special Disclosure Concerns" in this chapter.)

Patients Refusing Treatment and/or Near Death

The medical record plays a critical role in right-to-die situations. Whether it is the patient who makes the decision to withdraw or forgo life-sustaining medical treatment or someone designated to act on the patient's behalf, the medical record will be the primary if not sole source documenting the appropriateness of the decision. In either case, the patient's medical record should clearly set forth all relevant information concerning the patient's treatment decision and plan before the physician gives a directive to withdraw or forgo life-sustaining treatment for a patient. The following sections discuss some of the laws, regulations, and standards containing medical record requirements pertinent to end-of-life decision making.

Background

It is well established that competent adults have the right to refuse treatment unless state interests outweigh that right. Courts have long recognized that a patient's right to make decisions concerning medical care necessarily includes the right to decline medical care.[27]

A patient's ability personally to exercise the right to determine medical treatment does not exist if the individual is incompetent. Some patients who never have expressed their wishes regarding treatment become irreversibly incompetent and unable to communicate. Others never have had an opportunity to express their wishes because of youth or mental retardation. With increasing frequency courts are confronting these issues, and many have concluded that because competent adults have the right to refuse treatment, there must be a means for the same right to be exercised on behalf of incompetent patients.

---

[27]*See, e.g.,* White v. Chicago & N.W. Ry. Co., 124 N.W. 309 (Iowa 1910); State v. McAfee, 385 S.E.2d 651 (Ga. 1989); McKay v. Bergstedt, 801 P.2d 617 (Nev. 1990).

The U.S. Supreme Court addressed this issue in the well-publicized *Cruzan* case.[28] In that case, the parents of a young woman in a persistent vegetative state since her injury in an automobile accident in 1983 requested court authorization to remove the gastrostomy tube through which their daughter received life-sustaining nutrition and hydration. The Court recognized that a competent person has the right to refuse medical treatment, but that an incompetent patient is unable to exercise such a right. A state has the authority to set standards governing how this right may be exercised on behalf of the incompetent patient and how to ensure that the decision respects as much as possible the wishes expressed by the patient while competent, the Court ruled.

Both the federal and state legislatures have responded to the need to formalize the decision-making process for competent and incompetent patients who are faced with life-sustaining treatment decisions. As discussed next, legislation at the federal level imposes duties on health care providers to inform patients of their right to accept or refuse medical treatment, and every state has some type of statute that regulates patients' right to specify, in advance of incompetency, what medical measures should be used to sustain their lives. Moreover, the Joint Commission requires all health care organizations to have policies and procedures regarding decisions to forgo or withdraw life-sustaining procedures.

Patient Self-Determination Act

Legislation requiring that all federally funded facilities inform patients of their rights under state law to accept or refuse medical treatment was enacted as part of the Omnibus Budget Reconciliation Act of 1990, more commonly referred to as the Patient Self-Determination Act (PSDA).[29] Since December 1, 1991, when the PSDA took effect, health care providers and institutions that receive Medicare or Medicaid funding have been required to inform patients of their legal rights to accept or refuse medical or surgical treatment and the right to formulate advance directives.[30] "Advance directive" is defined as a written instruction, such as a living will or durable power of attorney for health care, recognized under

---

[28]Cruzan v. Director, Missouri Dep't of Health, 497 U.S. 261 (1990).

[29]*See* Omnibus Budget Reconciliation Act of 1990, Pub. L. No. 101-508, 104 Stat. 1388, codified at 42 U.S.C. § 1395cc(f).

[30]42 U.S.C. § 1305(b)(1)(a)(1)(A)(i).

state law and relating to the provision of medical care when the individual is incapacitated. Covered providers include, but are not limited to, hospitals, clinics, rehabilitation facilities, long-term care facilities, home health care agencies, hospice programs, and HMOs. Under the PSDA, each state must prepare a written description of the law in that state on advance directives and distribute this information to hospital patients, residents in a skilled nursing facility, HMO enrollees, or recipients of home health care and hospice program services.

In accordance with the law, health care facilities must develop written policies requiring that patients receive legal information on the exercise of their rights as well as information about the facility policy itself. Written information distributed by the health care provider must have two components: (1) a summary of individual rights under state law and (2) the written policy of the provider itself as to implementation of those rights. The summary of state law ultimately should be furnished by the appropriate state agency to facilitate uniformity among institutions. The provider itself is required to draft a written policy and provide a copy of it to patients at the time of admission. The PSDA requires only that a patient's medical record indicate whether or not the individual has an advance directive, and does not specifically require that a copy of the directive be obtained and made part of the medical record; state law, however, may otherwise impose this duty on attending physicians or hospitals. In general, health care organizations would be well advised to require that the advance directive be made a part of the medical record, with provisions for confirming its continued validity upon any readmission or renewal of services.

Joint Commission standards require that health care organizations be in compliance with the PSDA, and that their policies and procedures describe the means by which patients' rights under the PSDA are protected and exercised.[31] A patient's rights as defined in these standards include the opportunity to create advance directives, the access to information necessary to make informed decisions about medical treatment, and the right to participate in discussions of the ethical issues that may arise during the individual's care. According to the intent of the Joint Commission's standard on advance directives, if the actual advance directive is not placed in

---

[31]JOINT COMMISSION ON THE ACCREDITATION OF HEALTHCARE ORGANIZATIONS, 1997 COMPREHENSIVE ACCREDITATION MANUAL FOR HOSPITALS, Standards RI.1.2.4, RI.2.5 & RI.2.6; JOINT COMMISSION ON THE ACCREDITATION OF HEALTHCARE ORGANIZATIONS, 1998 COMPREHENSIVE ACCREDITATION MANUAL FOR HEALTH CARE NETWORKS, Standards RI.3, RI.3.1, RI.3.2 & RI.3.3.

the patient's medical record then the substance of that directive should be documented in the record;[32] moreover, the directive should be reviewed periodically with the patient or the surrogate decision maker.

Living Will Legislation

The most widely available instrument for recording future health care-related decisions is the living will. The vast majority of states have enacted legislation recognizing the right of a competent adult to prepare a document providing direction as to medical care if the adult becomes incapacitated or otherwise unable to make decisions personally. Many states' living will laws encompass "natural death acts" or statutory provisions allowing a living will to be specifically applied if the patient is suffering from a terminal condition or is irreversibly unconscious.[33]

Living will legislation covers a variety of topics, including procedures for executing such a document, physician certification of terminal illness or irreversible coma, immunity from civil and criminal liability for providers who implement the decisions, and the right to transfer a patient to another facility if a provider cannot follow the directive for reasons of conscience. As a general rule, the more precise and exact the directions in the living will are, the more likely it is that health care providers will comply with it.

Although some state laws used to contain statutorily dictated wording for written directives, the trend has been away from mandating the contents of living wills toward requiring that they contain "substantially" or "essentially" the same information as the statutory model. North Carolina law states that the statutory form "is specifically determined to meet the [legislative] requirements," implying that other forms would be acceptable if they rigidly met the same requirements.[34] West Virginia law states that a directive can be in "essentially" the same form as the one in the statute but may include other specific directions.[35] Arkansas provides that

---

[32]Joint Commission on Accreditation of Healthcare Organizations, 1997 Comprehensive Accreditation Manual for Hospitals, Standard RI.2.4.

[33]The terminology varies from state to state. *See, e.g.*, Cal. Health & Safety Code § 7185.5 ("permanent unconscious condition"); Ark. Code Ann. § 20-17-201(11) ("permanently unconscious"); N.M. Stat. Ann. § 24-7-2(B) ("irreversible coma"); N.C. Gen. Stat. § 90-321(a)(4) ("persistent vegetative state").

[34]N.C. Gen. Stat. § 90-321(d).

[35]W. Va. Code § 16-30-3(e).

in the absence of knowledge to the contrary, a health care provider may presume that a declaration complies with the law and is valid.[36]

State legislation also specifies the formality with which the directive must be executed. All of the acts require witnesses, and some disqualify certain people from being witnesses—such as relatives, those who will inherit the estate, those who have claims against the estate, the attending physician, and employees of the physician or hospital. Normally, the qualifications of the witnesses are not of concern to the hospital or physician because the directive usually includes a certification by the witness that they are not disqualified.

State laws also specify the means to revoke a directive. Written revocations generally must meet minimal requirements: they must be signed, dated, and communicated to the attending physician. In most states, any verbal revocation is effective upon communication to the attending physician.[37] If a copy of the directive is in the medical record, and the health care organization receives notice of revocation, a note should be entered on the directive stating that the patient has revoked it. If the original directive is in the record, a patient cannot revoke it by physical destruction. The effect of the directive also is defined in state law. The majority of statutes specify that any physician may decline to follow the directive but must make an effort to transfer the patient to a physician who will follow it.[38] Some states provide that a directive shall not apply while the patient is pregnant.[39]

State legislation generally makes it a crime to interfere with the proper use of directive forms. Unauthorized cancellation or concealment of a directive in order to interfere with a patient's wish not to be treated may constitute a criminal misdemeanor or grounds for professional disciplinary action. Falsification or forgery of a directive or withholding knowledge of revocation in order to cause actions contrary to the patient's wishes when those actions hasten death is a felony under state law.

---

[36]ARK. CODE Ann. § 20-17-211.

[37]*See, e.g.*, CAL. HEALTH & SAFETY CODE § 7188; W. VA. CODE § 16-30-4(3).

[38]*See, e.g.*, TEX. HEALTH & SAFETY CODE ANN. § 672.016; W.VA. CODE § 16-30-7; OR. REV. STAT. § 127.625 (physician must notify health care representative, who must make a reasonable effort to transfer the patient).

[39]*See, e.g.*, CAL. HEALTH & SAFETY CODE § 7189.5; KAN. STAT. ANN. § 65-28,103(A); TEX. HEALTH & SAFETY CODE ANN. § 672.004.

Durable Power of Attorney

A power of attorney is a written document that authorizes an individual, as an agent, to perform certain acts on behalf of and according to the written directives of another—the person executing the document—from whom the agent obtains authority. The agent is called the attorney-in-fact and the person executing the document is called the principal. Most states have adopted the Uniform Durable Power of Attorney Act,[40] which provides that the subsequent disability or incompetence of the principal does not affect the attorney-in-fact's authority. For the power of attorney to have any legal effect, however, the principal must be mentally competent when executing the instrument. The requirements governing witnesses and notarization of the instrument typically vary with state law.[41]

Such legislation is general in nature, however, and is not tailored to health care decision making. For this reason, the vast majority of states have gone further to provide for durable powers of attorney specifically for health care decisions.[42] Under that type of legislation, the state authorizes the appointment of an individual who is specifically empowered to make personal health care-related decisions for another person in the event the latter becomes incapacitated. Many state legislatures have provided model forms in their laws that include specific choices for the conditions under which life-sustaining treatment may be withdrawn.

The exact wording of durable powers of attorney for health care varies from state to state and, like that of living wills, is dictated largely by models contained in the statutes. In general, these documents grant agents full power and authority to make health care decisions for principals to the same extent as principals themselves would if they were competent. In exercising this authority, the agent must, to the extent possible, make decisions that are consistent with the principal's desires using the substituted

---

[40]8 U.L.A. 74.

[41]Because of the lack of uniformity in state laws, it is possible that a power of attorney valid in one state may not be enforceable in other jurisdictions. Health care providers should always seek legal counsel to determine the validity of an out-of-state power of attorney, and health care organizations should specifically require such consultation in relevant policies.

[42]*See, e.g.*, 755 ILL. COMP. STAT. ANN. 45/4-1 through 45/4-12; ARIZ. REV. STAT. §§ 36-3221 through 36-3224; CAL. PROB. CODE §§ 4600 through 4806; D.C. Code §§ 21-2205 through 21-2210.

judgment doctrine[43] or that are based on what the agent believes to be the principal's best interests.[44] The power of attorney can enumerate specifically the principal's desires as to different types of life-sustaining measures, admission or discharge from facilities, pain relief medication, and anatomical gifts. It also should allow the agent to gain access to the principal's medical records to be able to make informed decisions.

Of paramount importance is the actual determination of the principal's disability or incompetence. The durable power of attorney should state who will determine the principal's incompetence and should set the standards to be used in making that determination. It is best for one or more physicians, named in the document or chosen according to a procedure established in the document, to determine incompetence.[45] Disability and incompetence should be defined in the durable power of attorney and should be mutually acceptable to the principal and physicians involved. Copies of the durable power of attorney should be given to the attorney-in-fact, the principal's physician, and close family members. As an additional safeguard, the document also should be included in the patient's medical record.

A competent principal can revoke the durable power of attorney at any time. The instrument also may be terminated if it contains an expiration clause. Some state legislatures stipulate a maximum duration for durable powers of attorney, providing that unless a shorter period is defined in the document, it will expire automatically at the end of a given number of years.[46] An expiration clause allows the principal periodically to reconsider the directives in the writing.

As with living will legislation, state statutes governing durable power of attorney for health care usually impose criminal penalties for failing to conform with the health care agency provided for under the statutes. Falsi-

---

[43]Substituted judgment means that the decisions of the surrogate should be based on what the patient would have decided if the patient were able to do so at the time; in most states, it is the legal standard that applies in the absence of an explicit statement of desires in an advance directive. *See, e.g.,* IDAHO CODE § 39-4505.

[44]The American Bar Association, Commission on Legal Problems of the Elderly, has adopted a model Health Care Powers of Attorney containing this broad grant of authority.

[45]The ABA model suggests that incapacity should be determined by the agent and the attending physician.

[46]*See, e.g.,* CAL. PROBE CODE § 4654. To accomplish the purpose of a durable power of attorney for health care, given that the patient's incompetence may be for an indefinite period of time, an attorney may include a provision that extends the period of time it is effective in the event the principal is incompetent, disabled, unconscious, or hospitalized.

fication or forgery of a health care agency with the intent to cause withholding or withdrawal of life-sustaining or death-delaying procedures contrary to the intent of the principal, which thereby causes the death of the patient to be hastened, may be subject to felony charges.[47]

Health care providers view the durable power of attorney for health care as a more flexible instrument than a living will. The scope of a living will generally is limited to situations where the patient is either terminally ill or permanently unconscious. The power of attorney, on the other hand, can apply to a wider range of situations in which the patient is unable to communicate a choice regarding a health care decision. In addition, the power of attorney allows the agent to make any decision regarding an incapacitated patient's health care and is not limited to specific life-sustaining measures.

Do-Not-Resuscitate Orders

The term "cardiopulmonary resuscitation" (CPR) describes a procedure developed over the last two decades to reestablish breathing and heartbeat after cardiac or respiratory arrest. The most basic form of CPR, which is being taught to the public, involves recognizing the indications for intervention, opening an airway, initiating mouth-to-mouth breathing, and compressing the chest externally to establish artificial circulation. In hospitals, and in some emergency transport vehicles, CPR also can include the administration of oxygen under pressure to the lungs, the use of intravenous medications, the injection of stimulants into the heart through catheters or long needles, electric shocks to the heart, insertion of a pacemaker, and open-heart massage. Some of these procedures are highly intrusive and even violent in nature.

To ensure that CPR is not initiated where it is not indicated, it is common practice to write "Do not resuscitate" (DNR) or "No CPR" on the orders for treatment of the patient. The order is directed to on-call staff members who, because of the urgency of cardiac arrest, are unable to consult with the patient or primary care physician as to the desired course of treatment. Many institutions call the CPR team by announcing "Code Blue," so the order might read "No Code Blue." DNR orders provide an exception to the universal standing order to provide CPR. For prehospital and emergency department care, consent for cardiopulmonary resuscita-

---

[47]*See, e.g.*, 755 ILL. COMP. STAT. ANN. 45/4-6.

tion is implied unless a valid, written advance directive states otherwise. With respect to emergency care, the presumption at law is that the patient would choose to be resuscitated were the patient able to express such an opinion. Moreover, the American Medical Association (AMA) Council on Ethical and Judicial Affairs has stated that "[e]fforts should be made to resuscitate patients who suffer cardiac or respiratory arrest except when circumstances indicate that administration of cardiopulmonary resuscitation (CPR) would be futile or not in accord with the desires or best interest of the patient."[48]

Joint Commission standards require that health care organizations establish policies and procedures regarding the decision to withhold resuscitative services.[49] Moreover, state statutes in this area typically require that DNR orders be written by the physician who is primarily responsible for the patient's care and inscribed in the patient's medical record.[50] An appropriate consent form or refusal of treatment form should also be signed by the patient, the patient's family, or the patient's surrogate or proxy; a physician must obtain the informed consent of a competent patient or of an incompetent patient's family or other representative before entering a DNR order. Typically, hospital policies require daily review of DNR orders to determine if they remain consistent with the condition of the patient, as well as the desires of the patient or patient's representative.

If the patient is incompetent, any health care provider should proceed with caution before placing a DNR order in the medical record or in failing to respond in the event of cardiopulmonary arrest, unless a written advance directive such as a living will clearly indicates the patient's choice. In one leading case, a court ruled against a physician who concluded that a patient was incompetent and issued a no-code order in response to a relative's request.[51] Although a nurse gave evidence that the patient was able to communicated coherently up to a few minutes before his death, the physician relied on the patient's sister, who requested the DNR order. No efforts were made to resuscitate the patient when he stopped breathing. The court held that the patient should have been consulted before the

---

[48]AMERICAN MEDICAL ASSOCIATION, CURRENT MEDICAL OPINIONS A-96 (June 1994).

[49]JOINT COMMISSION ON ACCREDITATION OF HEALTHCARE ORGANIZATIONS, 1997 ACCREDITATION MANUAL FOR HOSPITALS, Standard RI.2.5; JOINT COMMISSION ON ACCREDITATION OF HEALTHCARE ORGANIZATIONS, 1998 ACCREDITATION MANUAL FOR HEALTH CARE NETWORKS, Standard RI.3.2.

[50]See, e.g., ALASKA STAT. §18.12.010(b); GA. CODE ANN. § 31-39-4; MD CODE ANN., HEALTH-GEN. §5-602(f)(2).

[51]Payne v. Marion Gen. Hosp., 549 N.E.2d 1043 (Ind. Ct. App. 1990).

physician gave the DNR order. In addition, the court noted that a year prior to the incident, the patient had suffered from the same type of illness and recovered. Thus, there was a good possibility that the patient would have survived if there had been concerted resuscitation efforts.

Moreover, a physician must explain the nature of the treatment to be withheld from an incompetent patient before obtaining consent from the patient's family or other representative. The necessity of obtaining genuinely informed consent from the patient's representative was upheld in a 1981 Minnesota case in which the court ordered the cancellation of a DNR order upon the determination that the parents and guardians of an incompetent patient were unaware of the nature of the treatment to be denied and did not demonstrate sufficient consideration of what the patient would have wanted.[52] Thus, the court ordered the patient's name to be taken off the hospital's DNR list until the parents gave "knowledgeable approval" to reinstate the DNR order. It is worth noting, however, that a physician is not required to obtain court approval before entering a DNR order.[53]

Although some states have enacted statutes that prohibit the use of DNR orders outside the hospital setting, at least 35 other states have advance directive legislation that either specifically permits emergency medical personnel to honor certain out-of-hospital DNR orders or leaves open the opportunity for the state's medical community to develop standards in this area.[54] In many of these states, statutes, regulations, or medical society standards provide that, if certain conditions are met by physician and patient, DNRs in these situations will be recognized and honored by emergency medical services (EMS) personnel responding to calls for patients suffering cardiopulmonary arrest. In Wisconsin, for example, a recently enacted statute allows certain individuals to request a DNR bracelet from his or her physician; if the bracelet is found on the patient's wrist (and the bracelet is not defaced in any way), emergency health care per-

---

[52]Hoyt v. St. Mary's Rehabilitation Ctr., No. 77455S (Minn. Dist. Ct. Hennepin County Feb. 13, 1981) (unpublished).

[53]*See, e.g.*, In re Quinlan, 355 A.2d 647 (N.J. 1976), *cert. denied sub nom.*, Gayer v. New Jersey, 492 U.S. 922 (1976); In re Dinnerstein, 380 N.E.2d 134 (Mass. App. Ct.1978); In re J.N., 406 A.2d 1275 (D.C. 1979). *See also* Severns v. Wilmington Med. Ctr, Inc., 421 A.2d 1334 (Del. 1980) (court authorized DNR order but did not state whether court authorization always is required).

[54]In some states, such standards are considered to be medical protocols appropriately promulgated by the medical community, rather than enacted by the state legislature.

sonnel will not undertake CPR measures.[55] The statute also provides that no physician, EMS worker, or other health care professional may be held criminally or civilly liable, or otherwise disciplined, if they withhold or withdraw resuscitation from a patient with a DNR order. In New Jersey, recently released guidelines for out-of-hospital DNR orders provide that such orders will be considered valid only if the DNR form is completed, signed, and dated by both the patient and his or her physician, and displayed prominently in the patient's home or presented to medical personnel who respond to an emergency call.[56]

Deceased Patients and Autopsy Authorizations

Autopsies are the most frequent cause of litigation involving dead bodies and hospitals. Autopsies are performed primarily to determine the cause of a patient's death. This finding can be crucial in detecting crime or ruling out transmittable diseases that may be a threat to the public health. More frequently, the cause of death can determine whether death benefits are payable under insurance policies, Workers' Compensation laws, and other programs.

Community mores and religious beliefs have long dictated respectful handling of dead bodies. Societal views have evolved now to the point that a substantial portion of the population recognizes the benefit of autopsies. Out of respect for those who continue to find them unacceptable, the law requires appropriate consent before an autopsy can be performed, except when one is needed to determine the cause of death for public policy purposes. The consent to the autopsy, whether given by the decedent, by family members, or by other persons authorized to do so in the particular state, must be documented in the patient's medical record. A few states require that an autopsy be authorized in writing. Many states include telegrams and recorded telephone permissions as acceptable forms of authorization. Common law does not require that the authorization be documented in a particular way, so evidentiary considerations are the primary basis for deciding the appropriate form of consent. A written authorization or recorded telephone authorization obviously is the easiest to prove.[57]

---

[55]WIS. STAT. §§ 154-19-154-29. *See also* Fla. Stat. ch. 401.45; Fla. Admin. Code Ann. r. 10D-66.325.

[56]Medical Society of New Jersey, Out of Hospital DNR Order Guidelines (1997).

[57]*See, e.g.*, Lashbrook v. Barnes, 437 S.W.2d 502 (Ky. 1969).

Recording Disagreements Among Professional Staff

All members of the medical team have a duty to take reasonable actions to safeguard the lives of their patients. Physician assistants, nurse practitioners, nurses, and other health care professionals often are given the responsibility of monitoring and coordinating patient care. As a result, in the exercise of reasonable professional judgment and in order to minimize the possible liability for negligence, nonphysician medical professionals may be expected to intervene to clarify or object to physicians' orders they believe are improper. Courts have upheld such interventions,[58] and also have recognized that nurses and other nonphysician medical professionals, including pharmacists, have an independent duty to patients and thus can be held liable for failing to question physicians' orders.[59] Accordingly, it is essential that nurses and other medical professionals document their efforts to fulfill their duty to object to improper orders and their attempts to obtain responsible intervention to settle a professional disagreement. At the same time, it is important to create a medical record that is sufficiently objective and factual that it could not be used as evidence against the physician or the institution in a negligence action.

Although there are no clear answers to the medical records issues presented in instances of disagreements among physicians and other medical professionals, several suggested approaches may be helpful. If hospital policy requires that resolution of disagreements be documented in the medical record, all persons making entries in patients' medical records should be trained as to proper documentation in these situations. Entries in the medical record should be objective, concise, and completely factual rather than judgmental. The more complex the intervention, the more care the nurse or other professional must take in documenting the facts. Statements such as "Dr. Smith is negligent again" or "Dr. Smith's order is incorrect" are unnecessary and inappropriate and, in the event of any legal action, may be used as evidence against the nurse or other nonphysician health care provider, the physician, and the health care institution.

---

[58]*See, e.g.*, Carlsen v. Javurek, 526 F.2d 202 (8th Cir. 1975).

[59]*See, e.g.*, Gassen v. East Jefferson Gen. Hosp., 628 So. 2d 256 (La. Ct. App. 1993) (holding pharmacist liable for failing to contact the prescribing physician when the physician made clear mistakes in prescription); Riff v. Morgan Pharmacy, 508 A.2d 1247 (Pa. Super. Ct. 1986) (holding pharmacist liable for failing to warn patient or inform her physician of inadequacies in prescription's instructions); Norton v. Argonaut Ins. Co., 144 So. 2d 249 (La. Ct. App. 1962) (holding nurse liable for administering fatal dose to patient as result of not contacting physician about apparently erroneous medication order).

There are varying opinions among health care professionals concerning whether these kinds of professional discussions and disagreements should be documented in a medical record, and, if so, in what manner. Regardless of the position one takes on the issue, it is clear that a health care organization must have a policy covering the question.[60] Otherwise practitioners are left to work out their differences on their own, and this inevitably leads to inconsistent patient care and record documentation practices, and may result in vindictive or otherwise "dangerous" medical records entries made in the heat of anger.

SPECIAL DISCLOSURE CONCERNS

Records Sought By Managed Care Organizations

In today's health care environment, health care organizations must regularly respond to requests for access to patient health care record information from managed care organizations (MCOs). In responding to these requests, health care organizations may trigger potential liability risks stemming from the inappropriate generation and use of and access to health care record information. Managed care and the growth of integrated health care delivery systems have created greater challenges with respect to protecting unauthorized disclosure and preserving the confidentiality of patient health care information. It has become increasingly difficult, for example, to identify all the possible sites where a particular medical record, or a segment of that record, may be located. Where formerly such documentation may have been located at various locations but within only one institution (e.g., within a number of hospital departments), now, in addition to these sources, parts of the patient's medical record information may be found at numerous other sites, including managed care organizations, utilization management companies, and various member-health care providers of integrated delivery networks.

While legislation, regulations, and contracts readily acknowledge that patients have a right to privacy of their health care information, the degree of control individuals exercise over this data is limited. Although state law

---

[60]Disagreements among health care professionals have not generated cases on documentation issues, but have resulted in cases involving employment issues. *See* Kirk v. Mercy Hosp. Tri-County, 851 S.W.2d 617 (Mo. Ct. App. 1993), in which the court ruled that a hospital wrongfully discharged a nurse for complaining to other hospital employees about the level of care given by a physician to a hospital patient.

typically recognizes that patient health care record information must be maintained in a confidential manner, and that access to it or disclosure of it is quite restricted, most states also have statutes carving out exceptions that permit access without a patient's permission; such exceptions usually permit health care providers the opportunity to review and use patient information for public health reasons,[61] or for purposes of research,[62] or for peer review and quality improvement activities.[63] State law and regulations also contain numerous exceptions, such as mandatory reporting laws, that allow the disclosure of confidential information with or without patient consent. (For a more detailed discussion of exceptions relating to both access and confidentiality, see Chapters 6 and 7.)

Notwithstanding these exceptions, the general principle is that patient records are to be generated and used in a manner that encourages the maintenance of confidentiality, and this principle applies to all health care institutions, including MCOs. Federal and state laws discussed throughout this book impose confidentiality and/or disclosure requirements for certain types of medical records, and MCOs are generally subject to these laws. In addition, several other laws obligate MCOs to maintain the confidentiality of health care record information; for example, MCOs may fall within the purview of the National Association of Insurance Commissioners Insurance Information and Privacy Protection Model Act, enacted in some form in many states,[64] which prohibits insurers from disclosing confidential information about individuals without statutorily-prescribed written authorization of the individual. Accreditation standards[65] and state utilization review statutes,[66] as well as state HMO Acts,[67] also typically contain provisions relating to the protection of confidential information and the MCO's obligation to ensure such protection.

Moreover, in managed care settings, contractual obligations often impose a duty to maintain patient information in confidence. Because contracts for managed care services are frequently a controlling source in the

---

[61]*See, e.g.*, Mo. Ann. Stat. § 191.656; N.D. Cent. Code § 23-07.5.

[62]*See, e.g.*, Neb. Rev. Stat. § 71-3402; N.M. Stat. Ann. § 14-6-1.

[63]*See, e.g.*, Haw. Rev. Stat. § 622-58.

[64] *See, e.g.*, Ariz. Rev. Stat. §§ 20-2101 through 20-2120; Cal. Ins. Code §§ 791.01 through 791.27; Conn. Gen. Stat §§ 38a-975 through 38a-998.

[65]*See* Joint Commission on Accreditation of Healthcare Organizations, 1998 Comprehensive Accreditation Standards for Health Care Networks, Standard IM.2.

[66]*See, e.g.*, Ark Code Ann. § 20-9-913; Ala. Code § 27-3A-5(a)(7).

[67]*See, e.g.*, Ga. Code Ann. § 33-21-23(a).

uses and format of managed care information, health care administrators reviewing such contracts (in consultation with legal counsel) should devote special attention to avoiding the inclusion of clauses in provider contracts that are contrary to state or federal requirements regarding confidentiality and access to health care record information. Legal counsel should be consulted whenever a managed care arrangement or provision within a managed care provider contract gives rise to any concerns regarding the negligent granting of access to unauthorized persons; this includes sharing or disseminating information to MCOs or other non–health care-related institutions (e.g., employers, utilization management and insurance companies) without patient permission and for uses other than patient care or quality research.

MCOs often have a legitimate purpose for obtaining access to patient health care records, such as monitoring discharge planning, case management, or utilization review, or the accreditation or credentialing of a physician who has applied to become a member-provider. To avoid disputes that may arise between the health care facility and the MCO requesting patient health care information,[68] health care records managers should develop policies and procedures for dealing with such requests.

One approach is to designate specific individuals to undertake the duties of (i) requesting access to information and (ii) responding to such requests. The health care facility may want to create a list of authorized users, which should include the names of MCO-designated representatives who will be informed about whom to contact at the facility regarding access to records and about the types of information they may access either with or without permission from the patient.[69]

The health care facility should also designate its own managed care coordinator or facilitator whose job is to field record access requests from managed care entities. Additionally, the health care facility should consider the benefits to be gained by establishing a managed care relations team comprising individuals, such as the coordinator responsible for records requests, who will receive special training in handling potential conflicts with managed care representatives; all members should ulti-

---

[68]For example, the frustrated managed care representative may demand access, and threaten to alert the CEO that the health care organization has technically breached its contract with the MCO by denying access to such information.

[69]A similar approach could be taken with respect to access requests involving medical staff files.

mately know the applicable laws relating to access to confidential patient information and medical staff records.

Other policies that might be developed in this area include:

- annual review of health care record information policy and procedures to make certain that it continues to comply with all applicable federal and state laws
- education for those responsible for generating and using managed care medical record information, with particular reference to how they should record information so as not to trigger needless denials of claims
- training for all staff members offered by risk manager(s) and legal counsel on issues related to the protection of patient health care information

To avoid potential liability for negligent granting of access to unauthorized persons or for unauthorized disclosure of information, both health care facilities and MCOs should have policies and procedures governing this area.

Records Sought by Parties to Adoption

For the most part, general rules on patient access to medical records do not resolve the competing policy interests that arise when one of the parties to an adoption attempts to access either the original birth records or the medical records of the biological parents. In this area, the issues are more complicated given that all 50 states have adoption laws that generally cover adoption procedures, the rights of all parties, and the process by which an adoption is accomplished. In almost all instances, court action of one form or another is involved in some aspect of the adoption process, and many state statutes provide that court records on adoption and the adoptee's original birth certificate can be placed under seal and made confidential by court order. Until the 1980s, when new adoption legislation was enacted in many states, the majority of states prohibited access to these adoption records unless a party, generally the adoptee, could demonstrate "good cause" to access the record based on medical or psychological needs. (For a discussion of court decisions in this area, see " 'Good Cause' to Obtain Adoption Record Information," below.)

Although current adoption statutes in many states still have provisions restricting inspection of adoption records except upon court order for good cause shown,[70] most states now require that the adoptive parents receive, at the time of placement for adoption, specific health-related information on the adoptee. Moreover, as discussed later in this section, many states allow individuals who are parties to an adoption (i.e., biological parents, adoptive parents, and adoptees) to access certain information via avenues other than court order, including direct requests by adult adoptees who meet specified statutory conditions, mutual consent registries, and confidential intermediary search programs.[71]

In addition to specifically authorizing the direct disclosure of nonidentifying health-related information to adult adoptees who request such information,[72] most state adoption statutes now require that certain background physical and mental health information be provided to the adoptive parents when the child is placed for adoption.[73] In some states, however, the decision as to whether to disclose information is left to the discretion of the state or private adoption agency.[74] In South Carolina, for example, the release of nonidentifying health information to adoptive parents, biological parents, or adoptees is left to the sole discretion of the chief executive officer of the adoption agency if that individual perceives that the release would serve the best interests of the persons concerned.[75] Some states have chosen to leave the decision to the judiciary, requiring a court order before information can be released.[76]

Although state adoption statutes generally provide for the sealing of original birth certificates, many states now also specify circumstances

---

[70] See, e.g., ALA. CODE § 26-10A-31(a) & (c); CAL. HEALTH & SAFETY CODE § 102705; COLO. REV. STAT. § 19-1-309.

[71] Note that, even under these newer statutes, parties to adoptions continue to challenge, on constitutional grounds, statutory provisions limiting access to information. See, e.g., Griffith v. Johnston, 899 F.2d 1427 (5th Cir. 1990), cert. denied, 498 U.S. 1040 (1991), wherein the court dismissed constitutional challenges to a Texas adoption statute in a case involving adoptive parents who contended that they could not provide necessary care and treatment for their adopted children with special needs because they were denied access to certain background information.

[72] Many of these statutes require that adoptees be 18 years of age or older to obtain such information, although some states impose no age restrictions on the adoptee's right of access. See, e.g., CONN. GEN. STAT. § 45a-746(c) (adult); 750 ILL. COMP. STAT. ANN. 50/18.4(c) (18 or older); N.D. CENT. CODE § 14-15-16 (adult); OR. REV. STAT. § 109.342(4) (age of majority); WIS. STAT. § 48.432(3)(a)(1) (18 or older). But see NEB. REV. STAT. § 43-146.02 (no age provision) and VT. STAT. ANN. tit. 15, § 461(a) (no age restriction).

[73] See, e.g., ALA. CODE § 26-10A-31; COLO. REV. STAT. § 19-5-207; CONN. GEN. STAT. § 45a-746; GA. CODE ANN. § 19-8-23; HAW. REV. STAT. § 578-14.5; 750 ILL. COMP. STAT. ANN. 50/18.4(c).

[74] See, e.g., DEL. CODE ANN. tit. 13, § 924; N.M. STAT. ANN. § 32A-5-40.

[75] S.C. CODE ANN. § 20-7-1780(D).

[76] See, e.g., D.C. CODE ANN. § 16-311; TENN. CODE ANN. § 36-1-138.

when the adopted person, or a designated representative for the adopted person, may be allowed access to birth certificate information, as well as other identifying information regarding the biological parents.[77] In addition, many states have amended their adoption statutes to establish mutual consent voluntary registries, which allow biological parents and adopted individuals to register to indicate their willingness to have their identity and whereabouts disclosed to each other under specified circumstances.[78]

Some adoption statutes also provide for obtaining background information by enlisting the services of a "confidential intermediary" who is authorized to contact one or both of the adoptee's biological parents and request information sought by the adoptee.[79] It is worth noting, however, that under some of these statutes, authorized confidential intermediaries are allowed access only to court records, not medical records; under Colorado's "confidential intermediary" provision, for example, if a health care provider receives a request from a confidential intermediary for medical records, the intermediary must provide a specific court order, signed by a judge, authorizing access to the medical records.[80]

"Good Cause" to Obtain Adoption Record Information

Courts have intervened on numerous occasions to determine whether "good cause" for the release of adoption records exists based on the medical need for such information. A medical necessity generally satisfies the "good cause" requirement of many statutes. In one case involving a female adoptee who was considering having children, a New York appeals court authorized the adoptee's access to any medical reports or nonidentifying related matter in the court records of her adoption, reasoning that "good cause" is demonstrated by concern about genetic or hereditary factors that might impact upon the decision to have children.[81] However, courts also have held that to satisfy the "good cause" requirement, the

---

[77]*See, e.g.,* OKLA. STAT. tit. 10, § 7505-6.6 (allowing adult adoptees to obtain, upon request to state registry, an uncertified copy of the original birth certificate, provided certain conditions are met).

[78]*See, e.g.,* 750 ILL. COMP. STAT. ANN. § 50/18.1; OKLA. STAT. tit.10, § 7508-1.2.

[79]*See, e.g.,* OKLA. STAT. tit.10, § 7508-1.3 (state-run confidential intermediary search program); 750 ILL. COMP. STAT. ANN. § 50/18.3a (court-appointed confidential intermediaries may contact adoptee's biological parents either to seek consent to release of identifying information or to ascertain willingness to meet or otherwise communicate information about any physical or mental condition).

[80]COLO. REV. STAT. § 19-5-304.

[81]Chattman v. Bennett, 93 N.Y.S.2d 768 (App. Div. 1977).

need to obtain information on hereditary or genetic diseases must be supported with detailed descriptions.[82]

Courts also have considered whether "good cause" for the release of adoption records exists based on the psychological need for such information, but generally have been less sympathetic to adoptees' requests for information in these cases than in those involving a request based on medical needs. In one New York case, for example, the adoptee sought both the records of her adoption and the sealed Board of Health records on her birth.[83] She asserted that because she did not know who her biological parents were, she was experiencing psychological problems that impaired her musical skills, was fearful of entering into an incestuous marriage, and was unable to establish her religious faith. The court held that the plaintiff had only demonstrated curiosity about the identity of her biological parents, and curiosity would not satisfy the good cause requirement.[84]

In recent years, some states have begun to enact legislation specifying what types of information will demonstrate "good cause" for disclosure of, or access to and inspection of, sealed adoption records. For example, a New York statute provides that certification from a state-licensed physician must address a serious physical or mental illness to show "good cause," and must give a description of the illness and a statement explaining why the records are needed to treat the illness; the certification also must identify the illness as being a substantial or significant risk to life or health.[85]

Responding to Record Requests

Health care records personnel may not frequently encounter requests from individuals seeking to inspect a medical record where the request is either primarily or incidentally premised on a desire to obtain information about the adoptee's biological parents. Parties to an adoption more often

---

[82]*See, e.g.*, Rhodes v. Laurino, 444 F. Supp. 170 (E.D.N.Y. 1978), *aff'd*, 601 F.2d 1239 (2d Cir. 1979); Golan v. Louis Wise Serv., 507 N.E.2d 275 (N.Y. 1987).

[83]In re Linda M., 409 N.Y.S.2d 638 (N.Y. Sur. Ct. 1978), *aff'd*, 442 N.Y.S.2d 963 (App. Div. 1979).

[84]*See also* In re Assalone, 512 A.2d 1383 (R.I. 1986) (curiosity to discover biological identity insufficient to establish "good cause" where adoptee's need to know did not arise from any mental or physical ailments); In re Dixon, 323 N.W.2d 549 (Mich. Ct. App. 1982) (denial of access to adoptee claiming "good cause" based on depressive illness). *But see* Mills v. Atlantic City Dep't of Vital Statistics, 372 A.2d 646 (N.J. Super. Ct. Ch. Div. 1977) (psychological need to know may establish "good cause," and thus adoptee's request for certain background information should be granted absent compelling reasons to withhold such information).

[85]N.Y. DOM. REL. LAW § 114(4).

address such requests to either the agency that handled the adoption or the court that entered the adoption order. Requests are also directed to the health care institution, however, and health care records managers should recognize that disclosure of such information must be handled carefully to assure protection of patient privacy and compliance with state law. Because of the policy conflict between laws that permit patient access to medical records and adoption laws that may require the sealing of court records to protect the privacy of the biological parents, health care organizations responding to a request for information relating to adoption may be presented with dilemmas requiring a difficult weighing of competing interests. To assist in the formulation of an appropriate response to such requests, health care records managers in consultation with legal counsel should develop policies and procedures to address disclosure of adoption information.

In developing policies and procedures in this area, health care records managers may be interested in relevant recommendations from the American Health Information Management Association (AHIMA), a national professional organization specializing in health information management issues.[86] With respect to disclosure of adoption record information, AHIMA suggests that health care records managers consider the following policies:

- Refer requests for record information from biological parents to the agency that handled the adoption; biological parents of a child placed for adoption relinquish their right to inspect their child's medical record after the adoption.
- If allowing adoptive parents to inspect the adoptee's medical records for health-related record information, implement a mechanism for ensuring that all identifying information pertaining to the biological parents has been excluded before the medical record is made available to the adoptive parents.
- Refer minor adoptees trying to trace their biological parents to the agency that handled the adoption. Although adult adoptees (i.e., age 18 or older) have the right to inspect their medical records (sans information identifying the biological parents), adopted children seeking such information do not have the same right. The health care provider

---

[86]*See,* American Health Information Management Association, "Practice Brief: Disclosure of Health Information," *Journal of American Health Information Management Association* 67, no. 9 (1996).

should inform the adopted child who is seeking medical history information that such information can only be disclosed in accordance with a court order.[87]

In addition, AHIMA suggests that, if the state operates an adoption history program such as a confidential intermediary search program, health care records personnel should always encourage requesters, particularly adopted children and biological parents, to contact that program for further assistance.

Records Indicating Child Abuse

Most states have enacted mandatory reporting laws obligating health care personnel who have reason to believe that a child has been abused to report their findings to a designated state agency. These reporting requirements specify the nature and content of the information provided to the state agency. Most state laws require that a health care organization's staff member covered by the statute who suspects child abuse notify the person in charge of the institution, who in turn makes the necessary report. Also common to many of these statutes is a grant of immunity to persons who make reports in good faith.[88] (For a more detailed discussion of child abuse reporting requirements, see Chapter 7.)

A typical child abuse statute authorizes a designated state agency to intervene for the child's protection and to assist the person committing abuse in finding appropriate counseling or treatment. As the known incidence of child abuse has increased with better reporting, the public's interest in its prevention has grown. As a result, some laws now declare that any evidence of a child's injuries may be admitted in any legal proceeding arising from the alleged abuse.[89] The public policies supporting child abuse reporting statutes are for the protection of children and the reduction of abuse through appropriate counseling.

The reporting requirements of these statutes, however, may conflict with other statutes protecting patient confidentiality. Federal and state

---

[87]An adopted child's request for such information should be given some consideration only in a situation involving emergent circumstances in relation to continued patient care (and therefore time does not allow for obtaining a court order); even then, the information disclosed should be abstracted from the record, providing only the essential medical information and excluding all identifying information regarding the biological parents.

[88]*See, e.g.,* 325 ILL. COMP. STAT. ANN. § 5/9.

[89]*See, e.g.,* 325 ILL. COMP. STAT. ANN. § 5/10.

statutes addressing disclosure of medical records information in a variety of contexts support the general rule that information in a patient's medical record may not be disclosed without the individual's consent. The evidentiary statutes of many states, for example, establish a privilege that protects statements made in the course of treatment by a physician where a physician-patient relationship exists. This privilege enables a patient (and, in some states, a physician or hospital) to object to any attempt to introduce such statements in a court proceeding.[90] Some states also have enacted statutes that prohibit or restrict disclosure of certain types of patient information in court or elsewhere. The Illinois Mental Health and Developmental Disabilities Confidentiality Act,[91] for example, prohibits the disclosure of information concerning a person undergoing treatment for mental illness or developmental disabilities (as defined by the Act) except under certain circumstances. The statute states that all records kept by a therapist or agency in the course of providing mental health or developmental disabilities services to a patient that concern the patient and the service are confidential and may not be disclosed, except as provided in the Act.[92]

Courts have long struggled with the conflicting public policies that underlie state mandatory child abuse reporting statutes and state and federal statutes prohibiting disclosure of certain medical records.[93] A typical dilemma might involve a situation where a patient discloses information in the course of treatment for mental illness or alcoholism that suggests or confirms that he or she abused a child. In response to this type of problem, state legislatures have incorporated waivers of the physician-patient privilege into child abuse statutes[94], and the courts increasingly favor disclosure in cases involving possible child abuse; the extent of disclosure remains ambiguous, however, in many jurisdictions.

The Supreme Court of Minnesota addressed this apparent conflict in a case involving a man charged with three counts of criminal sexual conduct involving his 10-year-old stepdaughter and his 11-year-old niece.[95]

---

[90]*See, e.g.*, 735 ILL. COMP. STAT. ANN. § 5/8-802; N.J. STAT. § 2A:84A-22.2.

[91]740 ILL. COMP. STAT. ANN. 110/1-110/17.

[92]740 ILL. COMP. STAT. ANN. 110/3.

[93]For a discussion of the requirements for a court order for disclosure in child abuse cases, *see* J. Tomes, *Healthcare Records: A Practical Legal Guide* (Westchester, Ill: Healthcare Financial Management Association, 1990), 203–218.

[94]*See, e.g.*, CAL. PEN. CODE § 1117(b); N.C. GEN. STAT. § 8-53.1; S.D. CODIFIED LAWS§26-8A-15.

[95]State v. Andring, 342 N.W.2d 128 (Minn. 1984).

State authorities had learned of the abuse from sources other than the defendant's medical records. After his release on bail, while undergoing treatment for depression and alcoholism at a crisis unit the defendant described his sexual contact with young girls. When state authorities sought to discover his medical records and statements made to the crisis unit, the defendant argued that such information was protected from disclosure under the federal Comprehensive Alcohol Abuse and Alcoholism Prevention, Treatment, and Rehabilitation Act, as well as the state's physician-patient privilege.

The court held that the federal alcoholism treatment act and regulations do not preempt the state's child abuse reporting law. Based on its review of the legislative history of both the state child abuse reporting law and the federal alcoholism treatment statute and regulations, the court concluded that Congress did not intend for state child abuse reporting laws to be preempted by the federal law. The Court ruled that the use of patient records in child abuse proceedings to the extent required by the state child abuse reporting statute is not precluded by the confidentiality of the patient records provision of the federal alcohol treatment statute. Emphasizing that the public policy underlying the child abuse reporting statute is to encourage child abusers to seek treatment voluntarily, the court also concluded that the child abuse reporting statute abrogates the physician-patient privilege, but only to the extent of permitting the use of information required to be contained in a maltreatment report.[96]

Other courts have held that the statutory waiver of the physician-patient privilege extends to criminal proceedings involving the prosecution of the child abuser. For example, a father who was accused of raping his two children attempted to exclude conversations that he had had with a nurse while seeking treatment for the symptoms of a sexually transmitted disease.[97] During the consultation, the patient had admitted to having had sex with both his son and daughter. The court declared that in accordance with child abuse reporting legislation, the physician-patient privilege did not apply to exclude the conversation from evidence. In adopting the

---

[96]Such information includes the identity of the child; the identity of the parent, guardian, or other person responsible for the child's care; the nature and extent of the child's injuries; and the name and address of the reporter.

[97]State v. Etheridge, 352 S.E.2d 673 (N.C. 1987). *See also* State v. Bellard, 533 So. 2d 961 (La. 1988) (waiver of physician-patient privilege in state's child abuse reporting statute applies to criminal proceedings against child abuser).

statute, the legislature balanced the need for confidential medical treatment against the need to protect child victims, and opted to provide the broadest possible exceptions to the physician-patient privilege, the court concluded.

Because of the importance of the public policy issues in child abuse reporting legislation, courts generally are reluctant to exclude medical record evidence on the basis of physician-patient privilege. Statutory waivers of the privilege, which frequently apply to any proceedings involving the abuse of a child, have been interpreted broadly. The cases indicate that states will be permitted to pierce the shield provided by both the federal alcoholism treatment act and state physician-patient privilege, at least to the extent necessary to protect the children involved.

Records Sought By Law Enforcement Agencies

As a general rule, health care organizations should not release medical records or other patient information to law enforcement personnel without the patient's authorization. In the absence of statutory authority or legal process, a police agency has no authority to examine a medical record. If, however, a law enforcement official provides the facility with a valid court order or subpoena (as discussed later), the health care organization, upon the advice of its attorney, should provide the information requested. Also on the advice of its counsel, health care administrators may determine that it would be in the community's best interest to release specific medical record information to law enforcement personnel; in such a situation, the administrator may rely on the doctrine of qualified privilege in releasing such information. Under this common law doctrine, a party (the health care organization) with a duty or a legitimate interest in conveying the information is permitted to engage in communication to a second party (the law enforcement agency) with a corresponding interest in receiving the particular information. The data transfer must be made in good faith and without malice, and based on reasonable grounds. [98] (For a more detailed

---

[98]*See* Tarasoff v. Regents of the Univ. of Cal., 551 P.2d 334 (Cal. 1976) where the court held that psychotherapists had an affirmative duty to report a patient to law enforcement agencies because the patient's medical or psychological condition represented a foreseeable risk to third persons. The therapists in this situation should have disclosed information that the patient had threatened to kill the eventual victim since the therapists are protected by the doctrine of qualified privilege. *See also* Hicks v. United States, 357 F. Supp. 434 (D.D.C. 1973), *aff'd*, 511 F.2d 407 (D.C. Cir. 1975).

discussion of this and other principles of the law of defamation, see Chapter 11.)

The doctrine of qualified privilege, however, only protects the health care organization if the law enforcement officer who receives the medical record information acts under the authority of law. Thus, before releasing information, health care records managers should determine that there is a basis for the request and that the officer requesting it is performing official duties. The information released should be limited to what is appropriate for the particular request; in other words, a patient's entire medical record should not be released unless there are reasonable grounds for doing so.

In addition to the doctrine of qualified privilege and cases involving court subpoenas (discussed later), there are statutory exceptions to the general rule requiring health care organizations to refrain from releasing patient information to law enforcement agencies in the absence of patient consent. State law varies widely regarding the release to government agencies of medical record information without patient authorization. Some state statutes allow certain patient records, such as those involving victims of crime or carriers of contagious disease not specifically designated by statute, to be revealed to government officials without the patient's consent in the course of routine police investigations or public health inquiries.[99] Moreover, many states have statutes imposing a duty upon physicians and/or health care organizations to report certain kinds of information, such as cases involving gunshot or knife wounds,[100] child abuse (see discussion earlier in this chapter), and disorders affecting a motorist's ability to drive safely.[101] In states having these types of reporting statutes, a patient's consent is not required in order to release the record. In fact, under some statutes health care facilities may be guilty of criminal misdemeanor if they fail to report certain cases. (For a more detailed discussion of such statutory reporting requirements, see Chapter 7.)

---

[99]*See, e.g.*, S.C. CODE ANN. § 44-22-100(A)(4) (allowing disclosure of medical record information without a patient's consent only in specified circumstances, including when disclosure is necessary in cooperating with law enforcement, health, welfare, and other agencies, or when furthering the welfare of the patient or the patient's family).

[100]*See, e.g.*, N.Y. PENAL LAW § 265.25. *See also* CAL. PENAL CODE § 11160.

[101]*See, e.g.*, 75 PA. CONS. STAT. § 1518(B). *See also* GA. CODE. ANN. §40-5-35(b) (physician *may* report).

Warrants And Searches

As discussed in the previous section, health care organizations have a strong interest in the privacy of their medical records, and as a general rule they may refuse to release records to law enforcement agencies that do not possess a valid subpoena or other court order for such records. This same rule applies to records sought by government officials, with one exception: government officials may be entitled to search and seize medical records if they first obtain a judicially issued search warrant. Because a search warrant requires the approval of a neutral magistrate and must state specifically the place to be searched, the objects to be seized, and the reason for the search, it effectively precludes general "fishing expeditions" by the government. In recent years, federal and state government officials conducting fraud and abuse investigations more frequently have arrived at a health care facility's door with a search warrant in hand, and subsequently seized a substantial portion of that facility's patient records and other documents. (For a more detailed discussion of such situations, see "Fraud and Abuse Investigations" later in this chapter.)

The Fourth Amendment to the United States Constitution is the source of the search warrant requirement, to protect persons and their houses, papers, and effects from unreasonable searches and seizures. The amendment is designed "to safeguard the privacy and security of individuals against arbitrary invasions by governmental officials."[102] Although the amendment was intended to apply primarily to private residences, its proscription of warrantless searches as presumptively unreasonable applies to commercial premises as well.[103] Generally, therefore, government access to medical records without a search warrant is presumptively unreasonable and violates the Fourth Amendment. Nevertheless, in some instances courts may determine that government officials are entitled to gain access to medical records even in the absence of a search warrant.

Although the search warrant requirement has been associated almost exclusively with criminal investigations, the U.S. Supreme Court has stated specifically that administrative or regulatory searches also come within the Fourth Amendment's scope.[104] Whether a court will impose a warrant requirement on an administrative search, however, depends on whether the search is designed to enforce a general regulatory scheme or

---

[102]Camara v. Municipal Court, 387 U.S. 523 (1967).

[103]*See* Marshall v. Barlow's, Inc., 436 U.S. 307 (1978).

[104]*See, e.g.,* See v. City of Seattle, 387 U.S. 541 (1967).

is aimed at specific licensed industries. The Supreme Court has imposed a warrant requirement when an administrative search is conducted pursuant to general regulatory legislation that applies to all residences, structures, or employers within a given jurisdiction. For example, the Court has required a warrant in situations involving routine commercial inspections of business premises not open to the public under the Occupational Safety and Health Act of 1970.[105]

The Supreme Court has treated searches of specific licensed industries differently, however, ruling that a warrant may not be required for searches of businesses that either are federally licensed or have a long history of supervision and pervasive regulation.[106] Lower federal and state courts also have recognized these two basic types of administrative searches (i.e., searches pursuant to general regulatory schemes and searches pursuant to specific licensed industries), and have analyzed situations involving government access to health care facilities generally and medical records specifically. After making the inquiry into the thoroughness of regulation and determining that the medical facility is not a pervasively regulated business, courts typically have decided whether a warrantless search is reasonable by balancing the privacy interests of the institution against the government interest in obtaining the desired information.

Only in certain narrowly defined situations, however, have courts authorized warrantless searches of health care facilities. In one case involving a skilled nursing facility, for example, a California appeals court upheld a warrantless inspection of business records.[107] A county health inspector routinely inspected the facility's records, without a search warrant, and discovered that the defendant, a licensee of the facility, had commingled patients' funds with his own. The court rejected the defendant's challenge to the warrantless search on the grounds that the health care industry in California had been pervasively regulated and that the state's interest in regulating the industry outweighed the facility's privacy interest. Similarly, a New York court upheld a state statute that authorized thorough warrantless inspections of hospitals, home health agencies, and nursing homes.[108] Because of the overriding interest of the state in protecting

---

[105]Marshall v. Barlow's, Inc., 436 U.S. 307 (1978).

[106]*See, e.g.*, United States v. Biswell, 406 U.S. 311 (1972).

[107]People v. Firstenberg, 155 Cal. Rptr. 80 (Ct. App. 1979), *cert. denied*, 444 U.S. 1012 (1980).

[108]Uzzilia v. Commissioner of Health, 367 N.Y.S.2d 795 (1975).

nursing home residents, and because of the thorough regulation of nursing homes in New York, the court concluded that such warrantless searches did not violate the Fourth Amendment.

Because hospital patients may be considered a less vulnerable population than nursing home residents, however, the cases described previously are not particularly strong precedent for challenging a warrantless search of medical records at hospitals. Moreover, hospital administrators involved in such a challenge may encounter difficulties in attempting to assert that the government has no interest whatsoever in medical records. Instead, hospitals may more effectively rely upon assertions that the government's interest is sufficiently protected by limits established by the warrant-obtaining procedure. Also, because the court's determination regarding the necessity of a warrant may rely on its assessment as to whether the burden of getting the warrant will negate the purpose of making the search, hospitals should consider emphasizing that there are no exigent circumstances that necessitate a warrantless inspection and that requiring the government to obtain a warrant will not in any way diminish the subsequent inspection of medical records.

Courts also have authorized warrantless searches of pharmacy records. In one case involving the warrantless search of pharmacy records by state health inspectors, the New York court noted that the search was pursuant to statute and upheld the search.[109] Refusing to impose a warrant requirement even though health inspectors had time and opportunity to procure a warrant, the court concluded that pharmacy records in New York are subject to inspection without warning because the pharmacist accepts a state license subject to the right of warrantless inspection, thereby consenting to warrantless searches.

Another category of medical facility for which courts have addressed the validity of warrantless searches comprises health care organizations or clinics that perform abortions. A number of federal courts have invalidated statutes allowing warrantless searches of such facilities, typically rejecting the contention that the performance of abortions is a pervasively regulated business.[110] Emphasizing the recognized need to privacy in the physician-patient relationship, such courts have determined that the pri-

---

[109]People v. Curco Drugs, Inc., 350 N.Y.S.2d 74 (Crim. Ct. 1973). *See also* Vermont v. Welch, 624 A.2d 1105 (Vt. 1992).

[110]*See, e.g.,* Akron Ctr. for Reproductive Health Inc. v. City of Akron, 479 F. Supp. 1172 (N.D. Ohio 1979); Margaret S. v. Edwards, 488 F. Supp. 181 (E.D. La. 1980); Marcowitz v. Dep't of Public Health, 435 N.E.2d, 1291 (Ill. App. Ct. 1982).

vacy interest in these cases far outweighs the minimal state interests in sanitary conditions and properly trained personnel.

From the cases discussed above, health care records personnel can take away some practical tips for responding to situations involving a request to review medical records pursuant to a search warrant. The health care records manager presented with a search warrant should carefully review the warrant to determine whether it states with requisite particularity the scope and place to be searched. A court cannot properly issue a warrant based on a government assertion of valid public interest; rather, the government must state specifically why it requires a search of specific medical records. If health care managers and other staff members responsible for keeping and maintaining medical records believe that a search warrant is insufficient in this respect, then they may want to consider affirmatively withholding consent to the search; it is important that these individuals understand that consent to an administrative search can be implied easily, and thus an affirmative statement may be necessary. However, health care records managers and other relevant personnel also should understand the mandatory nature of a valid search warrant, and the necessity of obeying a warrant that states in detail the time and place of the search and the specific records to be searched.

Responding to Subpoenas and Court Orders

Health care organizations may be required to release medical record information pursuant to "legal process," which generally refer to all of the writs that are issued by a court during a legal action, or by an attorney in the name of the court but without court review. In general, health care records managers should have some knowledge regarding how to deal with situations involving two types of legal process—the subpoena and the court order.

Subpoenas

Health care organizations customarily receive two types of subpoenas: (1) a subpoena *ad testificandum,* which is a written order commanding a person to appear and to give testimony at a trial or other judicial or investigative proceeding, and (2) a subpoena *duces tecum,* which is a written order commanding a person to appear, give testimony, and bring all documents, papers, books, and records described in the subpoena. These orders are used to obtain documents during pretrial discovery and to obtain testimony during trial. The form of the subpoena is prescribed by statute in certain states,[111] but generally a valid subpoena provides specifics such as the name of the court; the names of the plaintiff(s) and the defendant(s); the case docket number; the date, time, and place of the re-quested appearance; the specific documents sought (for a subpoena *duces tecum*); the name of the attorney who caused the subpoena to be issued; and the signature or stamp of the official authorized to issue the subpoena.

Those authorized to issue subpoenas vary from state to state, but in most states such persons include judges, clerks of court, justices of the peace, and other officials.[112] Many state statutes provide that any compe-tent person not less than 18 years of age may serve subpoenas,[113] but often subpoenas are served in person by local sheriffs (for state courts) or United States marshals (for federal courts). The manner of service varies from state to state; in some states the subpoena may be served by regis-tered or certified mail or delivery to counsel of record, while in others the subpoena must be physically handed to the subpoenaed person by the server. Usually, subpoenas must be served within a specified period of time in advance of the required appearance.[114]

Several cases have addressed the legitimacy of disclosing certain med-ical records in response to a grand jury subpoena. The state supreme court in Illinois, for example, has ruled that disclosure to a grand jury of the identities of abortion clinic patients does not violate the physician-patient privilege or the patients' constitutional right of privacy.[115] Similarly, a grand jury may gain access to information that psychiatric patients have consented to release from their medical records to insurers for reimburse-ment purposes, a federal circuit court has ruled, because such consent constitutes a waiver of any physician or psychotherapist privilege that

---

[111]*See, e.g.,* KAN. STAT. ANN. § 60-245a (c).

[112]In cases brought before federal courts, however, only clerks of the court have the authority to is-sue subpoenas. *See, e.g.,* FED. R. CIV. P. 45(a)(3).

[113]*See, e.g.,* GA. CODE ANN. § 24-10-23.

[114]In several states, statutes establish the advance-notice period with specific reference to medical records. In Connecticut, for example, subpoenas for hospital records must be served 24 hours in ad-vance of the time that they are to be produced, unless written notice of the intent to serve the subpoena has been delivered at least 24 hours in advance of the time for production to the person in charge of hospital records. CONN. GEN. STAT. § 4-104; *see also* N.Y. C.P.L.R. 2306.

[115]People v. Florendo, 447 N.E.2d 282 (Ill. 1983); *but see* People v. Smith, 514 N.E.2d 211 (Ill. App. Ct. 1987) (quashed subpoena *duces tecum* that sought information identifying abortion clinic's clients).

may exist, given the patients' expectation that confidentiality of these records might be compromised as a result of the reimbursement process.[116]

Courts also have addressed the issue of the appropriate means for responding to a subpoena for medical records, and have determined that certain responses violate the privacy rights of the person(s) whose medical records are at issue. In one case involving a pharmacy that received a subpoena *duces tecum* to appear in court and produce a customer's five-year prescription drug record, for example, the Supreme Court of Rhode Island held that, by mailing the customer's records directly to the requesting attorney, the pharmacy violated the customer's right to privacy under state law.[117] Although prescription drug information may be subject to disclosure within a legal proceeding, a subpoena alone does not cause the confidential nature of the information to "evaporate," the court cautioned. Rather, privileged health care records may only be released in strict compliance with legal process, and in this case, the court explained, the pharmacy's unilateral disclosure of the records to the attorney in advance of either court authorization or the customer's consent clearly did not comply with proper judicial process.

Court Orders

Occasionally, a state or federal court, or a state commission, orders a health care organization to release medical records or other confidential patient information or to produce patient records in court. Written court orders usually are served upon health care facilities in a manner similar to that of subpoenas, but also may be issued orally in court to an attorney representing the health care organization. Provided the court order does not violate a statute or regulation, the health care organization should make every effort to comply with it, although the organization does have the option to contest a court order and present its case to the court before

---

[116]In re Pebsworth, 705 F.2d 261 (7th Cir. 1983). *See also* In re Grand Jury Subpoena, 710 F. Supp. 999 (D.N.J.), *aff'd without op.,* 879 F.2d 857 (3d Cir., 1989) (unpublished) (upholding subpoena based on determination that psychotherapist-patient relationship must give way to government's interest in investigating criminal fraud); *but see* People v. Helfrich, 570 N.E.2d 733 (Ill. App. Ct. 1991) (subpoena quashed in homicide investigation in which government sought all medical record information pertaining to male tenants at treatment center for mentally ill).

[117]Washburn v. Rite Aid Corp., 695 A.2d 495 (R.I. 1997).

any sanctions for failure to comply are imposed. Failure to comply with a final, valid court order subjects either the person ordered to act or the health care organization's corporate officers, if the organization has been ordered to act, to a contempt-of-court citation. Such corporate officers are liable if the institution declines to follow the order even if a health care administrator or other staff member is the person who decides not to follow the order.

A court order requiring the disclosure of medical records will not violate the statutory physician-patient privilege if "sufficient steps" are taken to safeguard the identity of the patient involved, a state appellate court in Arizona has ruled.[118] Although the state supreme court had ruled previously that a trial court's order requiring physicians to disclose the names, addresses, and means of contacting patients they had treated undermined the purpose and intent of the physician-patient privilege, the question remained as to whether the removal of all information in medical records that tended to identify the patients would render the records discoverable. In this case, the appeals court, noting that the state supreme court had objected only to identification of the patients, ruled that the disclosure of anonymous records is permissible.

Compliance Requirements

A health care organization should comply with valid legal process, properly served upon it, in the manner prescribed by its state's statutes. In recent years, many states have enacted statutes establishing compliance procedures with specific reference to subpoenas of medical records.[119] In states that have not enacted such statutes, the subpoena of medical records is treated like any other subpoena. Health care records managers should be aware of current developments in their own states in this rapidly changing area of the law. Failure to comply correctly with a subpoena, without reasonable justification, is punishable as contempt of court.

The time permitted for compliance with subpoenas of medical records varies from state to state. In some states, for example, statutes require the health care organization to comply by the date specified on the subpoena.[120] Other state statutes provide for a specific time period for compli-

---

[118]Ziegler v. Superior Court, 656 P.2d 1251 (Ariz. Ct. App. 1982).

[119]*See, e.g.,* CONN. GEN. STAT. § 4-104; KY. REV. STAT. ANN. § 422.305; N.Y. C.P.L.R. 2306.

[120]*See, e.g.,* N.Y. C.P.L.R. 2306(b).

ance.[121] Generally, the records must be sealed, then enclosed in an envelope, and may be opened only with the court's authorization. Most states expressly permit copies to be submitted in lieu of the original documents. A few states specify that the court may subpoena the originals if the copies are illegible or if their authenticity is in dispute.[122]

In several states, records furnished in compliance with legal process must be accompanied by an affidavit from the health care organization's records custodian to certify the records' genuineness, attesting that any copy of a record is a true copy and that the records were prepared by personnel of the health care organization, staff physicians, or persons acting under control of either.[123] In addition, these statutes provide that if the hospital possesses none, or only part, of the records described in the subpoena, the custodian must make certification to this fact in the affidavit. A subpoena may also require the custodian to attend the proceeding for which the records are requested. In most cases, the director of the medical records department is served with a subpoena because he or she is deemed to have custody of the medical records. However, very few states define the term "custodian." Some states do specify that the custodian may be any person who prepares records, such as a physician, nurse, or therapist, or anyone entrusted with the care of the records.[124]

No health care organization is expected to respond to requirements that would be considered unreasonable, and, in consultation with legal counsel, health care records managers should develop appropriate responses under such circumstances. The health care organization certainly has no obligation to respond if it receives a subpoena after the date upon which it is required by statute to be served, or if the subpoena arrives after the designated response date that appears on the document. The health care organization also may claim unreasonableness if the subpoena commands presentation of records so voluminous or old that they cannot be reproduced by the return date given, or records that are not in the organization's possession.

Turning to the health care organization's legal counsel is usually the best course of action in any matter that requires dealing with other attor-

---

[121]See, e.g., VA. CODE ANN. § 8.01-413(B).

[122]See, e.g., ALA. CODE § 12-21-6; NEV. REV. STAT. ANN. § 52.355(1).

[123]See, e.g., MISS. CODE ANN. § 41-9-109; ARK. CODE ANN. § 16-46-305; NEV. REV. STAT. ANN. § 52.325(2).

[124]See, e.g., NEV. REV. STAT. ANN. § 52.260(6)(a).

neys who have made unreasonable demands for medical records. If the subpoena was initiated by a plaintiff in an action against the health care organization, the organization should consider not complying with the subpoena, and instead demanding that the plaintiff file a motion to produce the records; in so doing, the health care organization is provided with the opportunity to argue against disclosure. If the health care records manager believes that a subpoena is invalid or improper, the health care organization should consider having its attorney file a motion to quash the subpoena.

The person designated to process subpoenas of medical records should respond in accordance with a procedure established by the health care organization and approved by its attorney. The procedure should include at least the following steps:

- Examination of the record(s) subject to subpoena to make certain that it is complete, that signatures and initials are legible, and that each page identifies the patient and the patient's identification number.
- Examination of the record to determine whether the case forms the basis for a possible negligence action against the health care organization and, if so, to notify the appropriate administrators, legal counsel, or risk managers.
- Removal of any material that may not properly be obtained in the jurisdiction by subpoena, such as, in some cases, notes referring to psychiatric care, copies of records from other facilities, or correspondence.
- Enumeration of each page of the medical record, and marking of the total number of pages on the record jacket.
- Preparation of a list of the medical record contents to be used as a receipt for the record if the record must be left with the court or an attorney. (Most medical records departments use a standard form for this purpose.)
- Use of a photocopy of the record, whenever possible, rather than the original in responding to legal process.

With respect to the last step listed, if the original medical record(s) must be sent, a health care organization should have an established procedure for such deliveries to the court, including the designation of a person to deliver originals in person. Health care records managers should recognize that they lose all control over medical records that are placed in the mail, and that if original records are subsequently lost through the mail or otherwise, this may present a serious problem in the event of a negligence action brought against the health care organization.

Fraud and Abuse Investigations

Aggressive enforcement of health care fraud and abuse prohibitions on the part of the Department of Health and Human Services (HHS) through its Office of the Inspector General (OIG) have expanded the likelihood that health care facilities will one day confront this type of investigation. It is not uncommon for a health care facility to learn that it is the object of an OIG investigation when federal agents arrive at its place of business, brandishing search and seizure warrants and taking possession of a significant portion of the facility's internal documentation, including all active and inactive patient files. It is important for health information managers to understand the nature and scope of this type of government investigation, given the implications such an investigation can have for medical record integrity and confidentiality.[125]

Every federal agency has an Inspector General who is responsible for ferreting out waste, fraud, and abuse in that agency's programs. Although the Inspector General's offices in several other agencies are involved in health care fraud and abuse investigations, the Office of the Inspector General of the Department of Health and Human Services is the most significant player in this area because it oversees the largest federal government insurance programs. To exercise its authority, the HHS OIG has the right to subpoena documents[126] with respect to both civil and criminal investigations. The OIG subpoena represents one of the primary methods used by investigators and prosecutors to obtain information in health care fraud and abuse cases. These subpoenas may be used in OIG audits, evaluations, or investigations, and may be served on parties that have no immediate connection with the entity under investigation.[127]

---

[125]Note that fraud investigations (and search and seizure of patient records) may also be initiated by state government officials who are acting pursuant to state law, and have valid search warrants. *See, e.g.*, Brillantes v. Superior Ct. of Los Angeles County, 58 Cal.Rptr. 2d 770 (Ct. App. 1996) (patient records seized as part of a Medi-Cal fraud investigation).

[126]5 U.S.C. § 6(a)(4).

[127]*See* United States v. Art-Metal U.S.A., 484 F. Supp. 884 (D.N.J. 1980).

In addition to its subpoena authority, the OIG has "immediate access authority," which derives from its right to impose a permissive exclusion from the Medicare/Medicaid program against an individual or entity that fails to give the OIG immediate access to review any documents and data necessary to the performance of its statutory duties.[128] Regulations that implement this authority provide that the government must submit a reasonable request for the documents, signed by the OIG, to the provider.[129] The request must include:

- a statement of authority for the request
- the entity's or individual's rights
- the definitions of "reasonable request" and "immediate access"
- the penalties that would be imposed for failure to comply.

The request also must include information suggesting that the entity or individual has violated statutory or regulatory requirements under specific statutes relating to health care fraud.

A provider fails to grant immediate access if it does not produce or make available for inspection and copying all requested records within 24 hours of the request. If the government reasonably believes that the requested documents are at imminent risk of being altered or destroyed, it is not required to give the provider the 24-hour period prior to granting access. In addition, according to the preamble in the regulations, a provider does not have the right to learn about the nature of the allegations from the agents who arrive on site to conduct an immediate access investigation.

As a condition of their participation in the Medicare and Medicaid programs, all health care providers are required to provide to the government the records used in determining appropriate reimbursement,[130] and this requirement encompasses investigations conducted by the OIG within the scope of its fraud and abuse enforcement authority. A Medicare or Medicaid beneficiary essentially waives any state-established physician-patient privilege regarding his or her medical records. If the Medicare or Medicaid program requests the medical records relating to one of its beneficiaries, then those records must be turned over to the program.

---

[128]42 U.S.C. § 1320a-7(b)(12).

[129]42 C.F.R. § 1001.1301.

[130]42 C.F.R. § 482.24.

It is important for health care providers to be adequately prepared to respond to an OIG investigation. To protect legitimate business interests, personnel should be trained to respond properly to subpoenas, search warrants, and unannounced visits by government agents. Appropriate strategies include retaining outside counsel, maintaining the integrity of internal documentation, reviewing and negotiating the scope of the subpoena, negotiating the response period to produce the requested documents, collecting that documentation and forwarding it to counsel for review, and finally producing the documents for the OIG.

If the government mainly requests billing and medical records, an index can be created to assist in locating the documents. However, in tracking the particular billing practices that are usually the focus of government scrutiny, it is often helpful to create a database for cataloguing the documents produced to the government. This database could include the basic information related to each document, such as the author, the recipient, and a document description. A database is helpful in cataloguing documents because each document can be coded as relating to a particular issue and being responsive to one or more of the subpoena requests. Of course, the scope and efficiency of these cataloguing efforts depend in large part on the number of documents that have been produced and the types of documents requested by the OIG.

USE OF OUTSIDE TEST REPORTS IN HOSPITAL PATIENTS' RECORDS

Numerous hospitals permit the use of test reports from outside clinical laboratories and diagnostic centers to satisfy preadmission or preoperative test requirements, and such reports are entered into hospital patients' medical records. Hospital administrators and risk managers should be aware that the hospital's policies regarding the use of outside test reports may trigger special concerns, particularly in two areas: (1) licensure and accreditation and (2) antitrust law.

Licensure and Accreditation

The Joint Commission standards require that hospitals have a system that ensures that pathology and clinical laboratory services and consultation are readily available to meet patients' needs, and that provides for the prompt performance of adequate testing, either on site or in a reference/

contract laboratory.[131] Accordingly, while the patient is under the hospital's care, all laboratory testing must be done in the hospital's laboratories or approved reference laboratories. When outside laboratories are used for testing hospital patients, the Joint Commission requires that the hospital's director of pathology and clinical laboratory services recommend reference laboratory services to the medical staff for acceptance. If the hospital does not have centralized pathology and clinical laboratory services, the medical staff must establish a mechanism to identify acceptable reference and/or contract laboratory services; such laboratories must meet applicable federal standards for clinical laboratories (the Clinical Laboratory Improvement Amendments of 1988, otherwise known as CLIA '88).[132]

Some licensing acts also impose controls on the use of outside laboratories for testing of hospital patients. In Illinois, for example, a hospital may use outside laboratories only if three conditions are met: (1) the outside laboratory is either part of a hospital licensed under the Illinois Hospital Licensing Act or approved to provide these services as a laboratory under the Illinois Clinical Laboratory Act; (2) the original report from the outside laboratory is contained in the medical record; (3) the conditions, procedures, and availability of examinations performed in the outside laboratory are in writing and available in the hospital.[133]

In formulating a policy on outside testing sources, a hospital should assess the risk and likelihood of poor quality performance by outside testing sources as well as the ease of monitoring those sources' compliance with quality assurance standards of the hospital. The policy should require that the original report from the outside facility be placed in the hospital's

---

[131]JOINT COMMISSION ON ACCREDITATION OF HEALTHCARE ORGANIZATIONS, 1997 COMPREHENSIVE ACCREDITATION MANUAL FOR HOSPITALS, Standard PE.1.9 & PE.1.9.1. Note that the accreditation standards in this area apply only to hospitals that perform limited laboratory testing (otherwise referred to as waived testing), or that refer all testing to outside laboratories. Waived testing procedures are specifically defined in the standards as those that meet requirements to be classified as waived tests under CLIA '88, 42 U.S.C. § 263a(a)-(q), and 42 C.F.R. § 493.15 (federal regulations listing waived tests); JOINT COMMISSION ON ACCREDITATION OF HEALTHCARE ORGANIZATIONS, 1997 COMPREHENSIVE ACCREDITATION MANUAL FOR HOSPITALS, Standards PE-17 & PE-45 (noting that tests are constantly evaluated for inclusion in the waived-test category, and listing tests within that category as of Sept. 1997). Hospitals that perform moderate- or high-complexity testing are subject to different Joint Commission standards. *See, e.g.,* JOINT COMMISSION ON ACCREDITATION OF HEALTHCARE ORGANIZATIONS, 1997 ACCREDITATION MANUAL FOR PATHOLOGY AND CLINICAL LABORATORY SERVICES.

[132]JOINT COMMISSION ON ACCREDITATION OF HEALTHCARE ORGANIZATIONS, 1997 ACCREDITATION MANUAL FOR HOSPITALS, Standard PE.1.9.2, PE.1.9.2.1, & PE.1.9.2.2.

[133]Ill. ADMIN. CODE tit. 77, § 250.510(b) & (c)(3).

medical records, that the name of the outside source be placed in the report, and that there be some mechanism for ensuring that the outside source meets all relevant federal regulatory,[134] state licensing, and accreditation requirements.

Under circumstances demonstrating that quality assurance should be of concern, a hospital policy may allow for the exclusion of outside test reports from medical records and for the prohibition on the use of such reports to meet preadmission or preoperative testing requirements unless the outside source is recommended by the relevant department head, approved by the medical staff, and complies with all relevant laws, regulations, and accreditation standards. However, as discussed in the next section, refusal to accept outside test reports may give rise to antitrust concerns, and thus legal counsel should be consulted when drafting a policy in this area.

Antitrust Issues

Potential antitrust problems arise when a hospital proposes to exclude all outside test reports from its medical records. Such exclusionary conduct can create substantial antitrust risk, particularly if a competitor, such as an outside laboratory or diagnostic testing facility, can demonstrate that it was injured by that conduct and that the hospital had an anticompetitive intent in implementing a restrictive policy regarding outside test reports. A competitor could assert that the hospital unlawfully monopolized or attempted to monopolize the relevant market by implementing a blanket prohibition on outside test reports with the intent to use its existing market power to create barriers to the entry of additional competitors for diagnostic service.[135] By demonstrating that its ability to enter the market was reduced due to the hospital's exclusion of outside test reports, the competitor may sufficiently demonstrate economic harm resulting from the hospital's conduct, and therefore establish a prima facie claim of antitrust violation. A competitor also could assert that the hospital's exclusionary policy constitutes an illegal tying arrangement involving a tie-in between hospital services and diagnostic testing, and that, by this arrangement, the

---

[134]*See, e.g.*, 42 C.F.R. § 482.27 (requiring hospitals that participate in the Medicare program to ensure that all laboratory services provided to their patients are performed in Medicare-approved facilities).

[135]Such conduct would constitute a violation of Section 2 of the Sherman Act, which prohibits monopolization and attempted monopolization. *See* 15 U.S.C. § 2.

hospital unlawfully foreclosed competition in the market for diagnostic testing by exercising its power in the market for hospital services.[136]

Other less restrictive alternatives such as the imposition of strict guidelines for acceptable outside testing may be appropriate and may help avoid exposure to antitrust liability or the expense of antitrust litigation. Those guidelines should be uniform for all outside facilities whose test reports are included in the medical records. For example, outside laboratories could be required to meet the standards for a particular class of licensed laboratories under applicable state licensing laws, assuming that this requirement also is met by any other laboratories whose results would be included in medical records.

CHANGE OF OWNERSHIP OR CLOSURE: DISPOSITION OF RECORDS

The rapidly changing managed care environment has prompted many mergers[137] and acquisitions[138] as health care facilities strive to streamline their operations and improve their competitive positions. In this process, health care facilities are faced with a change of ownership or, in some cases, closure (for instance, where an unacquired facility is unable to compete with larger managed care networks). The management of health information is one of many critical issues to be considered when a health care organization undergoes a change of ownership via merger or acquisition or closes its doors and withdraws from the health care market. These circumstances should be significant to any health care records manager or risk manager because the health care organization's obligation to maintain

---

[136]Such conduct would violate Section 1 of the Sherman Act, which prohibits any contracts, combinations, or other conspiracies in restraint of trade. *See* 15 U.S.C. § 1. Courts have established key elements necessary for establishing a tying claim, and if these criteria are met, the tying of two products has been condemned as a per se violation of the Sherman Act.

[137]A merger is a corporate transaction that involves one corporation being absorbed into a second corporation (the "new entity"), which takes on all of the rights and obligations of the first corporation.

[138]There are two types of acquisitions: an asset acquisition and a stock acquisition. An asset acquisition is a corporate transaction that involves one corporation acquiring part or all of the assets of another corporation, and generally the acquiring corporation takes on agreed-upon rights and obligations of the selling corporation. A stock acquisition is a corporate transaction that involves one corporation acquiring part or all of the stock of another corporation, and generally the acquiring corporation assumes only the rights and liabilities of an owner of the stock in the acquired corporation and does not directly assume any of the acquired corporation's rights or liabilities.

the safety and confidentiality of its patient records continues after a change or ownership or closure.

The procedures for handling patient records in such situations are governed primarily by state law and regulations, which vary across the country. Health care records managers also can turn to various guidelines in this area published by national professional organizations.[139] In most cases, however, the better source of information is any applicable state law that covers the disposition of records in the event of change of ownership or closure,[140] and any additional guidance offered by state hospital associations or state health information groups.[141] There are several ways for a health care organization to handle the disposition of its records, depending on whether a change of ownership or closure is involved.

Change of Ownership

Some states have statutory or regulatory guidelines regarding the management of health information in the event of change of ownership (e.g., during the process of a merger or acquisition).[142] Most require that the new entity comply with all legal, regulatory, and accreditation requirements regarding the disposition, maintenance, and retention of health care records. Statutory and regulatory provisions in this area also may require the new entity to merge the old entity's active records with its records and prepare a retention schedule that meets the needs of patients and others who legitimately require access to these records. Accordingly, health care records managers and risk managers for facilities involved in a merger

---

[139]See, e.g., H. Rhodes, "Practice Brief: Managing Health Information in Facility Mergers and Acquisitions," *Journal of Health Information Management Association* 67, no. 10 (1996); P. Wanerus, "Managing Health Information through a Merger," *Journal of American Health Information Management Association* 65, no. 4 (1994): 55; American Hospital Association Ad Hoc Committee for Hospital Closures, *Guidelines for Managing Hospital Closures* (Chicago: American Hospital Association, 1990); M.D. Brandt, "Practice Brief: Protecting Patient Information after a Closure," *Journal of American Health Information Management Association* 67, no. 8 (1996).

[140]See, e.g., CAL. CODE REGS. tit. 22, § 70751(e); ILL. ADMIN. CODE tit. 77, § 250.120(f).

[141]See, e.g., Colorado Hospital Association, *Consent Manual and Guidelines for Release of Health Information* (Colorado Hospital Association, 1996); Iowa Health Information Management Association, *Guide to Medical Records Law* (Iowa Health Management Association, 1993).

[142]See, e.g., CAL. CODE REGS. tit. 22, § 70751(e); FLA. ADMIN. CODE ANN. r. 59A-3.153; MASS. GEN. LAWS ch. 111, § 70 (hospitals, institutions for unwed mothers, and clinics); N.C. ADMIN. CODE tit. 10, r. 3H.0607(b) (nursing homes); OR. ADMIN. R. 333-505-0050(14); S.C. CODE REGS. 61-16 § 601.7(c); 25 TEX. ADMIN. CODE § 115.13 (home and community support services); WASH. ADMIN. CODE § 246-318-440(11)(d).

and/or acquisition, or otherwise undergoing a change of ownership, should check with legal counsel to verify that health information arrangements within the merger transaction satisfactorily meet all federal and state law requirements,[143] as well as accreditation standards.[144] In addition, legal counsel should be consulted whenever a merger/acquisition arrangement or other network formation gives rise to any liability concerns in relation to protecting the confidentiality of patient health care record information. (For a more detailed discussion of these concerns, see "Records Sought by Managed Care Organizations" in this chapter.)

In general, when ownership changes and the facility remains open to patients, custody of the records should be transferred to the new governing body, but the files should remain stored at the health care organization. In some states, this arrangement is required by law.[145] In California, for example, before the change in ownership occurs, both parties must submit written documentation informing the Department of Health Services that the newly licensed facility will take custody of the prior licensed facility's patient records, or that some other arrangement has been made whereby the records remain available to both parties and other authorized persons.[146] Similarly, Washington requires that patient records, registers, indices, and analyses of hospital services be kept in the hospital building and maintained by the new owner in accordance with the law.[147]

After licensure, regulatory, and accreditation requirements have been evaluated, the newly formed health care organization must address the many operational issues that are involved with health information man-

---

[143]Aside from state licensing requirements, for example, many health care facilities will need to ensure compliance with the Medicare Conditions of Participation and Interpretive Guidelines, which provide that a medical record must be maintained for each inpatient and outpatient, and that records may be combined into a single unit record, or maintained in two different systems as long as an adequate cross-referencing mechanism is in place.

[144]*See, e.g.*, JOINT COMMISSION ON ACCREDITATION OF HEALTHCARE ORGANIZATIONS, 1997 ACCREDITATION MANUAL FOR HOSPITALS, Standard IM.7.9, which requires that health care organizations use a patient information system to quickly assemble all relevant information from components of a patient's record when a patient is admitted to a hospital or is seen for ambulatory or emergency care. The Joint Commission also requires notification from a health care facility if a change of ownership occurs before a facility's scheduled Joint Commission survey and this change has resulted in inaccuracies in the facility's previously submitted application form. *See, e.g.*, JOINT COMMISSION ON ACCREDITATION OF HEALTHCARE ORGANIZATIONS, 1997 COMPREHENSIVE ACCREDITATION MANUAL FOR HOSPITALS, AC-23.

[145]*See, e.g.*, OR. ADMIN. R. 333-505-0050(14); S.C. CODE REGS. 61-16 § 601.7(c).

[146]CAL. CODE REGS. tit. 22, § 70751(e).

[147]WASH. ADMIN. CODE § 246-318-440(11)(d).

agement in the context of mergers and acquisitions. In this respect, a critical consideration in any merger or acquisition is integration of the merging entities' information systems. The new health care organization will need to inventory existing information systems and technology, and then develop plans to consolidate these systems. According to AHIMA, significant savings may be realized through consolidating software licenses and maintenance contracts; however, careful advance planning and consultations with legal counsel are necessary to ensure compliance with the terms of such licensure agreements.[148]

If the consolidation of information systems results in the discontinuation of one or more existing systems, AHIMA recommends that health care records managers consult with legal counsel to obtain more information about precautions that should be taken under these circumstances, such as:

- Ensuring that all final data, including diagnostic and procedures codes and billing information, has been entered, and that all work, such as transcription of dictated reports, has been completed.
- Facilitating ongoing access to old files by saving and reformatting them for compatibility with any new system(s) and, with any such data transfer, implementing appropriate audit trails.
- Assessing the need for retaining and accessing existing databases, especially abstract databases.
- Assessing the need for archiving data in its original form or for retaining reports or records in hard copy, microfilm, or other media for future use.[149]

AHIMA makes a number of other recommendations in its practice brief on health information management in the context of merger and acquisitions. Some important objectives for health care personnel responsible for handling health information needs during a change-of-ownership process, or for facilitating the integration of health information during a post-merger or acquisition transition, include:

---

[148]*See* H. Rhodes, "Practice Brief: Managing Health Information in Facility Mergers and Acquisitions," *Journal of Health Information Management Association* 67, no. 10 (1996).

[149] *See* H. Rhodes, "Practice Brief: Managing Health Information in Facility Mergers and Acquisitions," *Journal of Health Information Management Association* 67, no. 10 (1996).

- Developing and implementing a records retention policy to meet the needs of patients and other legitimate users, and to ensure compliance with legal, regulatory, and accreditation requirements. This is particularly important with respect to merger and acquisitions resulting in the closure of health facilities.
- Assessing the compatibility and functionality of existing information systems, and formulating a plan that, to the greatest extent possible, allows for the integration of these systems.
- Ensuring the maintenance of existing databases in an accessible form if there is any anticipated need for that data in the future.
- Employing or contracting with health information management professionals to evaluate the options and implement plans for integrating information systems, as needed.

Closure

When a health care facility closes or a medical practice dissolves, there is a continuing obligation to maintain the confidentiality of patients' health care information and to assure that such information is available if it is needed in the future. Health care records managers should work closely with the state licensing agency when arranging for the preservation of medical records upon change in ownership or closure. Although some states do not have specific laws governing the disposition of records under these circumstances, the state licensing agency is likely to provide guidance for handling records in a manner that preserves confidentiality and ensures the availability of the records for access by patients.

In developing procedures for the disposition of patient records upon closure of the health care facility, health care records mangers must consider a number of statutory and regulatory requirements, including state licensing and record retention laws, as well as Medicare requirements and, if applicable, federal laws governing records of patients undergoing treatment for alcohol and drug abuse. Many states require approval from the state department of health or licensing authority before implementation of any plan regarding disposition of records upon closure.[150]

When a health care organization closes, the records usually must be transferred to another location. Most state laws do not specify where the

---

[150]*See, e.g.*, Wash. Admin. Code § 246-138-440(11)(e).

records should be kept; however, they require the health care organization to notify the licensing agency in writing about the arrangements made for safekeeping of the records.[151] This notification should include the location of the storage facility and the name of the person acting as custodian.[152] In some states the licensing agency will accept custody of the records after closure; in fact, at least one state requires the health care organization to index the records and deliver them to the agency for safekeeping.[153] Most states, however, encourage the closing health care organization to transfer its records to another health care facility in the area.[154] Nebraska requires the closing hospitals to transfer records to the licensed facility to which the patient is transferred; otherwise the closing hospital should dispose of all remaining records by shredding, mutilation, incineration, or other equally effective protective measure.[155] Utah regulations suggest returning the records to the attending physician if that person still is in the community.[156] Where no other facility is located nearby (for example, in remote rural areas) and no physician wants to keep the records, the files might be stored at the closest government office, a reputable commercial storage company, or a law firm.

In general, the closing health care organization must notify the licensing agency of its arrangements for recordkeeping before the closing is completed.[157] In addition, closing health care organizations should notify former patients as to how to obtain access to their records should the need arise.[158] In some states, before patients' records are transferred to an archive facility or another health care facility, patients must receive reasonable notification, if not by letter then by publishing a series of notices in the local newspaper.[159]

---

[151]See, e.g., CAL. CODE REGS. tit. 22, § 70751(d); KAN. ADMIN. REGS. 28-34-9a(d)(2); 902 KY. ADMIN. REGS. 20:016(3)(11)(3); N.J. ADMIN. CODE tit. 8, § 43G-15.1(c); N.D. ADMIN. CODE § 33-07-01.

[152]See, e.g., 25 TEXAS ADMIN. CODE § 115.21(b)(4)(k) (home and community support service agencies).

[153]See, e.g., TENN. CODE ANN. § 68-11-308.

[154]See, e.g., IND. ADMIN. CODE tit. 410, r. 15-1-9(2)(b)(2)I; MISS. CODE ANN. § 41-9-79.

[155]NEB. ADMIN. R. & REGS. tit. 175, ch. 9, § 003.04A6.

[156]UTAH ADMIN. CODE 432-100-35(6)(d).

[157]See, e.g., Ill. ADMIN. CODE tit. 77, ch. I § 250.120(k) (90 days notice); FLA. ADMIN. CODE ANN. r. 59A-3.153 (90 days notice); UTAH ADMIN. CODE 432-2-14 (30 days notice); CAL. CODE REGS. tit. 22, § 70751(d) (48 hours notice).

[158]See, e.g., Colo. Dept. of Health Standards for General Hospitals ch. IV, § 4.2.2; 28 PA. CODE § 115.24; Utah Dept. of Health Hospital Licensing Rules, Rule 7.406(D)(2).

[159]See, e.g., Utah Dept. of Health Hospital Licensing Rules, Rule 7.406(D)(2); WIS. STAT. § 146-819(2).

Contractual provisions regarding the disposition of records come into play when a health care facility closes as part of a sale of that facility to another health care organization. In this situation, patient records may be considered assets and included in the sale of the property.[160] AHIMA recommends that a sales agreement should contain a provision allowing the closing facility the right to access or obtain copies of patients' records, as needed. Another advisable provision is one that allows the facility the right to reclaim the patient records if the new owner later decides to sell to a third party.[161]

Contractual obligations will also likely arise when a facility closes without a sale. In this case, the facility must make arrangements to have patient records transferred to another health care facility or otherwise appropriately stored (for instance, archived with the state government or stored in a reputable commercial storage facility). Prior to transferring the records, a written agreement should be signed by the closing health care facility and the facility accepting transfer of the records; because the closing facility remains responsible for ensuring that records are stored safely for the required length of time, the agreement should thoroughly outline the terms and obligations of both facilities.

AHIMA advises that contractual provisions should be carefully drafted and very specific if a closing health care facility must transfer patient records to a storage firm. Among the provisions AHIMA recommends for inclusion in a written contract between the health care facility and the storage firm are the following:

- agreement to keep all information confidential and to disclose patient record information only to authorized representatives of the health care facility or upon written authorization from the patient or his or her legal representative
- prohibition against selling, sharing, discussing, assigning, transferring, or otherwise disclosing confidential information with any other individuals or business entities

---

[160]If the facility is sold to an organization other than a health care entity, patient records should not be included in the assets available for purchase, and the facility should take steps to transfer patients' records to an archive or to another appropriate health care provider. *See* M.D. Brandt, "Practice Brief: Protecting Patient Information after a Closure," *Journal of American Health Information Management Association* 67, no. 8 (1996).

[161] *See* M.D. Brandt, "Practice Brief: Protecting Patient Information after a Closure," *Journal of American Health Information Management Association* 67, no. 8 (1996).

- agreement to protect information against theft, loss, unauthorized destruction, or other unauthorized access
- return or destruction of information at the end of the agreed-upon retention period
- assurance that health care providers, patients, and other legitimate users will have access to the information, as needed[162]

Once the records of a closed health care organization are moved, they must be preserved safely for some time. In Pennsylvania, a special law requires that records be stored at least five years after a hospital discontinues its operations. After that time, a hospital wishing to destroy any remaining records may do so after notifying the public and providing opportunity for patients to claim their files.[163] In Tennessee, records may be destroyed ten years after the hospital closes.[164] Many state laws, however, do not specifically address the duration of the time period for record retention upon closure of a health care organization. Health care records managers also must be careful to ensure compliance with any applicable retention requirements under federal law; if the facility participates in the Medicare program, for example, it must retain records in their original or legally reproduced form for at least five years to comply with Medicare Conditions of Participation.[165] (For a more detailed discussion of record retention requirements, see Chapter 3.)

Health care records managers should be aware of one important consideration to be factored into any determination of how long records must be kept after a facility closes (assuming that no state law specifies the retention period): the state's malpractice statute of limitations for both adults and minors. The retention period should be at least as long as, and preferably longer than, the period of time specified by such statute-of-limitations provisions.[166] Also, according to AHIMA, the health care organiza-

---

[162]See M.D. Brandt, "Practice Brief: Protecting Patient Information after a Closure," *Journal of American Health Information Management Association* 67, no. 8 (1996).

[163]28 PA. CODE § 115.23(c).

[164]Tenn. Hospitals Rules & Regs. § 1200-8-4-03(1)(f).

[165]See 42 C.F.R. § 482.24(b)(1).

[166]AHIMA recommends a retention period longer than the state's malpractice statute of limitations because, in some cases, that statute will not begin to run until the potential plaintiff learns of the causal relationship between an injury and the care received. Moreover, the appropriate retention period for the records of patients who are minors is the period of time up to the patient's reaching the age of majority plus the period of the state's statute of limitations, unless otherwise provided by state law. M.D. Brandt, "Practice Brief: Protecting Patient Information after a Closure," *Journal of American Health Information Management Association* 67, no. 8 (1996).

tion should contact its malpractice insurance carrier regarding closure and disposition of records. Wherever the records are stored, the closing health care organization and the carrier must be provided with access after closure if a malpractice claim is later filed. (For a more detailed discussion of records retention and its importance for purposes of defending against malpractice claims, see "Developing a Record Retention Policy" in Chapter 3.)

After an established retention period has come to an end, the health care facility may consider giving original records directly to patients. AHIMA cautions, however, that original records should never be given out to patients during the required retention period, as the health care facility and other legitimate requesters may need access to these records for business reasons.

Finally, special issues related to disposition of records upon closure arise for facilities covered by the Confidentiality of Alcohol and Drug Abuse Patient Records regulations.[167] If a program covered by these federal regulations is "taken over or acquired" by another program, it must notify its patients of the change in ownership and obtain written consent to transfer custody of the records to the new owner or to another program designated by the patient; in the absence of such consent, the program must delete all patient identifying information from the records or destroy them.[168] This provision applies regardless of whether the physical site of the program changes or remains the same after the ownership change. Patients who refuse consent to transfer their records to the acquiring program or some other facility must withdraw from treatment. The original program then may edit or destroy the records pursuant to the regulations unless another legal requirement directs the facility to preserve the records for some additional period of time.[169]

Although the obligation to obtain consent from every patient may be burdensome for many facilities, the Department of Health and Human Services has determined that the burden is outweighed by the public policy to protect the confidentiality of substance abuse patients' records. When a substance abuse treatment program completely discontinues operations, it must destroy all medical records except those for any patients who consent to having their records transferred to another program, or un-

---

[167]42 C.F.R. §§ 2.1 through 2.67.

[168]42 C.F.R. § 2.19(a).

[169]42 C.F.R. § 2.19(a)(1) & (2).

less a different law requires the records to be maintained.[170] Records kept pursuant to another legal requirement must be sealed and labeled.[171] According to HHS, this other legal requirement may be a state law governing the disposition of medical records during a closure or change in ownership, or the applicable statute of limitations for malpractice claims. When the retention period expires, the federal regulations authorize destruction of the records.[172] Although the federal rules do not require the program to notify patients before destroying their records, other federal or state laws may contain such a notification requirement; thus, health care records managers uncertain of the law in this area should obtain legal counsel prior to destroying records for which the retention period has expired.

---

[170]42 C.F.R. § 2.19(a)(1) & (2).

[171]42 C.F.R. § 2.19(b)(1).

[172]42 C.F.R. § 2.19(b)(2).

9

HIV/AIDS: Mandatory Reporting and Confidentiality

Chapter Objectives

- Outline statutory/regulatory requirements for mandatory reporting of HIV/AIDS cases to state and local health departments.
- Describe restrictions contained in provisions of state HIV/AIDS statutes intended to protect the confidentiality of HIV/AIDS information.
- Discuss common exceptions specified in state HIV/AIDS statutes prohibiting the disclosure of HIV test results without the test subject's written informed consent.
- Explain the limits on disclosure of HIV/AIDS test results of the patient (in circumstances where exceptions apply), and of the health care provider.
- Describe statutory provisions allowing disclosure of HIV/AIDS information pursuant to a court order, and give examples of how courts respond to petitions for such orders.
- Describe civil and criminal liability provisions of state HIV/AIDS statutes, and compare with common law liability for unauthorized disclosure of HIV/AIDS information.
- Recommend steps to protect patient privacy and confidentiality of HIV/AIDS information.

INTRODUCTION

One of the more significant problems in medical records management is the treatment of records of patients who have acquired immune deficiency syndrome (AIDS) or are human immunodeficiency virus (HIV) positive. The complexity and variety of the laws governing these records can interfere with the ability of record managers to cope with the demands of government agencies, researchers, hospital administrators, and the patients themselves. It is important, therefore, for health care records managers to understand the laws applicable to such records and to keep abreast of legal developments as they occur.

The issues presented by records containing HIV- and AIDS-related information continue to complicate the operation of health institutions' medical record departments, particularly with respect to special confidentiality and reporting provisions. Most states impose a duty on physicians and/or health care facilities to report all cases of "contagious," "infectious," or "sexually transmitted" diseases to the department of health. The statutory or regulatory definitions of reportable diseases typically include AIDS, as all states must report AIDS cases to the federal Centers for Disease Control and Prevention (CDC). In addition to these general reporting laws, special reporting laws for AIDS and related conditions are in effect in the vast majority of states.

In conjunction with these reporting statutes, many states also have enacted special confidentiality statutes governing the disclosure of AIDS-related information in patients' medical records, which typically prohibit the attending physician and health care facility from releasing such information to persons other than the patient and the department of health. Most of these statutes, however, also list several exceptions that permit disclosure of AIDS-related information under specified circumstances to specified individuals or entities, including medical professionals, emergency assistance personnel, spouses, sexual and needle-sharing partners, epidemiologists and researchers, blood banks, medical facilities handling body parts of the deceased, funeral directors, correctional facilities, managed care and peer review organizations, employers, schools, and insurance companies (for reimbursement purposes). Courts also can order disclosure of AIDS patients' records in circumstances not addressed directly by legislation. These laws are important because they authorize the release of information in a patient's records without the individual's consent—and, in some cases, despite his or her protests.

The question of when AIDS-related information may be disclosed without consent is a particularly sensitive issue because of the strong interests involved. The patient wants to prevent any disclosure of information because of the personal nature of the disease and the stigma attached to it, and the public interest in fostering medical treatment and encouraging blood and organ donations is perhaps best served by the assurance of donor and patient confidentiality. Health care providers need to know the patient's condition in order to protect themselves from the virus while providing proper care to the patient. The government seeks access to AIDS-related information in order to conduct scientific research and monitor the spread of the disease. Finally, third parties, such as spouses, need to know whether their partners are carriers of the deadly virus. This chapter discusses the statutory and regulatory requirements in this area, with a focus on the difficult balancing of conflicting interests that often comes into play in disclosure determinations.

DUTY TO REPORT

All states have statutes and/or regulations requiring health care providers to report cases of AIDS to the state or local department of health, and a majority of states require HIV and/or ARC (AIDS-related complex) reporting as well.[1] The reporting laws and regulations vary widely as to who has the duty to report; some place the duty of reporting on the attending physician and/or the laboratory that performs a test which concludes with a positive result,[2] while others require hospitals, clinics, blood banks and plasma centers, and other facilities such as health maintenance organizations (HMOs) to report AIDS and/or HIV cases[3]; some states require reporting from a combination of all these sources.[4] Minnesota has enacted what appears to be the only state statute containing

---

[1]According to one recent survey, 41 states have statutes requiring the additional reporting of HIV infection. *See* L. Gostin, Z. Lazzarini, & K. Flaherty, Legislative Survey of State Confidentiality Laws, with Specific Emphasis on HIV and Immunization, Final Report (Presented to the U.S. Centers for Disease Control and Prevention, the Council of State and Territorial Epidemiologists, and the Task Force for Child Survival and Development—Carter Presidential Center, Georgetown University Law Center, July 1996).

[2]*See, e.g.*, ARK. CODE ANN. § 20-15-904 (physician); FLA. STAT. ANN. § 384.25(1) (physician and laboratory); KAN. STAT. ANN. § 65-6002(a) (physician and laboratory).

[3]*See, e.g.*, 410 ILL. COMP. STAT. ANN. 310/4(b); IOWA CODE § 141.8 (2)-(4).

[4]*See, e.g.*, COLO. REV. STAT. § 25-4-1402(1) & (2); MICH. STAT. ANN. § 333.5114 ("any person or governmental entity"); WIS. STAT. § 252.15(7)(b).

a self-reporting provision that requires health care workers diagnosed with HIV to report that information to the commissioner of health no more than 30 days after learning of the diagnosis or 30 days after becoming licensed or registered by the state.[5] The Minnesota law also requires health care workers who personally know of another health care worker's failure to comply with infection control procedures to report that to the appropriate licensing board or a designated hospital official within 10 days.[6]

Reporting laws governing HIV- and AIDS-related information also vary with respect to what information must be reported. Many states require the patient's name and address to be disclosed in the report, along with age, race, and sex,[7] while a few states prohibit the release of identifying information unless set criteria are met.[8] Some states have statutes that permit the test subject, upon request, to remain unknown—in other words, the patient who consents to testing has the right to anonymous testing.[9] Under these statutes, patients also may be permitted to execute an HIV test consent form in a manner that does not reveal their identity; for example, patients may choose not to execute the document by signing their names, but by using an alias or a coded number, which the health care provider must then use in identifying the test subject, the test sample, and the test results. In states with such anonymous testing programs, reported cases of AIDS and HIV-infection from anonymous testing sites usually do not include patient-identifying information.[10]

All of the laws distinguish between the forms of the disease for purposes of reporting. In many states, the identity of patients with full-blown AIDS cases is reportable while the identity of HIV-positive patients is exempt; state statutory provisions in this regard typically permit the names

---

[5]MINN. STAT. § 214.18, sub. 2.

[6]MINN. STAT. § 214.18, sub. 4.

[7]See, e.g., COLO. REV. STAT. § 25-4-14-2(4); IDAHO CODE § 39-606; MICH. COMP. LAWS § 333.5114(1); WIS. STAT. § 252.15(7)(b).

[8]See, e.g., OR. ADMIN. R. 333-018-0030(3)(a)(A)-(E) (anonymous reporting unless the HIV-infected person fits into specified categories, including persons who: have donated blood or tissue in the last year; have a criminal record involving sex offenses; are under six years of age; or request assistance in notifying partners). See also 410 ILL. COMP. STAT. ANN. 310/4 (registry of reported cases of AIDS and ARC to be identified by code rather than number).

[9]See, e.g., FLA. STAT. ANN. § 384.25(7)(a); 410 ILL. COMP. STAT. 305/6; ME. REV. STAT. ANN. tit. 5, § 19203-B. See also IND. CODE § 16-41-6-2.5 (applies to prenatal health care providers).

[10]MICH. COMP. LAWS § 333.5113(2)(b)(iii); W. VA. CODE § 16-3C-2(c).

of AIDS patients to be released while prohibiting the identification of persons who test positive only for HIV infection.[11] In Iowa, for example, the physician who orders an HIV test must report positive results to the department of health, but may not include the patient's name and address in the report without the person's written consent.[12] On the other hand, physicians must release patients' names and addresses to the health department, along with other information, when they diagnose AIDS or an AIDS-related condition or attend to patients who die from an AIDS-related condition.[13]

Mandatory disclosure laws in most states also require the attending physician and/or laboratory to submit a written report on a patient within a specified number of days after a reportable diagnosis is confirmed.[14] In Maryland, for example, the director of a medical laboratory in which serum samples are tested for HIV must submit a report within 48 hours of an HIV-positive test result, and the report must contain statistical data but no identifying information.[15] Other institutions that obtain or process semen, blood, or tissue must obtain a blood sample from all potential donors in order to test for HIV, and all positive test results must be reported to the department of health.[16]

A growing number of states require the identity of persons with either AIDS or HIV to be reported.[17] Michigan law, for example, requires all persons who obtain a positive HIV result for a test subject to report the name, address, age, race, and sex of the test subject within seven days.[18] Reports must be filed with both state and local health departments, and only licensed clinical laboratories are exempt from those requirements. However, patients who submit to HIV testing in a physician's private prac-

---

[11]*See, e.g.,* Iowa Code § 141.8(6); Kan. Stat. Ann. § 65-6002(a); Md. Code Ann., Health-Gen. § 18-205(b)(ii)(1) & (2).

[12]Iowa Code Ann. § 141.8(6). The same rules apply to directors of blood banks, plasma centers, and clinical laboratories.

[13]Iowa Code Ann. § 141.8(6).

[14]*See, e.g.,* Fla. Stat. Ann. § 384.25(1) (not to exceed 2 weeks); Iowa Code § 141.8(3) (7 days); Kan. Stat. Ann. § 65-6002(a) (1 week); Md. Code Ann., Health-Gen. § 18-205(a) (48 hours); Mich. Comp. Laws § 333.5114(1) (7 days). *See also* Cal. Health & Safety Code § 1603.1 (72 hours; applies to blood banks and plasma centers that have received tainted blood).

[15]Md. Code Ann., Health-Gen. § 18-205(a)(1) & (b)(2)(ii)(2).

[16]Md. Code Ann., Health-Gen. § 18-334(b)(2)(i).

[17]*See, e.g.,* Ala. Code § 22-11A-2; Ark. Code Ann. § 20-15-904(b); Colo. Rev. Stat. § 25-4-1402(1); Mich. Comp. Laws § 333.5114(1); Wis. Stat. § 252.15(7)(b).

[18]Mich. Comp. Laws § 333.5114(1).

tice office or the office of a physician engaged by an HMO may request their doctor not to reveal their name, address, or telephone number.[19]

In at least one state, a state supreme court has ruled that a mandatory disclosure statute that requires physicians to report the names and addresses of patients who are HIV-positive or suffer from AIDS to the state department of health is not unconstitutional.[20] An Alabama statute imposing this requirement was challenged by a physician who was willing to report certain statistical data but refused to provide the names and addresses of patients; the department of health sued to compel the physician's full compliance with the reporting statute. The physician argued that the statute violates the Equal Protection Clause because sellers of confidential HIV-testing kits and out-of-state laboratories that evaluate test results are not required to report the names and addresses of purchasers. In rejecting this argument, the court concluded that out-of-state testing labs and testing kit vendors are not similarly situated to those individuals required to report HIV and AIDS cases, and therefore ruled that the reporting requirement was constitutional. The labs do not know the identity of the persons who are being tested and the testing-kit vendors sell kits without knowing whether a particular purchaser is HIV-positive or suffers from AIDS, the court explained. The court thus affirmed a lower court decision ordering the physician to disclose identifying information as required by the statute.

PROTECTING CONFIDENTIALITY OF HIV-RELATED INFORMATION

In addition to protecting the confidentiality of medical records in general and medical records containing information about sexually transmitted diseases, many states have statutes specifically directed at protecting the confidentiality of HIV- or AIDS-related information and records. These confidentiality statutes usually provide that, except in specified circumstances, no person may disclose the identity of an HIV test subject,[21] and test results and individuals' HIV status must be kept confidential and recorded in a manner that does not reveal the test subject's identity.

---

[19]MICH. COMP. LAWS § 333.5114(3).

[20]Middlebrooks v. State Board of Health, No. 1961079 (Sup. Ct. Ala. Jan. 9, 1998).

[21]Confidentiality provisions in this area typically prohibit disclosure of the identity of a person who has undergone an HIV test regardless of the results of the test.

Many statutes also prohibit the disclosure of test results without the test subject's written informed consent.[22] Some statutes strictly limit the sharing of HIV test results to persons with a statutorily-defined "need to know," making distinctions among personnel within a single health care facility. Massachusetts prohibits disclosing HIV test results without the patient's written consent, and recognizes no exceptions.[23] Other states provide exceptions that specify when disclosure is permissible without the patient's written consent. New York, for example, prohibits the release of HIV-related information except with consent of the patient, but then specifies more than a dozen exceptions for disclosure without the patient's consent.[24] (For a more detailed discussion of disclosure exceptions, see "Statutory Provisions Regarding Disclosure," outlined next in this chapter.)

The first exception often listed in these confidentiality statutes permits access to test results to the person obviously most interested in such information: the test subject or the subject's legally authorized representative.[25] A second common exception permits disclosure of test results to any person(s) designated in a written authorization or otherwise legally effective release executed by the test subject or the subject's authorized representative.[26] (For a more detailed description, see "Disclosure to Third Parties with Patient Authorization" in this chapter.) Thus, a health care provider who orders an HIV test for a patient may inform the patient or his or her representative of the results without liability.[27] While these confidentiality statutes create special civil and criminal liability for unauthorized disclosures (e.g., where none of the exceptions apply), they are not intended to discourage health care practitioners from indicating the results of an HIV test in a patient's file.[28]

---

[22]See, e.g., FLA. STAT. ANN. § 381.004 (f)(2); 77 ILL. ADMIN. CODE. tit. 77 §697-140 (a)(2); LA. REV. STAT. ANN. § 40:1300.16; R.I. Code R. 14-040-006, §15.1.

[23]MASS. GEN. LAWS ch. 111, § 70F.

[24]N.Y. PUB. HEALTH LAW § 2782(1)(a)-(o). *See also* CAL. HEALTH & SAFETY CODE §§ 121015 & 121035 through 121070.

[25]*See, e.g.,* DEL. CODE ANN. tit. 16, §1203(a)(1); 410 ILL. COMP. STAT. ANN. 305/9(a); N.Y. PUB. HEALTH LAW § 2782(1)(a); ME. REV. STAT. ANN. tit. 5, § 19203(1).

[26]*See, e.g.,* DEL. CODE ANN. tit. 16, §1203(a)(2); 410 ILL. COMP. STAT. ANN. 305/9(b); N.Y. PUB. HEALTH LAW § 2782(1)(b); ME REV. STAT. ANN. tit. 5, § 19203(3).

[27]However, a patient may sue a health care provider for negligently advising the patient that he or she has tested HIV-positive. *See* Johnson v. United States, 735 F. Supp. 1 (D.D.C. 1990).

[28]*See, e.g.,* N.Y. PUB. HEALTH LAW § 2782(8) ("confidential HIV-related information shall be recorded in the medical record of the protected individual").

In a small office setting, such as a physician's or group practice's office, test results can be maintained in a separate confidential file, with access limited to the patient's physician. In a larger institutional setting, however, protecting confidentiality of test results is more problematic. Establishing separate confidential files may not be feasible. Recognition of this problem underlies the provisions in some state HIV confidentiality statutes that permit HIV test results to be recorded in a patient's medical record.[29] Some states elaborate further by providing that, if HIV test results are recorded in patients' medical records, this must be done in a manner that does not permit a person to learn a patient's HIV status by some means other than reading the record. Regulations promulgated under the Illinois AIDS confidentiality statute, for example, require that "[a]ny procedure utilized to maintain [AIDS-related information] in a patient's medical record must be uniform and consistent for all patient records"; a practice is considered uniform and consistent if the records containing the confidential information cannot be distinguished from other medical records, unless the record is assessed and read.[30] Accordingly, records containing AIDS-related information should not bear distinguishing labels or marking; for instance, the health care records manager should avoid placement of such information in a separate, distinctive colored document or file within the patient's medical record.

STATUTORY PROVISIONS REGARDING DISCLOSURE

Disclosure to Third Parties with Patient Authorization

Many of the HIV confidentiality laws allow the patient to authorize release of test results to third parties.[31] This provision permits a health care practitioner to release confidential information to persons who otherwise are precluded from access to the patient's records. A patient might authorize release to any insurance company, employer, or school. The practitioner should require that such release be in writing and signed by the patient or the patient's representative. A copy of the release should be attached to the patient's records.

---

[29]See, e.g., CAL. HEALTH & SAFETY CODE § 120985(a); N.Y. PUB. HEALTH LAW § 2782(8).

[30]ILL. ADMIN. CODE tit. 77, § 697.140(c)(2).

[31]See, e.g., DEL. CODE ANN. tit. 16, § 1203(a)(2); 410 ILL. COMP. STAT. ANN. 305/9(b); N.Y. PUB. HEALTH LAW § 2782(1)(b); ME REV. STAT. ANN. tit. 5, § 19203(3); VA. CODE ANN. § 32.1-36.1(2).

Disclosure to Health Care Workers

Most confidentiality laws, whether general or AIDS-specific, allow information to be released to medical personnel involved in the patient's care and without the patient's consent.[32] Under these circumstances, authorizing the disclosure of HIV- and AIDS-related information can serve several purposes. To facilitate proper medical treatment for AIDS victims, many statutes authorize release of AIDS information to the patient's medical provider, who is thereby authorized to place the results of an HIV test directly into the patient's record.[33] Physicians often are authorized to reveal information directly to other health care providers for purposes of treating the patient.[34] In addition, the laws reflect a concern for the safety of medical workers who are at risk for HIV infection during performance of their duties. Several statutes authorize the attending physician to reveal an HIV patient's identity to other health care workers who come into contact with body fluids or body parts of the patient, or who work directly with HIV patients.[35]

Some statutes permit disclosure upon finding that the health care worker has a "reasonable" or "medical" need to know the information to provide proper care. Other laws allow disclosure whenever generally relevant to the patient's treatment. Many of the laws are unclear, however, as to whether the authorized disclosures are permissive or mandatory. This question bears on the ability of a concerned worker to demand that a physician confirm the test results of a patient who the worker suspects is positive for the virus. Many statutes also are unclear as to whose interests must be analyzed for purposes of disclosure—the worker's or the patient's. For example, a "need to know" for purposes of providing patient care may refer to the worker's need to take precautions to prevent

---

[32]*See, e.g.*, CAL. CIV. CODE § 56.10 (c)(1); *see also* N.C. GEN. STAT. § 130-143(3). According to one survey, 43 states allow for some form of disclosure of HIV-related information to health care providers. *See* L. Gostin, Z. Lazzarini, & K. Flaherty, Legislative Survey of State Confidentiality Laws, with Specific Emphasis on HIV and Immunization, Final Report (Presented to the U.S. Centers for Disease Control and Prevention, the Council of State and Territorial Epidemiologists, and the Task Force for Child Survival and Development—Carter Presidential Center, Georgetown University Law Center, July 1996).

[33]*See, e.g.*, CAL. HEALTH & SAFETY CODE § 120985(a); W.VA. CODE § 16-3c-3(a)(5).

[34]*See, e.g.*, CAL. HEALTH & SAFETY CODE § 120985(a); HAW. REV. STAT. § 325-101(a)(10); IOWA CODE § 141.23(1)(d); ME. REV. STAT. ANN. tit. 5, § 19203(2); MICH. COMP. LAWS § 333.5131(5)(a)(iii); W. VA. CODE § 16-3c-3(a)(5).

[35]*See, e.g.*, CAL. HEALTH & SAFETY CODE §§ 120985(a) & 121010(b) through (e); KAN. STAT. ANN. § 65-6004(a); 410 ILL. COMP. STAT. ANN. 305/9(h).

becoming infected while rendering treatment to the patient; on the other hand, the "need to know" might relate to special treatments available only for AIDS patients.

Not every health care worker involved with the patient has a legitimate need to know that the person has been tested for HIV; only a limited class of medical practitioners have access to such information under HIV confidentiality statutes. In California, for example, the results of an HIV test may be recorded in the subject's record and otherwise revealed without the patient's consent to providers of care for purposes of "diagnosis, care, or treatment of the patient."[36] Accordingly, the results of an HIV test may be disclosed to an agent or employee of the health care provider who provides "direct patient care and treatment."[37] Similarly, Maine authorizes disclosure of HIV test results to the health care provider designated by the patient, and the patient's physician then may make results available only to other providers working directly with that person, and only for the purpose of providing direct patient care.[38] These provisions appear to be permissive, and it is unclear whether a provider of direct care could demand successfully that the physician confirm that a suspected AIDS patient had indeed tested positive for the HIV infection.

In Delaware and Iowa, HIV confidentiality statutes provide that no person may disclose the identity of any subject of an HIV test, or the results thereof, in a manner that permits identification of the test subject except, among other circumstances, to an authorized agent or employee of a health care provider if: (i) that provider is authorized to obtain the test results, (ii) the agent or employee provides patient care or handles or processes specimens of body fluids or tissues, and (iii) the agent or employee has a medical need to know such information to provide health care to the patient.[39] These statutes seem to reflect concern for the patient, rather than for the safety of health care workers, because the third prong of the test—the employee's medical need to know—must be tied into the purpose to provide health care to the patient. Thus, the medical aspect of the need to know refers to the patient's medical interests, not the employee's own health concerns.

---

[36]CAL. HEALTH & SAFETY CODE § 120985(a).

[37]CAL. HEALTH & SAFETY CODE § 121010(c).

[38]ME. REV. STAT. ANN. tit. 25, § 19203(2).

[39]DEL. CODE. ANN. tit. 16, § 1203(a)(3); IOWA CODE § 141.23(1)(c).

Illinois has adopted a similar three-part test for disclosing AIDS information to other health care providers; however, the third prong of that test requires only that the employees have a need to know the information.[40] Similarly, Missouri allows the release of HIV test results to "health care personnel working directly with the infected individual who have a reasonable need to know the results for the purpose of providing direct patient health care."[41] Again, it is unclear whether the "reasonable need to know" relates to the worker's safety or the patient's proper care. In either case, the Missouri law is fairly typical in limiting the circle of disclosure to persons directly involved with the patient. New Hampshire's HIV confidentiality statute also is concerned for the patient's treatment; the relevant provision of that statute provides that a physician or other health care provider may disclose information pertaining to the identity and test results of the person tested to other physicians and health care providers directly involved in that person's health care when the disclosure of such information is necessary to protect the health of the person tested.[42]

In contrast, Kentucky and Hawaii have HIV confidentiality statutes that allow for much greater discretion on the part of the physician. While Kentucky law authorizes the release of medical information only to the physician retained by the person infected with AIDS or another sexually transmitted disease, the statute is silent on the extent to which the physician may release such information to co-workers involved in the patient's care, except in the case of an emergency when information may be released to protect the life or health of the patient.[43] Hawaii allows disclosure of AIDS, ARC, and HIV information by the patient's health care provider to another health care provider "for the purpose of continued care of [or] treatment of the patient."[44] These broadly written provisions defer to the judgment of the physician on the question of disclosure, but allow release of the information in an emergency to the extent necessary to protect the life or health of the patient.

Other states' HIV confidentiality statutes demonstrate more concern for persons other than the patient and those that provide direct care for the patient, such as other health care professionals. In Texas, the HIV

---

[40]410 ILL. COMP. STAT. ANN. 305/9(c).

[41]MO. REV. STAT. § 191.656(2)(b).

[42]N.H. REV. STAT. ANN. § 141-F:8(IV).

[43]KY. REV. STAT. ANN. § 214.420(3)(e).

[44]HAW. REV. STAT. § 325-101(a)(10).

confidentiality statute is permissive but provides that results of an HIV test may be released to a physician, nurse, or other health care personnel who have a "legitimate" need to know the results to provide for their protection and the patient's health and welfare.[45] The New York confidentiality provision authorizes release of confidential HIV-related information only to an agent or employee of a health facility or health provider if three conditions are met: (i) the agent is permitted to access medical records, (ii) the facility is authorized to obtain HIV information, and (iii) the agent either provides health care to the protected individual or maintains medical records for billing or reimbursement.[46] The statute then provides that a provider or facility is authorized to receive HIV-related information when knowledge of such material is "necessary to provide appropriate care or treatment to the protected individual or a child of the individual."[47]

Like the New York law, Utah's statute in this area provides for disclosure to a health care provider, health care personnel, and public health personnel with a "legitimate need to have access to the information in order to assist the patient, or to protect the health of others closely associated with the patient."[48] The statute expressly notes that the above language does not create a duty to warn third parties, but is designed to assist providers in treating and containing AIDS, HIV, and other infectious diseases.[49] This provision clearly authorizes disclosure to certain medical personnel working closely with the patient, but also extends to family members, sexual partners, and needle-sharing partners.[50] (For a more detailed discussion of other state statutes addressing this subject, see "Disclosure without Consent to Spouse or Needle-Sharing Partner" in this chapter.) Many laws also permit disclosure of a patient's identity to facili-

---

[45]TEX. HEALTH & SAFETY CODE ANN. § 81.103(b)(5); *see also* IDAHO CODE § 39-610.

[46]N.Y. PUB. HEALTH LAW § 2782(1)(c).

[47]N.Y. PUB. HEALTH LAW § 2782(1)(d).

[48]UTAH CODE ANN. § 26-6-27(2)(h); *see also* IDAHO CODE § 39-610.

[49]UTAH CODE ANN. § 26-6-27(2)(h); *see also* CAL. HEALTH & SAFETY CODE § 121015(c).

[50]While the state legislation authorizes disclosure to health care workers treating the patient, it is possible that courts will impose a duty on patients to reveal whether they have AIDS. *See, e.g.,* Boulais v. Lustig, No. BC038105 (Cal. Super. Ct. 1993), (unpublished) in which a surgical technician successfully sued a patient for fraudulently concealing the fact that she had AIDS when filling out forms before undergoing surgery. After the technician was cut with a scalpel while removing sutures, the patient revealed her HIV-positive status. The technician had not been wearing gloves at the time of the exposure, and although the technician consistently tested negative for HIV post-exposure, the court awarded her damages for fraud but refused to award her damages for negligent infliction of emotional distress.

ties that procure, process, distribute, or use blood, other body fluids, body parts, tissues, or organs.[51]

The statutes discussed above govern the release of all HIV-related information. Others focus directly on disclosure of the reports submitted to the department of health. Colorado, as described above, has a mandatory AIDS and HIV reporting law applicable to health care workers,[52] which provides that reports containing HIV-related information held by a health care provider or facility, physician, clinic, blood bank, or other agency shall be strictly confidential and shall not be released, shared, or made public except as provided.[53] Louisiana has a special law requiring a hospital to notify a nursing home of an HIV patient's condition when the hospital transfers the patient to the home. A similar duty is placed upon a nursing home transferring an HIV patient to a hospital.[54]

Disclosure without Consent to Emergency Medical Personnel

Many confidentiality statutes allow the release of HIV-related information without the patient's consent to medical technicians who provide emergency care to an HIV-positive patient.[55] The statutes vary, however, in the purpose for such disclosure. Some link disclosure to the health of the patient; others indicate a concern for the safety of the emergency workers, and many reflect an ambiguous balance between the two concerns.

In some states, for example, confidential HIV-related information may be released to medical personnel in a "medical emergency" to the "extent necessary to protect the health or life of [the patient]."[56] The relevant statutory provision in Hawaii defines "medical emergency" as any disease-related situation that threatens life or limb.[57] Other states authorize disclosure to health care providers rendering medical care when knowledge of HIV test results is "necessary" to provide "appropriate emergency

---

[51]*See, e.g.*, N.Y. Pub. Health Law § 2782(1)(e); Va. Code Ann. § 32.1-36.1(A)(8); Wis. Stat. § 252.15(5)(a)(4).

[52]Colo. Rev. Stat. § 25-4-1402.

[53]Colo. Rev. Stat. § 25-4-1404(1).

[54]La. Rev. Stat. Ann. § 40:1099(B)(2); Miss. Code Ann. § 41-23-1(5).

[55]*See, e.g.*, Cal. Health & Safety Code § 121010(e); Colo. Rev. Stat. § 25-4-1404(1)(c); Del. Code Ann. tit. 16, § 1203(a)(4); Fla. Stat. ch. 384.29(1)(d); Wis. Stat. § 252.15(5)(11).

[56]*See, e.g.*, Colo. Rev. Stat. § 25-4-1404(1)(c); Fla. Stat. ch. 384.29(1)(d); Iowa Code § 141.10(1)(c); Kan. Stat. Ann. § 65-6002(c)(4); Ky. Rev. Stat. Ann. § 214.420(3)(e).

[57]Haw. Rev. Stat. § 325-101.

care or treatment" to the patient.[58] These laws demonstrate concern for the patient's treatment.

Other state statutes in this area reflect a predominant concern for the safety of rescue workers. For example, Illinois allows release of the identity of the subject of an HIV test to "[a]ny health care provider or employee of a health facility, and any firefighter or any EMT-A or EMT-I, involved in an accidental direct skin or mucous membrane contact with the blood or bodily fluids of an individual which is of a nature that may transmit HIV, as determined by a physician in his medical judgment."[59] Similarly, the Wisconsin HIV confidentiality statute permits the release of HIV-positive test results to persons who, in rendering care to the victim of an emergency or accident, are significantly exposed to the victim, provided that a physician certifies in writing that the emergency caregiver has been significantly exposed, and that this certification accompanies any request for disclosure.[60]

A few states impose an affirmative duty on an attending physician or health care facility to respond to inquiries by emergency rescuers regarding contact with a patient later diagnosed with a contagious disease or virus including HIV;[61] under such statutes, rescuers entitled to receive such information include paid or volunteer firefighters, emergency medical technicians, rescue squad personnel, and law enforcement officers. Such statutes typically require that the rescue worker be notified within 48 hours after confirmation of the patient's diagnosis, and that the information be communicated in a manner that protects the confidentiality of both the patient and rescuer. In Maryland, each medical care facility must develop and disseminate written procedures for exposure notification. A facility or provider acting in good faith under this section is not liable for failure to give notice of exposure where the rescuer does not properly initiate the process as developed.[62] Other statutes in this area are permissive; Washington law, for example, authorizes certain emergency rescuers and other health care workers who come into significant contact with the blood and/or other body fluids of another person to request that an HIV

---

[58]See, e.g., DEL. CODE ANN. tit. 16, § 1203(a)(4).

[59]410 ILL. COMP. STAT. ANN. 305/9(h).

[60]WIS. STAT. § 252.15(5)(11). See also CAL. HEALTH & SAFETY CODE § 121135 (outlining procedure for requesting disclosure of patient's HIV status in the event of significant exposure).

[61]See, e.g., LA. REV. STAT. ANN. § 18-213(e); MICH. COMP. LAWS § 333.20191(5).

[62]MD. CODE ANN., HEALTH-GEN. § 18-213(i)(1).

test be performed on that person; the requester is then entitled to know the results.[63] California outlines detailed procedures to follow under circumstances where an exposed worker requests an evaluation of the exposure by a physician, including measures to be taken in relaying information regarding HIV status to the exposed worker.[64]

Disclosure without Consent to Spouse or Needle-Sharing Partner

Many states have confidentiality statutes that provide for notification of an HIV patient's spouse, needle-sharing partner, or other "contact" at risk for the infection.[65] A small minority of states authorizes the release of HIV test results to the spouse of the test subject, but not to other sexual partners.[66] These provisions usually are permissive and do not create a duty on the part of the physician to warn all third parties.[67] Thus, a contact who develops the virus but who was not informed of risk by the partner's physician cannot bring a lawsuit against the physician under the statute. On the other hand, a physician who reveals the risk to a contact as authorized is not liable to the patient for breach of confidentiality.[68] This exception in South Carolina's disclosure law, for example, simply states that a physician or state agency identifying and notifying a spouse or known contact of a person having HIV infection or AIDS is not liable for damages resulting from the disclosure.[69]

---

[63]WASH. REV. CODE § 70.24.105(2)(h).

[64]CAL. HEALTH & SAFETY CODE § 121135.

[65]*See, e.g.*, CAL. HEALTH & SAFETY CODE § 121015 (spouse, sexual partner, or needle-sharing partner); HAW. REV. STAT. § 325-101(a)(4) (sexual or needle-sharing contact); 410 ILL. COMP. STAT. ANN. 305/9 & 325/5.5(b) (spouse and contacts); KAN. STAT. ANN. § 65-6004(b) (spouse or partner); MICH. COMP. LAWS § 333.5131(5)(b) (contacts); N.Y. PUB. HEALTH LAW § 2782(4) (contact); W. VA. CODE § 16-3C-3(d) (sex and needle-sharing partners and other contacts). One survey estimates that the HIV confidentiality statutes in 39 states contain statutory exceptions allowing disclosures to spouse, needle-sharing partners, or other contacts (*e.g.*, sexual partners). *See* L. Gostin, Z. Lazzarini, & K. Flaherty, Legislative Survey of State Confidentiality Laws, with Specific Emphasis on HIV and Immunization, Final Report (Presented to the U.S. Centers for Disease Control and Prevention, the Council of State and Territorial Epidemiologists, and the Task Force for Child Survival and Development—Carter Presidential Center, Georgetown University Law Center, July 1996).

[66]*See, e.g.*, TEX. HEALTH & SAFETY CODE ANN. § 81.103(b)(7); VA. CODE ANN. § 32.1-36.1(A)(11).

[67]*See, e.g.*, CAL. HEALTH & SAFETY CODE § 121015(c); 410 ILL. COMP. STAT. ANN. 305/9(c); KAN STAT. ANN. § 65-6004(c); N.Y. PUB. HEALTH LAW § 2782 (4)(c); W. VA. CODE § 16-3C-3(e).

[68]*See, e.g.*, CAL. HEALTH AND SAFETY CODE § 121015(a); 410 ILL. COMP. STAT. ANN. 305/9(a).

[69]S.C. CODE ANN. § 44-29-146; *see also* W.VA. CODE § 16-3C-3(d).

State statutes containing mandatory HIV notification provisions do exist, although they are few in number.[70] Such statutes require either the health department or the health care provider to notify persons at risk, and typically specify the circumstances when the requirement applies. Oregon, for example, requires health care providers to report the names of HIV-infected persons to the health department specifically for purposes of partner notification in two circumstances: (i) when the patient requests assistance in notifying partners and (ii) without the patient's consent, when the patient's partner is not a member of certain population groups who may have high risk of HIV infection (i.e., hemophiliacs, prostitutes, intravenous drug users, homosexuals).[71] Before notifying the health department, however, the health care provider must have tried and been unable to persuade the patient to voluntarily notify his or her partners.

Under North Carolina's notification scheme, patients are required to notify all past (since the date of infection, if known) and future sexual partners of their infection.[72] If a physician knows the identity of the spouse of an HIV-infected patient, and has not notified the spouse after obtaining the patient's consent, then the physician must report the identity of the spouse to the department of health. In doing so, the physician fulfills the statutory requirement to notify exposed and potentially exposed persons.

Whether mandatory or permissive, these notification laws usually require the physician to protect the identity of the patient when making such disclosures.[73] For example, California provides that a physician or surgeon having the results of a confirmed positive HIV test of a patient under his or her care cannot be held criminally or civilly liable for disclosing to a person reasonably believed to be the spouse, sexual partner, or needle-sharing partner, or to the county health officer, the patient's test result; in disclosing that information to sexual partners who are not spouses, however, the health care provider must not disclose any identifying informa-

---

[70]*See, e.g.*, MICH. COMP. LAWS § 333.5131(5)(b); OR. ADMIN. R. 333-019-0030.

[71]OR. ADMIN. R. 333-018-0030 (3)(a) (D) & (E).

[72]N.C ADMIN. CODE tit. 15A, r. 19A.020 (1)(e).

[73]According to one estimate, only two states specifically permit disclosure of the name of the HIV-positive patient by the health department. *See, e.g.*, OHIO REV. CODE ANN. § 3701.243 (B)(1) (a) (authorizing disclosure of HIV test results and the identity of person tested to spouse or any sexual partner); MICH. COMP. LAWS § 333.5114a (5) (b) (allowing disclosure of identity of person tested but only if that person consents to such disclosure).

tion about the individual believed to be infected.[74] Further, before any disclosure, the physician must discuss the importance of notification with the patient, attempt to obtain the patient's voluntary consent for notification of any contact(s), and, regardless of whether consent is granted, inform the patient of the physician's intent to notify the patient's contact(s).[75]

A physician who wishes to notify a contact under one of these laws should discuss such plans in depth with the patient. The physician should remind the patient of the moral obligation to disclose the condition to third parties at risk. In addition, patients should be aware that some states impose criminal liability on an HIV carrier who knowingly engages in activities likely to spread the virus.[76] The physician should fully document the discussion in the patient's record. If after this consultation the patient still refuses to reveal the condition to sexual partners or others at risk, the physician then may contact the third parties directly; however, the physician should not proceed in a manner that identifies the patient. The physician also should be sensitive to the effect of the notification on a third party that may be completely unaware of the situation. While HIV notification provisions in most state statutes do not create a duty to warn third parties, other federal or state laws may impose such an obligation.[77]

Moreover, case law in a few states appears to create a duty to warn for health care providers, and there is no statute protecting them from liability for failure to warn. In Vermont, for example, the state supreme court has imposed a "duty to warn" on mental health professionals who know or should know that a patient poses a serious risk of danger to an identifiable victim,[78] and this ruling could be extended to other health care professionals, particularly with respect to notifying spouses of known HIV-positive

---

[74]CAL. HEALTH & SAFETY CODE § 121015(a). The provision is permissive, however, and thus imposes no duty on the part of the physician to notify any of these contacts. *See, e.g.,* CAL. HEALTH & SAFETY CODE § 121015(c).

[75]CAL. HEALTH & SAFETY CODE § 121015(b).

[76]*See, e.g.,* FLA. STAT. ANN. § 384.24.

[77]For example, one federal law that might be relevant in this respect comprises regulations effective as of November 1996 which amend the laboratory Medicare and Medicaid Conditions of Participation to require hospitals to take action when they learn that they have received a blood product at increased risk of transmitting HIV. *See* 42 C.F.R. § 482.27(c). Under these regulations, if a blood bank notifies a hospital that a previous blood donor has tested HIV-positive, the hospital must dispose of the donor's blood or blood products and follow specified procedures to notify patients who received blood or blood products derived from the donor.

[78]Peck v. Counseling Serv. 499 A. 2d 422 (Vt.1985). *See also* Tarasoff v. Regents of Univ. of Calif., 551 P.2d 334 (Cal. 1976).

patients. Two other courts have found a duty to warn a partner of a patient where the hospital knew that the patient received HIV-infected blood as result of undergoing a blood transfusion at the hospital. In Texas, for example, an appeals court ruled that a hospital can be liable for failing to warn a former patient's wife that the patient may have contracted AIDS from contaminated blood products used for the patient's blood transfusions.[79] The hospital did not notify the patient or his wife of its discovery of contamination in some of the blood products used at the time the patient had received blood transfusions. The wife sued the hospital for failing to inform, and one of the hospital's defenses was that it had no duty to warn the wife. The appeals court ruled that where a health care professional discovers that its services or products likely caused a medical condition that may endanger a readily identifiable third party, the health care professional has a duty to warn that party of the danger.[80]

In at least one state, however, a court has held to the contrary on the issue of whether there is a duty to warn the spouse of a hospitalized patient who has tested positive for HIV where no blood transfusion is involved; a District of Columbia appeals court ruled that hospital employees owed no duty to warn the husband of such a patient.[81] The husband, who was separated from his wife when she was hospitalized but later reunited with her, sued the hospital for emotional distress, arguing that he had suffered psychologically upon learning at least one year after the hospitalization that his wife had tested HIV-positive at that time. The court dismissed the suit, finding that the hospital did not owe the husband any duty to disclose his wife's test results, but rather that a duty was owed to the wife to not disclose the information to anyone without her written consent.

Other Permissible Disclosures without Consent of Patient

In addition to the common exceptions described in the previous sections, disclosure of HIV-related information is permitted, under many statutes, to numerous other parties, including blood banks and organ donors, epidemiologists or other researchers, correctional facilities,

---

[79]Garcia v. Santa Rosa Care Corp., 925 S.W.2d 372 (Tex. Ct. App. 1996).

[80]*See also* Reisner v. Regents of Univ. of Cal., 37 Cal. Rptr. 2d 518 (Ct. App. 1995) (HIV-infected person who contracted virus from his girlfriend can sue hospital for failing to inform girlfriend that she had received HIV-tainted blood transfusion at hospital).

[81]N.O.L. v. District of Columbia, 674 A.2d 498 (D.C. 1995).

schools, HMOs or other health care facilities, and insurance companies.[82] Most states allow, rather than require, release of this information; some states, however, mandate that HIV test results be disclosed to school officials, blood donors, correctional officials, and law enforcement authorities who are investigating criminal offenses that may have resulted in HIV transmission.[83] (See "Duty to Report," discussed previously in this chapter.) Some confidentiality statutes also permit release of information to health facility staff committees, accreditation committees, and oversight review organizations.[84] In addition, New York allows disclosure to an authorized agency in connection with foster care or adoption of a child, to insurance companies or their agents to the extent necessary to reimburse health care providers for health services, and to the medical directors of correctional facilities.[85] Wisconsin authorizes release to a funeral director or person who performs an autopsy on an HIV patient, a coroner, and a sheriff or keeper of a prison.[86]

Disclosure of Health Care Provider's Status to Patients

Health care facilities also must confront the difficult issue of whether to reveal a health care worker's HIV status to patients. In this regard, it is important to distinguish between disclosure before treatment and disclosure after treatment. Guidelines issued by the CDC address both situations;[87] the Guidelines recommend that HIV-positive workers notify prospective patients of the worker's HIV status before the patients

---

[82]One survey estimates the following with respect to statutory exceptions authorizing disclosure of HIV-related information: blood bank and/or donors, 22 states; epidemiologists and researchers, 22 states; correctional facilities, 14 states; schools, 12 states; HMOs and other health care facilities, 14 states; and insurance companies, 8 states. *See* L. Gostin, Z. Lazzarini, & K. Flaherty, Legislative Survey of State Confidentiality Laws, with Specific Emphasis on HIV and Immunization, Final Report (Presented to the U.S. Centers for Disease Control and Prevention, the Council of State and Territorial Epidemiologists, and the Task Force for Child Survival and Development—Carter Presidential Center, Georgetown University Law Center, July 1996).

[83]*See, e.g.*, CAL. HEALTH & SAFETY CODE §§ 121055, 121060 & 121070; N.Y. PUB. HEALTH LAW § 2782(1)(l)-(o).

[84]*See, e.g.*, DEL. CODE ANN. tit. 16, § 1203(a)(7); 410 ILL. COMP. STAT. ANN. 305/9(f); N.Y. PUB. HEALTH LAW § 2782(1)(f); W. VA. CODE § 16-3C-3(a)(8).

[85]N.Y. PUB. HEALTH LAW § 2782(1)(h), (i) & (n). *See also* HAW. REV. STAT. § 325-101(a)(6)-(10).

[86]WIS. STAT. § 252.15(5)(a)(7), (12) & (13).

[87]*See, e.g.*, Centers for Disease Control and Prevention, Morbidity and Mortality Weekly Report (July 12, 1991).

undergo exposure-prone invasive procedures, and that disclosure after treatment should be decided on a case-by-case basis. More specifically, the CDC describes the case-by-case approach to decisions as to whether patients should be notified of possible exposure as a determination involving the "assessment of specific risks, confidentiality issues, and available resources." The CDC also recommends that decisions regarding notification and follow-up studies should be made in consultation with state and local public health officials.

Some states also require health care workers who perform exposure-prone procedures to notify prospective patients of their seropositive status and obtain written consent from patients before patients undergo exposure-prone procedures.[88] A New Jersey court has upheld a hospital's requirement that an HIV-positive surgeon disclose his HIV status to prospective patients as part of the informed consent procedure.[89] In Maryland, an appeals court has allowed two patients of a surgeon who died of AIDS to sue his estate based on the claim that he had failed to inform them before surgery that he was infected with HIV.[90] A physician's duty of care must include disclosure that an operating surgeon's HIV-positive status poses a risk, however minimal, of transmission of the AIDS virus during surgery, the court concluded.

With respect to disclosure after exposure, a hospital may make the decision to inform patients that a provider who treated them is HIV-positive. Some states allow notification of an individual who may have been exposed to HIV through contact with an HIV-infected provider, as well as an investigation of the health care provider.[91] In states that have HIV confidentiality statutes that forbid such disclosure, however, the hospital would need to obtain court authorization before disclosing such information. In a Pennsylvania case, for example, the high court allowed

---

[88]*See, e.g.*, TEX. HEALTH & SAFETY CODE ANN. § 85.205(c).

[89]*See* Estate of Behringer v. Medical Ctr. at Princeton, 592 A.2d 1251 (N.J. Super. Ct. Law Div.1991). *See also* Doe v. Noe, 690 N.E. 2d 1012 (Ill. Ct. App. 1997).

[90]Faya v. Almaraz, 620 A.2d 327 (Md. 1993). *See also* Kerins v. Hartley, 21 Cal. Rptr. 2d 621 (Ct. App. 1993) (when patient asked about surgeon's health, she conditioned her consent on being operated on by healthy surgeon, and thus nondisclosure of HIV-positive status established cause of action for battery).

[91]410 ILL. COMP. STAT. ANN. 325/5.5(b) & (c). *See also* Estate of Doe v. Vanderbilt Univ., Inc., 824 F. Supp. 746 (M.D. Tenn. 1993) (when hospital becomes aware that an HIV-positive worker participated in exposure-prone procedures, it has duty to decide whether to initiate a "look-back" program, and attempt to inform patients who may have been exposed to HIV).

a hospital to disclose the identity of an AIDS-infected obstetrics-gynecology resident to patients who had been treated by the resident.[92] Two hospitals where the physician had worked requested court permission to disclose the physician's name and medical information to more than 200 patients who had been associated to some degree with the physician in the course of their treatment. Under Pennsylvania law, information derived from HIV testing must remain confidential, but courts may authorize disclosure of such information if there is a compelling need to do so. The court emphasized in this case that the physician was involved in invasive surgical procedures where the risk of sustaining cuts and exposing patients to tainted blood was high. His medical problem became a matter of public concern the moment he picked up a surgical instrument and became involved in surgical procedures, the court declared. After weighing the physician's privacy interests against the interests of public health, the court concluded that the latter should prevail, given the potential risks for transmission of the disease.

Disclosure by Court Order

Many confidentiality statutes include standards by which a court may authorize disclosure of the results of a patient's HIV test. Some statutes allow disclosure under a "lawful court order";[93] others require the person seeking access to show a "compelling need," with no other means of acquiring the information.[94] In determining whether a compelling need exists, the court must balance the petitioner's interest against the patient's privacy interest and the public interest.[95] The public interest will not be served if disclosure deters future testing, fosters discrimination,[96] or discourages donations of blood, organs, or semen.[97] The petitioner may be required to show that other ways of obtaining the information are not

---

[92]In re Milton S. Hershey Med. Ctr. of Pa. State Univ., 634 A.2d 159 (Pa. 1993).

[93]Wis. Stat. § 252.15(5)(a)(9).

[94]*See, e.g.*, 35 Pa. Cons. Stat. § 7608 (A); Iowa Code § 141.23(1)(g)(1). *See also* Haw. Rev. Stat. § 325-101 (a)(11) (court order upon showing of good cause).

[95]*See, e.g.*, Del. Code Ann. tit. 16, § 1203(a)(10)(a); W.Va. Code § 16-3C-3(a)(9)(i).

[96]*See, e.g.*, Del. Code Ann. tit. 16, § 1203(a)(10)(a).

[97]*See, e.g.*, Fla. Stat. Ann § 381.004 (3)(f)(9)(a); Ky Rev. Stat. Ann. § 214.181 (5)(c)(9)(a); S.C. Code Ann. § 44-29-136 (A).

available or would not be effective.[98] Many statutes also provide that the patient's true name may not be included in any documents filed with the court—a pseudonym must be substituted. The test subjects must be given notice and opportunity to participate in the proceedings if not already a party. All proceedings are conducted in camera unless the test subject agrees to a hearing in open court, or the court determines that a public hearing is necessary to the public interest and proper administration of justice.[99]

Court Orders and Disclosure in Blood Donor Cases

Even in the absence of such statutory directives, courts have struggled to balance the interests involved when one person requests disclosure of medical information relating to another person. Numerous cases in this area have involved claims by patients who contracted AIDS through blood transfusions and who request the facility that provided blood to produce a list of donors' names and addresses. Such cases generally involve malpractice claims against a hospital or blood supplier or both, in which a patient attempts to discover the identity of the donor who provided the contaminated blood. The patient frequently alleges that access to the blood donor's identity is necessary to establish whether the hospital or supplier used proper screening and testing procedures when they accepted the blood.

Courts are divided on the issue of whether a donor's right to privacy outweighs an individual patient's need to prove negligence on the part of a health care provider in a malpractice suit. Some courts that have considered the issue have refused to order blood collection facilities to reveal the identities of donors. The Florida Supreme Court, for example, ruled that the privacy interests of donors and society's interest in maintaining a strong volunteer blood donation program outweigh a patient's need to prove the source of his AIDS contamination in a personal injury suit.[100] The court ruled that the release of the blood donor's records would result in an undue invasion of privacy, and added that discovery should be denied so that donors would not be deterred from donating blood for fear that someone would be able to inquire into their private lives by obtaining

---

[98]*See, e.g.*, DEL. CODE ANN. tit. 16, § 1203(a)(10)(a); MICH. COMP. LAWS ANN. § 333.5131(3)(a)(ii).

[99]*See, e.g.*, DEL. CODE ANN. tit. 16, § 1203(a)(10)(d); HAW. REV. STAT. § 325-101 (a)(11); W.VA. CODE § 16-3C-3(a)(9)(iv).

[100]Rasmussen v. South Florida Blood Serv., 500 So. 2d 533 (Fla. 1987).

their blood records. Similarly, a federal trial court in South Carolina ruled that a patient who sued a blood bank after she acquired HIV from a blood transfusion was not entitled to discover the identity of the donor because the donor's interest in privacy and public interest in protecting voluntary blood programs outweighed the patient's interest in the case.[101]

However, other courts have held that the patient's interest in discovering the identity of the donor outweighs the donor's privacy rights. The Louisiana Supreme Court allowed a patient who tested HIV-positive after a blood transfusion to discover the identity of a donor who tested HIV-positive.[102] The court ruled that the patient's interest in discovering the identity of the donor outweighed both the donor's privacy interest and public policy considerations favoring nondisclosure. The court emphasized that the donor already had tested HIV-positive, that the patient sought only to identify the donor of one specific unit of blood, and that the patient needed to identify the donor to evaluate the blood center's screening process.[103] One court has allowed a patient to sue a blood donor identified through information inadvertently provided by the Red Cross.[104] The court held that the patient's right to litigate her claim against the donor substantially outweighed the individual privacy rights and public interest in maintaining a safe and adequate blood supply, especially in light of evidence suggesting donor misconduct.

Some courts have resolved blood donor cases by allowing, but limiting, disclosure, such as by requiring the blood collection agency to reveal the name of the infected donor to the court, which then relays relevant communications between the patient and the donor.[105] One court that adopted this method also directed that communications between the donor and that person's lawyer and the court be maintained with redacted signatures in a sealed envelope marked "Confidential."[106] Another court that permitted

---

[101]Doe v. American Red Cross Serv., 125 F.R.D. 646 (D.S.C. 1989).

[102]Most v. Tulane Med. Ctr., 576 So. 2d 1387 (La. 1991).

[103]*See also* Sampson v. American Nat'l Red Cross, 139 F.R.D. 95 (N.D. Tex. 1991); Tarrant County Hosp. Dist. v. Hughes, 734 S.W.2d 675 (Tex. Ct. App. 1987); Long v. American Red Cross, 145 F.R.D. 658 (S.D. Ohio 1993).

[104]Coleman v. American Red Cross, 979 F.2d 1135 (6th Cir. 1992), *complaint dismissed on other grounds*, 145 F.R.D. 422 (E.D. Mich. 1993).

[105]Belle Bonfils Mem'l Blood Ctr. v. District Court, 763 P.2d 1003 (Colo. 1988). *See also* Watson v. Lowcountry Red Cross, 974 F.2d 482 (4th Cir. 1992).

[106]Watson v. Lowcountry Red Cross, 974 F.2d 482 (4th Cir. 1992).

discovery of donors' identities ordered the plaintiff not to communicate with the donors or undertake further discovery.[107]

Liability for Unauthorized Disclosure of HIV-Related Information

Health care providers' unauthorized disclosure of information relating to a patient's HIV status can lead to liability based on violation of HIV confidentiality or other relevant statutes. Liability provisions of most HIV confidentiality statutes create special civil and criminal liability for persons who make unauthorized disclosures of HIV test results. Civil liability gives the test subject a private cause of action for damages against the person who disclosed the information; criminal liability, on the other hand, allows the state attorney to prosecute the offender and impose fines and/or a jail sentence.

In most states, a person who consciously disregards the statute is subject to harsher penalties than one who is negligent. In California, for example, any person who negligently discloses the results of an HIV test to any third party in a manner that identifies or provides identifying characteristics of the person to whom the test results apply is liable to a civil penalty of up to $1,000 (to be paid to the test subject); the civil penalty to be assessed for willful disclosure, however, is up to $5,000 (to be paid to the test subject).[108] In Virginia, any person who willfully or through gross negligence makes any unauthorized disclosure is liable for a civil penalty of up to $5,000 per violation payable to a special state fund,[109] and the person who is the subject of an unauthorized disclosure may recover actual damages or $100, whichever is greater, plus reasonable attorneys' fees and court costs.[110] Wisconsin provides for actual damages and costs, plus exemplary damages of up to $5,000 for an intentional violation.[111] In addition to receiving damages and attorneys' fees, an aggrieved party in Illinois may request other appropriate relief, including an injunction.[112] Colorado provides for a criminal penalty only, imposing misdemeanor fines

---

[107]Tarrant County Hosp. Dist. v. Hughes, 734 S.W.2d 675 (Tex. Ct. App. 1987).

[108]CAL. HEALTH & SAFETY CODE § 120980.

[109]VA. CODE § 32.1-36.1(B).

[110]VA. CODE § 32.1-36.1(C).

[111]WIS. STAT. § 242.14(4).

[112]410 ILL. COMP. STAT. ANN. 305/13.

not less than $500 or greater than $5,000, and/or by imprisonment not less than 6 months or greater than two years.[113]

Health care providers may also be sued for unauthorized disclosure of information relating to a patient's HIV status based on common law grounds. In one California case, for example, a state appeals court allowed a patient to sue a health care provider for disclosing his HIV status to an insurance carrier based on the state's constitutional right to privacy.[114] After receiving treatment for injuries sustained at work, a patient told the physician's nurse to be careful because he was HIV positive, but made it clear that he was disclosing the information solely for the purpose of protecting health care professionals. The physician's report mentioning AIDS as a possible source of the patient's symptoms was sent to the insurance company, the insurance carrier, and the Workers' Compensation Appeals Board. The court found that the circumstances surrounding the patient's disclosure clearly demonstrated his anticipation that the information would remain private. Enforcing such reasonable expectations of privacy fosters disclosure of HIV-positive status only when necessary and protects against misuse of information, the court held, concluding that the disclosure was protected under the constitutional right to privacy.

In another case, a New Jersey hospital was found liable for failing to protect the confidentiality of a diagnosis of AIDS in a staff physician who had been treated at the facility.[115] The test results were placed in the physician's medical chart, which was kept at the nurses' station on the floor where the physician was an inpatient. There were no restrictions on access to the record. Within hours of the diagnosis, the physician's condition was widely known within the hospital. The court found the hospital negligent for failing to take reasonable precautions regarding access to the physician's record. (For a more detailed discussion of liability arising from improper disclosure of medical record information, see Chapter 10, DISCOVERY AND ADMISSIBILITY OF HEALTH CARE RECORDS.)

---

[113]COLO. REV. STAT. § 25-4-1409(2).

[114]Estate of Urbaniak v. Newton, 277 Cal. Rptr. 354 (Ct. App. 1991).

[115]Estate of Behringer v. Medical Ctr. at Princeton, 592 A.2d 1251 (N.J. Super. Ct. Law Div.1991). *See also* Goins v. Mercy Ctr. for Health Care Servs., 667 N.E.2d 652 (Ill. App. Ct. 1996) (hospital security officer exposed to HIV-positive patient's blood can sue hospital for breach of confidentiality based on hospital's failure to keep secret the officer's HIV testing and results).

RECOMMENDED POLICIES AND PROCEDURES

Health care providers frequently encounter situations requiring them to balance their duty to protect third parties from the spread of the disease with their duty to protect the privacy of individuals who are infected with HIV. Individuals tested for HIV and/or treated for AIDS must be assured that information shared with health care professionals will remain confidential. Without such assurance, patients may withhold critical information that could affect the quality and outcome of care, safety of health care workers, and reliability of the information. In developing policies and procedures to safeguard patient privacy and the confidentiality of information relating to HIV infection, health care records managers may want to consider guidelines in this area issued by the American Health Information Management Association (AHIMA),[116] which recommends implementation of the following measures:

- Develop screening programs to provide confidential testing of individuals and communication of their test results.
- Implement a system that ensures that specific, written informed consent is obtained from the individual or his or her legal representative prior to voluntary testing,[117] followed by post-test counseling provided by a qualified health care professional.
- Maintain health records of patients infected with HIV with other patients' records in a secure area with restricted access; segregation of records based on HIV status should be avoided, as such a system may call attention to the patient's HIV status.[118]
- Manage HIV-positive health care workers according to guidelines outlined by the CDC and state and federal laws. The health care worker's privacy must be balanced against the risk of transmission to patients, employees, and others. If questions arise, the facility's legal counsel should be involved in resolving the related questions.

---

[116]M. D. Brandt, "Practice Brief: Managing Health Information Relating to Infection with the Human Immunodeficiency Virus (HIV)," *Journal of American Health Information Management Association* 68, no.2 (1997).

[117]State law may permit testing of a patient without consent if a health care worker has been exposed to the patient's blood or body fluids; in such cases the exposure incident and the need for HIV testing should be discussed with the patient or his or her legal representative before the test is made.

[118]In some states, the law may require that HIV antibody test results be maintained in a special manner, in which case health care information managers should develop procedures for marking such records in an obscure manner to prevent the inadvertent disclosure of HIV test results.

In addition, AHIMA emphasizes that health care facilities must implement clear policies and procedures for disclosure of health information related to HIV/AIDS, and for continual monitoring of such procedures to ensure consistent compliance. Depending on state law, the facility may be required to report the name of the person tested or other identifying information to local health authorities, but within the facility, a patient's serologic status should be disclosed only as needed for diagnosis, management, or treatment. Others who may review patient health records for administrative purposes (such as quality improvement, billing, and risk management) must ensure that this information is handled in a confidential manner. Information should be disclosed to other legitimate users only with specific written authorization of the patient or his or her legal representative or upon receipt of a valid subpoena.[119] Information disclosed to authorized users should be limited strictly to that required to fulfill the purpose stated on the authorization. Authorizations for release of "any and all information" without specifically mentioning HIV or AIDS should not be honored. Due to the sensitivity of this information, it should not be transmitted via facsimile machine or disclosed over the telephone unless urgently needed for patient care. Redisclosure of information relating to HIV/AIDS should be prohibited, unless otherwise required by state law.

---

[119]Some states require a court order for release, thus protecting the records of HIV/AIDS patients from discovery by subpoena.

10

Discovery and Admissibility of Medical Records

Chapter Objectives

- Distinguish between discoverability and admissibility.
- Define the physician-patient privilege and discuss its effect on discovery and admissibility.
- Describe the health care provider's role in protecting health information from discovery.
- Explain waiver of the physician-patient privilege and give examples of how the privilege may be waived.
- Define hearsay.
- Define the business record exception and its application to medical records.
- List other types of records containing patient information that may be sought in discovery.
- Describe the peer review privilege and what types of records it protects from discovery.
- Recommend steps to protect peer review records from discovery.
- Outline the factors that affect whether incident reports are protected from discovery.

INTRODUCTION

Medical records often play a crucial role in legal actions. For example, medical record information is central to workers' compensation claims, disability insurance claims, personal injury suits, and medical malpractice suits. Consequently, patients and other parties to legal actions typically seek every record that may be relevant to their controversy, including patient medical records, quality assurance and other committee records, hospital incident reports, and other types of documents that may contain information about patients.

Whether records are discoverable by parties to a legal proceeding or admissible during the course of proceedings may significantly affect the outcome of the claim. At the outset, it is important to distinguish between the discoverability and admissibility of evidence.

- Discoverability refers to access to documents or witnesses by parties to a legal proceeding. A document or information is discoverable if it must be produced to the party who requests it.
- Admissibility concerns whether documents, objects, or testimony may be admitted formally into evidence. The judge, jury, arbitrator, or other decision maker may only consider evidence that has been admitted.

The legal standard for determining whether something is admissible is more stringent than the standard for discoverability. Thus, health information may be discoverable by parties in advance of a legal proceeding, but not admissible into evidence during the proceeding itself. The judge, administrative hearing officer, or panel will apply the rules of evidence to determine whether a record is discoverable or admissible. Since these rules vary from state to state, it is extremely important for health care administrators and health information professionals to refer questions on this subject to their legal counsel. Counsel will interpret applicable rules and help prepare appropriate arguments for or against discoverability or admissibility.

DISCOVERABILITY OF MEDICAL RECORDS

Discovery is pretrial access to either witnesses or documents, allowing parties to a suit to discover facts and possible evidence in the case. The standard for what information and documents must be revealed is broad, allowing parties to obtain most items reasonably calculated to lead to the discovery of admissible evidence. There are a variety of methods of discovering information, including:

- Conducting an oral deposition (a question and answer session) of a party or witness
- Obtaining court permission to examine documents or other objects
- Sending written requests for copies of documents
- Sending written lists of questions, known as interrogatories, to parties and other witnesses

Because the confidentiality of medical information is important, courts sometimes require an "in camera" inspection of patient records during discovery, rather than allowing records to be freely copied and distributed to the parties. In this type of inspection, the judge will personally review the medical records requested, determining what information should be revealed.

Medical record professionals may receive a request to examine or copy patient records from the patient, the patient's attorney, or another party to a lawsuit involving a patient. A subpoena or court order to produce documents might also be served on a health care provider, facility, or organization, perhaps requiring the medical records "custodian" to appear in person with the requested records. Federal fraud or other investigators may appear without advance notice and demand to examine patient records. (For further discussions of search warrants and other legal authority for inspecting records, see Chapter 8, DOCUMENTATION AND DISCLOSURE: SPECIAL AREAS OF CONCERN.) Policies and procedures should specify how to respond to each type of request for access to records. The procedures should be clearly written and consistent with the legal and ethical duties of health care providers.

Physician-Patient Privilege

One way patients or health care practitioners may seek to shield health information from discovery is to assert the physician-patient privilege. Even if a court, hearing officer or other decision maker rules that a medical record is discoverable, the physician-patient privilege may later preclude admissibility, under the more stringent standard for admitting records into evidence. Nearly every state has a statute that protects communications between a patient and a physician from disclosure in judicial or quasi-judicial proceedings under specified circumstances. While the physician-patient privilege is often a creation of statute, a few courts in jurisdictions in which no statutory privilege exists have created one.[1] The purpose of this privilege is to encourage the patient to tell the physician all the information necessary for treatment, no matter how embarrassing.[2]

Statutory provisions vary. Four aspects to examine when assessing the privilege conferred in a state law are

1. the categories of health care providers that are covered by the statute;
2. the scope and extent of the patient's privilege to prevent disclosure by the health care provider;
3. the extent to which the provider may exercise the patient's privilege; and
4. the nature of the proceedings in which the privilege may be raised.

In Illinois, for example, a state law says that no physician, surgeon, psychologist, nurse, mental health worker, therapist, or other healing art practitioner may disclose information acquired while professionally attending a patient, if the information was necessary to serve the patient, except in specified circumstances. The circumstances include:

- homicide trials
- malpractice actions against the health care practitioner
- actions where the patient's physical or mental condition is an issue, including any action in which the patient seeks damages for personal injury, death, pain and suffering, or mental or emotional injury[3]

Virginia's privilege statute protects the information a licensed practitioner of any branch of the healing arts acquires in treating a patient in a professional capacity if the information is necessary to treat the individual. However, the Virginia law states that the information may be disclosed when the physical or mental condition of a patient is at issue, when a patient unlawfully attempts to procure a narcotic, when necessary for the care of the patient, to protect the practitioner's rights, in connection with the operations of a health care facility or health maintenance organization (HMO), or to comply with state or federal law.[4]

---

[1]*See* Wanda Ellen Wakefield, Annotation, *Physician-Patient Privilege as Extending to Patient's Medical or Hospital Records,* 10 A.L.R.4th 552.

[2]*See* Wanda Ellen Wakefield, Annotation, *Physician-Patient Privilege as Extending to Patient's Medical or Hospital Records,* 10 A.L.R.4th 552.

[3]735 ILL. COMP. STAT. ANN. 5/8-802.

[4]VA. CODE ANN. § 8.01-399.

In suits between the patient and others, it is not the health care provider's concern or right to assert the privilege, or to oppose a records subpoena. However, the court may order the provider to permit examination of medical records without disclosing confidential communications.[5]

When a patient seeks to discover the medical records of other patients who are not parties to the legal action, a health care provider may be able to assert the physician-patient privilege on behalf of the nonparty patients.[6] The effectiveness of the provider's assertion depends on the governing state statute. Health care providers and medical records professionals must proceed carefully, with the advice of counsel, as courts have ruled on the discovery of these records based on a variety of grounds:

- In a Georgia case, the court allowed evidence of orthodontic treatment provided by a dentist to patients other than the person suing.[7] The court stated that the evidence was admissible to contradict any possible testimony by the dentist that, in similar cases, similar treatment had not resulted in the same unfortunate results.
- The highest court in Maryland has ruled that a physician being sued for malpractice could not challenge a second physician who was serving as an opposing expert witness by introducing the expert's patients' records.[8] Although state law allows a health care provider to release the records of any patient if the records will assist in defending a lawsuit, that statute did not apply in this case, because the provider defending the suit did not wish to disclose his own patients' records.
- A Florida court allowed an obese patient suing for malpractice to obtain the records of other obese patients treated by her obstetrician.[9] Although a state law requires notice to nonparty patients before their records can be disclosed, the patients' names and addresses would have to be divulged to implement that requirement. The court ruled that redacting the identifying information made the notice requirement inapplicable and ordered the physician to produce the records.

---

[5]*See* In re D.M.C., 331 N.W.2d 236 (Minn. 1983); In re Larchmont Gables, Inc., 64 N.Y.S.2d 623 (Sup. Ct. 1946).

[6]*See* Dag E. Ytrebert, Annotation, *Discovery, in Medical Malpractice Action, of Names of Other Patients to Whom Defendant Has Given Treatment Similar to that Allegedly Injuring Plaintiff,* 74 A.L.R. 3d 1055.

[7]Gunthorpe v. Daniels, 257 S.E.2d 199 (Ga. Ct. App. 1979).

[8]Warner v. Lerner, No. 69, Sept. Term 1997 (Md. Feb. 19, 1998).

[9]Amente v. Newman, 653 So.2d 1030 (Fla. 1995).

Unless applicable law requires health care providers to disclose medical records information of nonparty patients under the circumstances, they should attempt to assert the confidential communications privilege on behalf of the patient if the patient is not a party to the lawsuit. A physician who asserts the privilege improperly and refuses to provide records when required to do so, however, may be held in contempt of court and fined or jailed. Thus, the advice of counsel should be sought whenever a broad request for nonparty patient records is received.

Waiver of the Physician-Patient Privilege

The physician-patient privilege belongs to the patient, not the physician. The patient may waive this privilege expressly or impliedly. What constitutes a waiver has been a matter of litigation. Most courts will hold that an individual who files a suit that places his or her own physical or mental health in issue impliedly waives the physician-patient privilege.[10] For example, a patient who seeks compensation for physical injuries or "pain and suffering" generally must allow opposing parties to review medical record information pertinent to the evaluation and treatment of those injuries. As mentioned above, state statutes may also specify that the privilege is waived under those circumstances.[11] Even if a patient waives the physician-patient privilege by putting his physical or mental condition at issue in a lawsuit, however, the scope of the waiver is limited to relevant information. For example, a patient who alleged medical malpractice during her pregnancy did not waive her privilege as to medical records outside of that pregnancy.[12] At least one court has ruled that a patient suing for medical malpractice only waives the physician-patient privilege as to information exchanged between the patient and the physician sued, not between the patient and subsequent physicians.[13]

A number of courts have ruled that the privilege is not waived unless it is evident that the patient intended to waive it.[14] In one case, for example, a court ruled that a patient had not waived his privilege by turning his

---

[10]Carr v. Schmid, 432 N.Y.S.2d 807 (Sup. Ct. 1980); J.R. Kemper, Annotation, *Commencing Action Involving Physical Condition of Plaintiff or Decedent as Waiving Physician-Patient Privilege as to Discovery Proceedings*, 21 A.L.R.3d 912.

[11]*See, e.g.,* 735 ILL. COMP. STAT. ANN. 5/8-802.

[12]Murphy v. LoPresti, 648 N.Y.S.2d 169 (Sup. Ct. App. Div. 1996).

[13]Acosta v. Richter, 671 So. 2d 149 (Fla. 1996).

[14]*See, e.g.,* Schaffer v. Spicer, 215 N.W.2d 134 (S.D. 1974).

records over to his insurer. The court held that doing so was not an unequivocal demonstration that the patient intended to abandon the privilege.[15] Rather, it was an act consistent with the intention to reveal confidential information only to the extent necessary to obtain treatment and payment. On the other hand, once the privilege is truly waived in one context, a patient may be precluded from asserting it in another context. For example, one court held that a patient who disclosed his medical records in a suit against him (alleging that he injured a young child in a car accident) may not object to discovery of the same records in a later suit against his physicians.[16]

Physician-Patient Privilege vs. the Public Interest

Some courts have held that the physician-patient privilege may give way to an important public interest.[17] For example, when dealing with a child care or custody case, courts are likely to find that the interest of the child outweighs the parents' interest in keeping their medical records confidential.[18] This balance may be struck at the legislative level, also. The Illinois confidential communications statute specifically provides that the privilege does not apply in civil or criminal actions arising out of the filing of a report under Illinois' Abused and Neglected Child Reporting Act.[19] In this situation, a court may attempt to partially protect the physician-patient privilege by allowing a private examination of medical records by the court and other parties, rather than admitting entire records into evidence.

Another important public interest is the prosecution of a crime.[20] In the modern health care industry, courts have generally permitted the broad-scale discovery of patient records in the context of fraud investigations. In a New York case, a trial court ruled that a hospital under investigation for Medicare violations was required to turn over the billing and medical

---

[15]State ex rel. Gonzenbach v. Eberwein, 655 S.W.2d 794 (Mo. Ct. App. 1983).

[16]Landelius v. Board of Regents, 556 N.W.2d 472 (Mich. 1996).

[17]*See, e.g.,* People v. Doe, 435 N.Y.S.2d 656 (Sup. Ct. 1981); Wanda Ellen Wakefield, Annotation, *Physician-Patient Privilege as Extending to Patient's Medical or Hospital Records,* 10 A.L.R.4th 552.

[18]*See, e.g.,* Bieluch v. Bieluch, 462 A.2d 1060 (Conn. 1983); In re Baby X, 293 N.W.2d 736 (Mich. Ct. App. 1980); In re Doe Children, 402 N.Y.S.2d 958 (Fam. Ct. 1978); Wanda Ellen Wakefield, Annotation, *Physician-Patient Privilege as Extending to Patient's Medical or Hospital Records,* 10 A.L.R.4th 552.

[19]735 ILL. COMP. STAT. ANN. 5/8-802(7).

[20]*See* Wanda Ellen Wakefield, Annotation, *Physician-Patient Privilege as Extending to Patient's Medical or Hospital Records,* 10 A.L.R.4th 552.

records of 96 former patients to the grand jury. Noting that "the privilege was never intended to prevent disclosure of evidence of a crime," the court refused to grant the hospital's request to quash the grand jury's subpoenas.[21] Similarly, a California court ruled that a physician whose records were seized as part of a Medi-Cal fraud investigation was not entitled to a hearing to assess whether the physician-patient privilege protected the records. Allowing a physician accused of fraud to assert the privilege would serve the physician's rather than the patients' interest, the court found.[22] In an Ohio fraud investigation, a court ruled that a physician could not assert the physician-patient privilege as a shield from criminal prosecution. Although the records seized from the physician's office were admissible, they must be redacted by erasing or concealing the patients' names, the court cautioned.[23]

ADMISSIBILITY OF MEDICAL RECORDS

Although historically there was a diversity of opinion, most modern courts hold that medical records are admissible into evidence.[24] Admissibility is of great importance to the health care provider being sued for medical malpractice, because the records may contain information damaging to the provider. When the health care provider is not a party, medical records should be produced in accordance with the law. The rules of evidence govern the admissibility of all evidence, including medical records.

All evidence, including medical record information, must be relevant, material, and competent before it can be admitted. Although these three terms often are used as synonyms, they have distinct meanings.

1. Evidence is relevant if it tends to prove or disprove a fact at issue in the case.

---

[21]People v. Doe, 435 N.Y.S.2d 656 (Sup. Ct. 1981). *See also* In re Pebsworth, 705 F.2d 261 (7th Cir. 1983).

[22]Brillantes v. Superior Ct., 51 Cal. App. 4th 323 (Ct. App. 1996).

[23]Ohio v. McGriff, 669 N.E.2d 856 (Ohio Ct. App. 1996).

[24]*See generally* Annotations, James D. Lawlor, *Admissibility under Uniform Business Records as Evidence Act or Similar Statute of Medical Report Made by Consulting Physician to Treating Physician*, 69 A.L.R.3d 104; James D. Lawlor, *Admissibility under Business Entry Statutes of Hospital Records in Criminal Case*, 69 A.L.R.3d 22; *Admissibility of Hospital Record Relating to Cause or Circumstances of Accident or Incident in which Patient Sustained Injury*, 44 A.L.R.2d 553; Donald M. Zupanec, *Admissibility under State Law of Hospital Record Relating to Intoxication or Sobriety of Patient*, 80 A.L.R.3d 456; Jean F. Rydstrom, *Admissibility of Hospital Records under Federal Business Records Act* (28 USC § 1732(a)), 9 A.L.R. Fed. 457.

2. Evidence is material if it is important to an issue in the case.

3. Evidence is competent if it is fit and appropriate proof.

Thus, a party who seeks to admit medical records into evidence must show that the record meets all three tests—unlike in discovery, where a party seeking access to medical records need only argue that the record might be admissible, or might lead to the discovery of admissible evidence.

Medical Records as Hearsay

Hearsay is a statement made out of court that is introduced into a court proceeding for the purpose of proving the truth of the facts asserted in that statement. Under traditional rules of evidence, a patient care record is hearsay. Generally, hearsay is not admissible into evidence because the person who actually made the statement is not there to be cross-examined. Consider the example of a nurse who has made an entry regarding the patient's blood pressure. The following problems may result if the record is admitted into evidence as proof of that blood pressure:

- The opposing side cannot ask the nurse about mistakes the individual may have made in transcribing the record.
- The jury cannot observe the nurse's demeanor and judge the nurse's veracity.
- The jury will be unable to check the records as it would if the record were part of the nurse's testimony in the courtroom.

Business Record Exception to the Bar on Hearsay

Although medical records are hearsay, they may be admitted into evidence on other grounds. In states that have enacted an exception to the bar on hearsay for business records, for example, medical records may be admissible if they qualify as business records. Business records are typically defined as documents that are made in the regular course of business at or within a reasonable time after the event recorded occurred and under circumstances that reasonably might be assumed to reflect the actual event accurately.[25] Other documents retained by health care providers, facilities, and organizations that may qualify as business records include billing records, discharge summaries, and record extracts.[26]

---

[25]*See, e.g.,* FLA. STAT. ch. 90.803; N.D. CENT. CODE § 31-08-01.

[26]Sandegren v. State, 397 So. 2d 657 (Fla. 1981).

Even if a medical record qualifies as an admissible business record, other standards of admissibility may preclude *information in the record* from being entered into evidence. Observations in a patient care record that health care providers are trained to make and that they routinely make in the course of treating patients will be admissible. In one case, for example, a physician's observation that the patient was intoxicated on arrival at the hospital was held admissible.[27] In another, statements regarding the cause of a construction worker's crushed foot were admissible because the information was helpful to diagnosis and treatment.[28] Generally, information in the medical record will be inadmissible if it is not relevant to the patient's diagnosis or treatment. For example:

- A statement in a hospital discharge summary that a patient had fallen from a catwalk around an oil tank was not admissible because the summary was not made at or near the time of the injury, the information was not used to diagnose or treat the patient, and the record didn't indicate who gave the physician the information or when it was given.[29]
- A statement that an injured bicyclist was not wearing a helmet and accidentally ran into a stationary car was not admissible because the evidence did not indicate who made the statement and someone other than the bicyclist could have given the information to the hospital staff.[30]
- A statement by a truck driver that she slipped on diesel fuel and fell was not admissible, because the driver had no motivation to tell the truth, since the information was not necessary to her diagnosis or treatment.[31]

Other Exceptions to the Bar on Hearsay

Even if a medical record does not qualify as a business record, it may be admissible if it qualifies under another exception to the hearsay rule. Because statements in certain categories are considered to be free of the untrustworthiness and inaccuracy that underlie most out-of-court assertions,

---

[27]Rivers v. Union Carbide Corp., 426 F.2d 633 (3d Cir. 1970).

[28]Santucci v. Govel Welding, Inc., 564 N.Y.S.2d 518 (App. Div. 1990).

[29]Benson v. Shuler Drilling Co., 871 S.W.2d 552 (Ark. 1994).

[30]Barrera v. Wilson, 668 A.2d 871 (D.C. 1995).

[31]Carton v. Missouri P.R. Co., 798 S.W.2d 674 (Ark. 1990).

they may be admitted into evidence even when the person making the statements is unavailable to testify. (For example, statements made in a moment of surprise are considered trustworthy because the person had no time to fabricate a false statement.) Such exceptions include:

- declarations against interest
- spontaneous exclamations
- statements made for medical diagnosis and treatment
- dying declarations
- admissions of a party [32]

State statutes also may make medical records admissible under hearsay exceptions for public or official records. This is especially true when state statutes require public hospitals to keep records. The rationale is that the requirement that the record be kept ensures that the information in the record will be reliable. Hospital records also may be admissible under Workers' Compensation laws. Under Illinois law, for example, medical records, certified as true by a hospital officer and showing medical treatment given to an employee in the hospital, are admissible as evidence of the medical status of the Workers' Compensation claimant.[33]

OTHER HEALTH CARE DOCUMENTATION

Aside from patient records, there are many types of documentation that a health care facility, organization, or provider may wish to keep confidential. By the same token, patients and others may seek these documents in the course of a malpractice or other lawsuit. Examples include:

- credentialing committee records and reports
- Joint Commission on Accreditation of Healthcare Organizations (Joint Commission) and other accreditation surveys and recommendations
- state inspection reports and recommendations
- mortality committee records
- incident reports
- grand rounds presentations
- surgical reviews
- infection control committee records

---

[32]*See generally, e.g.,* FED. R. EVID. 803; OKLA. STAT. 12 § 2803.
[33]820 ILL. COMP. STAT. ANN. 305/16.

- evaluations of health care providers
- peer review records
- deselection documentation
- medical call center protocols
- care protocols
- practitioner training materials
- licensing applications and documents
- operating room records, such as logs
- risk management data
- patient representative/ombudsman records
- patient complaints
- profiling data
- utilization review reports

Generally, these types of records are discoverable unless they are specifically shielded by a state statute. Admissibility, however, may hinge on whether the records fall within an exception to the bar on hearsay. The state statutes that may create a privilege for these categories of records are too various to discuss here. However, two types of documents with a well-established history regarding discovery and admissibility serve as examples: peer review documents and incident reports.

Peer Review Records

Health care facilities and organizations are required by a variety of authorities to establish and maintain programs to monitor and improve the quality of the patient care they provide. Quality assurance and peer review programs rely on committees that collect data and generate records on the performance of individual physicians or the treatment of patients. Hospital medical staffs, for example, generally have a medical executive committee, a credentials committee, and various performance evaluation committees to carry out their functions. The importance of peer review is well-established. In a Connecticut case, the court said "[t]he overriding importance of these review committees to the medical profession and the public requires that doctors have unfettered freedom to evaluate their peers in an atmosphere of complete confidentiality. No chilling effect can be tolerated if the committees are to function effectively."[34]

---

[34]Morse v. Gerity, 520 F. Supp. 470 (D. Conn. 1981).

The potential value of records generated by such committees to a person suing for negligence is clear, and the demand for access to them has created a substantial body of law.

The first step in determining whether a peer review record is discoverable or admissible is to examine state statutory and case law. Although there is a great deal of variety between states, similar issues should be considered when analyzing a peer review confidentiality statute:

- Whose communications are protected? Does the statute create a privilege only for peer review committee members, for example, or also for individuals who make reports to the committee? Is the peer review protection limited to physicians, or are other health care practitioners included?

- What committees are protected? Some statutes protect the activities of hospital medical staff committees, while others might include other quality assurance, peer review, and utilization review committees individually or generally. The activities of ad hoc committees or individuals, acting outside of bylaws or other established parameters, are not likely to be protected.

- What is the subject of the communication at issue? Generally, statutes require that a committee activity be motivated by patient care concerns to be protected.

- Who is seeking the peer review records? Some statutes specifically allow physicians challenging peer review decisions (on antitrust or defamation grounds, for example) to obtain committee records.

- What communications and information are protected? Some statutes designate as confidential official committee proceedings and reports, but allow independent discovery of information provided to the committee. The identities of committee members and witnesses might also be subject to discovery. State laws might allow discovery of communications volunteered to a committee, but disallow as confidential information developed at the request of the committee.

- Are there other laws that might create a privilege? Federal laws create a privilege for information provided to qualified Peer Review Organizations (PROs), with some exceptions.[35]

---

[35]42 U.S.C. § 1320c-9.

- On what authority are the records sought? Some state statutes protect peer review records from subpoena, discovery, or disclosure; other laws simply declare the records confidential or privileged.

Some recent cases illustrate the high degree of variability in court decisions regarding the discovery of peer review records:

- The Pennsylvania peer review privilege does not apply to physician credentialing records created by an independent practitioner model HMO, according to the high court in that state.[36] An independent practice association (IPA) HMO does not come within the definition of health care provider in the peer review statute because it is neither a direct provider, nor an administrator of a health care facility.
- Physician credentialing documents were discoverable in a physician's suit against a hospital for discriminating against him in violation of the Americans with Disabilities Act (ADA), a Louisiana court ruled.[37] Although a state law peer review privilege existed, the court ruled that federal law, which provides no similar privilege, applied.
- The statutory peer review privilege in North Dakota applies only to those committees mandated by the statute, the high court in that state ruled.[38] The court rejected the argument that the activities of all committees performing quality assurance functions are privileged, limiting coverage to committees specifically enumerated in the statute.

Admissibility of Peer Review Records

Even if they are not protected from discovery by state law, peer review and quality assurance committee records may be inadmissible as hearsay. Unlike patient records, committee minutes and reports often do not meet the formal requirements of the business records exception to the hearsay rule. Peer review and quality assurance committees do not generate records at or reasonably soon after the time at which the events discussed occurred. Moreover, committee records usually contain conclusions or opinions that generally are inadmissible.

Another option for a party seeking to admit medical staff committee records into evidence is to obtain the records and allow an expert witness

---

[36]McClellan v. Health Maintenance Org., 686 A.2d 801 (Pa. 1996).

[37]Robertson v. Neuromedical Ctr., 169 F.R.D. 80 (M.D. La. 1996).

[38]Trinity Med. Ctr. v. Holum, 544 N.W.2d 148 (N.D. 1996).

to review them before trial. Under the federal rules of evidence, the expert witness may be able to testify as to the content of the records, by expressing an opinion based, in part, on information "perceived by or made known to him at or before hearing."[39] Further, an expert witness may be able to testify concerning the contents of medical records even though the records are found to have been admitted improperly.[40]

Practical Tips

Since state statutes and court decisions on the protection of peer review and quality assurance activities from discovery vary considerably, participants should review carefully and understand thoroughly the applicable law. Health care administrators should organize and operate peer review and quality assurance activities in a manner designed to obtain the greatest possible protection available, in consultation with legal counsel. Once policies for committee records are in place, all personnel involved in committee activities should be educated as to the importance of following meticulously those policies. All peer review committee minutes and reports should be prepared carefully and should demonstrate that the committee performed an objective, considered review. Committee minutes should document actions taken on the matter discussed and not the details of the actual discussion or personal comments made by committee members. Administrators should limit distribution of and access to committee minutes and reports to as few individuals and files as possible.

Incident Reports

Incident reports are another type of document likely to be sought during health care litigation, but potentially protected from discovery. A health care facility or office generates incident reports to document the circumstances surrounding an incident, to alert its insurer or defense counsel to a potential liability situation, and to create data with which to monitor the number and type of incidents occurring in the institution. Incident reports are an essential part of good risk and claims management programs and, like other records, can be a fertile source of information for parties in litigation.

---

[39]Fed. R. Evid. 703.

[40]*See, e.g.*, Wilson v. Clark, 417 N.E.2d 1322 (Ill.), *cert. denied*, 102 S. Ct. 140 (1981).

In many states, incident reports are protected from discovery primarily under the attorney-client privilege and the attorney work product rule. Where legal advice is sought from an attorney, communications between the attorney and the client are privileged and may not be disclosed by the attorney unless the client waives the privilege.[41] Therefore, an incident report made to an attorney for purposes of obtaining legal advice based thereon may not be discovered.[42] Because dissemination of incident reports can waive the protection of the attorney-client privilege, it is imperative that the circulation of the reports be strictly limited.

The scope and application of any privilege that may protect incident reports from discovery is highly dependent on state law, the allegations in the lawsuit, the job duties of the individuals developing and reviewing the reports, and the surrounding circumstances. The following decisions illustrate the variability of court rulings and the importance of specific, strictly implemented procedures regarding incident reports:

- An Illinois court ruled that a report written by a coordinator in a hospital's risk management department is not discoverable in a malpractice suit against the hospital.[43] The court observed that the hospital relied on the coordinator's advice and opinions in its decision to settle or litigate matters. The coordinator therefore was entitled to the protection of a privilege when communicating with hospital counsel.

- In a New York case, a federal court ruled that a state confidentiality law did not prevent discovery of hospital incident reports in a civil rights lawsuit involving the kidnapping of an infant on hospital premises.[44] The parents sued the hospital under federal civil rights laws and sought to discover incident reports prepared about the kidnapping. Although under state law incident reports are protected from release in medical malpractice lawsuits, the court ruled that the hospital's interests must give way when violations of constitutional law are involved.

- The Iowa Supreme Court ruled that statements prepared by nurses shortly after an incident and in anticipation of litigation were discov-

---

[41]*See* Alexander C. Black, Annotation, *What Corporate Communications Are Entitled to Attorney-Client Privilege—Modern Cases,* 27 A.L.R.5th 76.

[42]*See* Sierra Vista Hosp. v. Superior Ct., 56 Cal. Rptr. 387 (Ct. App. 1967).

[43]Mlynarski v. Rush Presbyterian-St. Luke's Med. Ctr., 572 N.E.2d 1025 (Ill. App. Ct. 1991).

[44]White v. New York City Health and Hosp. Corps., No. 88 Civ. 7536 (LBS) (S.D.N.Y. Mar. 19, 1990) (unpublished).

erable because two years had elapsed between the incident and the nurses' depositions and the nurses were able to recall very little of the event.[45]

- A New York court permitted discovery of postincident investigation reports.[46] A patient alleging that she was misdiagnosed attempted to discover statements and records relating to an investigation of her case. The court found that the reports were not protected from discovery within a New York statute prohibiting disclosure of records relating to medical review functions. Although peer review investigations are protected by the statute, the hospital could not establish that the incident reports constituted a medical review function.

Admissibility of Incident Reports

Since incident reports constitute hearsay, they are inadmissible in evidence unless they fall within one of the exceptions to the hearsay rule. The hearsay exception most frequently cited for the purpose of admitting incident reports into evidence is the business records exception, particularly where the party seeking the reports can show that the report was made in the routine course of business at or near the time of the occurrence reported under circumstances that would indicate a high degree of trustworthiness.[47] Although some courts have interpreted "business" narrowly, the trend is toward admitting incident reports that meet the requirements of the business record exception.

Practical Tips

Although it is becoming difficult in some jurisdictions to prevent discovery and admission of incident reports, a health care facility, office, or organization that has established incident-reporting procedures should take specific actions to protect its reports. It should

- treat incident reports as confidential documents, clearly marked as such;

---

[45]Berg v. Des Moines Gen. Hosp. Co., 456 N.W.2d 173 (Iowa 1990).
[46]Wiener v. Memorial Hosp. for Cancer and Allied Diseases, 453 N.Y.S.2d 142 (Sup. Ct. 1982).
[47]*See* Fagan v. Newark, 188 A.2d 427 (N.J. Super. Ct. App. Div. 1963).

- limit strictly the number of copies made and the distribution of the reports in the institution;
- not place a copy of the report in the patient's medical record or in a file on the patient care unit, although it may retain copies with other quality assurance records;
- limit the content of the report to facts, not conclusions or assignment of blame, and place analyses of the cause of an incident in a separate document;
- address the report and any separate analysis of an incident to the attorney or claims manager by name;
- train personnel to complete incident reports with the same care used in completing a medical record; and
- treat incident reports generally as quality assurance records and subject them to the same stringent policies as are applied to other quality assurance records.

11

Legal Theories in Improper Disclosure Cases

Chapter Objectives

- Describe how state statutes affect liability for releasing medical record information.
- List the elements of a defamation claim and describe when releasing patient information might constitute defamation.
- Discuss the privileges against liability for releasing patient information.
- Describe the effect of a patient's consent to release information.
- Distinguish between a defamation claim and an invasion of privacy claim.
- List the types of invasion of privacy claims and give examples in the health information context.
- Discuss the potential liability for publishing patient photographs, releasing patient information to obtain reimbursement, and divulging patient information to the news media.
- List the elements of a breach of confidentiality claim and give examples in the health care context.

INTRODUCTION

Health care providers and institutions may face civil and criminal liability for a release of medical records information that has not been authorized by the patient or that has not been made pursuant to statutory, regulatory, or other legal authority. State statutes and regulations may provide for criminal or professional disciplinary sanctions for violating statutory confidentiality requirements, as discussed in examples throughout this book. State laws and regulations may also expressly grant individuals the ability to file civil suits and recover particular damages under specified circumstances. Unlike a criminal proceeding, which is initiated by government officials, a civil lawsuit must be instituted by a private individual, who usually seeks an award of monetary damages. Civil liability also may be grounded in "common law," as established by court decisions.

STATUTORY BASES FOR LIABILITY

State statutes may impose both criminal sanctions and civil liability on health care providers that disclose medical records information without authorization. A Tennessee law, for example, addresses both types of consequences for breaching confidentiality, making a willful violation of the medical records confidentiality statute a misdemeanor. In addition, hospitals (and their employees, medical and nursing personnel, and officers) in that state may be held liable for civil damages for "willful or reckless or wanton" violations of the confidentiality statute.[1] The Illinois Mental Health and Developmental Disabilities Confidentiality Act more specifically lists the civil remedies available to the patient: "Any person aggrieved by a violation of this Act may sue for damages, an injunction, or other appropriate relief. Reasonable attorney's fees and costs may be awarded to the successful plaintiff in any action under this Act."[2]

In some states, statutes impose specific criminal and/or civil penalties for revealing particular types of medical information, such as a patient's human immunodeficiency virus (HIV) status. For example, in Wisconsin, an individual who negligently discloses a patient's HIV status may be liable for actual damages (which compensate for losses suffered and proved by the patient), as well as $1,000 in punitive, or exemplary, damages (which are intended to punish the violator). An individual who intention-

---

[1] Tenn. Code Ann. § 68-11-311.
[2] 740 Ill. Comp. Stat. Ann. 110/15.

ally discloses a patient's HIV status may be liable for up to $5,000 in punitive damages. If the disclosure causes bodily or psychological harm to the patient, the violator may be fined up to $10,000 and sentenced to nine months in jail in a criminal proceeding.[3] Additional examples of statutes prescribing remedies for improper disclosure of particular types of medical information are included throughout this book. The remainder of this chapter discusses civil liability for improper disclosure of medical information.

THEORIES OF LIABILITY

Whether a patient suing to recover monetary damages for release of confidential medical information cites statutory or common law authority to pursue a claim, the patient must state a valid legal theory, or cause of action. The patient must then prove the required "elements" of the cause of action to establish that a compensable injury occurred. Three legal theories pertinent to medical information liability are discussed below: defamation, invasion of privacy, and breach of confidentiality.

Defamation

Defamation is one legal theory under which patients may file civil lawsuits for unauthorized disclosure of medical information. To prevail in a suit for defamation, the patient must prove the following:

- a false and defamatory statement about the patient
- "publication" of the statement to a third party
- fault on the part of the publishing person
- either injury caused by the statement, or that the statement falls into a category not requiring proof of injury[4]

A communication is defamatory if it "tends so to harm the reputation of another as to lower him in the estimation of the community or to deter third persons from associating or dealing with him."[5] If the individual bringing the defamation suit is a public official or public figure, that indi-

---

[3]WIS. STAT. § 252.15(8).
[4]RESTATEMENT (SECOND) OF TORTS § 558.
[5]RESTATEMENT (SECOND) OF TORTS § 559.

vidual must also prove that the speaker knew the statement was false or acted with reckless disregard of its truth or falsity.[6]

There are two types of defamation. Traditionally, libel is the written form of defamation, while slander is oral. A libel suit may be pursued without proof of actual damages, although slander suits ordinarily require actual damages, unless the statement falls into a special class of defamatory comments.[7] Thus, even oral disclosure of medical record information by a health care provider to an unauthorized person could result in an action for defamation, if the information is false and would affect a person's reputation adversely in the community.

However, a patient's chance of obtaining a recovery against a health care provider for defamation for release of medical records information is slight. Medical records entries ordinarily are true. As a general rule, truth of the published statement is an absolute defense to a civil cause of action for libel or slander, irrespective of the publisher's motive. Although the rule has been modified in some states to allow application of the truth defense only where the publisher's motive was good, the traditional rule, even as modified, provides substantial protection for health care providers.

Patients who sue health care providers for defamation must prove that the defamatory statement was published—that is, that it was revealed to someone other than the patient or health care provider. For example, a state appeals court affirmed a judgment in favor of two physicians when the allegedly libelous statement was contained in a letter that the physicians mailed to the patient.[8] The physicians prepared a letter containing the results of a patient's physical examination, including a statement that the patient had had gonorrhea during the patient's marriage. The statement was not true. When the letter arrived at the patient's home, the patient's wife opened it and read it to him over the telephone. The patient and his wife sued the physicians for libel, claiming that the defamatory contents of the letter caused marital discord. The court rejected the patient's suit because the letter was sealed and addressed only to the patient. The letter was not published to the patient's wife, except by the patient, who had asked her to read it to him over the phone.

---

[6]*See, e.g.,* New York Times Co. v. Sullivan, 376 U.S. 254 (1964); McKinnon v. Smith, 275 N.Y.S.2d 900 (Sup. Ct. 1966), *aff'd*, 300 N.Y.S.2d 520 (App. Div. 1969).

[7]RESTATEMENT (SECOND) OF TORTS § 568. An individual suing for slander need not prove that he suffered actual harm if the statement imputes a criminal offense, a loathsome disease, a matter compatible with his profession, or serious sexual misconduct. *See also* RESTATEMENT (SECOND) OF TORTS § 570.

[8]Dowell v. Cleveland Clinic Found., No. 59963 (Ohio Ct. App. 1992) (unpublished).

Privileges against Defamation

Two privileges may serve as a defense for health care providers sued for defamation, even if the patient proves the elements of a defamation claim. These are absolute privilege and qualified privilege. The absolute privilege protects publications made in legislative, judicial, and administrative proceedings. Thus, statements made in those contexts ordinarily do not serve as the basis for a defamation suit. In a Maryland case, for example, a psychologist's courtroom statements during custody proceedings that a father sexually abused his child were absolutely privileged, although they were defamatory.[9] There are limits to the scope of absolute privilege, however. One court has stated that a physician who discloses medical records information in connection with a court proceeding may lose the protection of absolute privilege upon disclosing information unrelated to the court action.[10]

The second type of privilege, known as conditional, or qualified, privilege, provides protection from defamation liability if the person who publishes the statement reasonably believes that

- the information affects a sufficiently important interest of the publisher and
- the recipient's knowledge of the information serves the lawful protection of that interest.[11]

Thus, a court examining whether a statement is protected by qualified privilege will examine the publisher's motive and interest in disclosing the information. The extent of the qualified privilege is uncertain and impossible to reduce to a formula. The disclosure must be justified by the importance of the interest served, and it must be called for by a legal or moral duty, or by generally accepted standards of decent conduct.

For example, a hospital was not liable for defamation for indicating on an insurance claim form that an unmarried 14-year-old was pregnant because the institution had acted within its qualified privilege.[12] The hospital

---

[9]Rosenberg v. Helsinki, 616 A.2d 866 (Md. 1992). *See also* O'Barr v. Feist, 296 So. 2d 152 (Ala. 1974) (letter from physician to probate judge absolutely privileged); Bond v. Pecaut, 561 F. Supp. 1037 (N.D. Ill. 1983), *aff'd*, 734 F.2d 18 (7th Cir. 1984) (letter from psychologist relevant to custody proceedings and within judicial privilege).

[10]Moses v. McWilliams, 549 A.2d 950 (Pa. Super. Ct. 1988).

[11]Restatement (Second) of Torts § 594.

[12]Edwards v. University of Chicago Hosp., 484 N.E.2d 1100 (Ill. App. Ct. 1985).

was required to provide a diagnosis to the insurance company in order to receive compensation for its services. Although the diagnosis of pregnancy was incorrect, the court ruled that the hospital was shielded from liability by a qualified privilege. Specifically, the hospital had acted in good faith and in pursuit of its valid business interest in obtaining compensation. In addition, the statement was limited in scope to the proper purpose, occasion, manner, and parties, having been disclosed only as required on the standard insurance claim forms. As illustrated by this case, the qualified privilege provides important protection against defamation liability for health care providers who release potentially defamatory information to insurers, health plans, utilization reviewers, and others with control over payment for medical services. However, health care personnel are cautioned to consider other legal theories and statutes, discussed throughout this chapter and elsewhere in the book, that may create liability.

Courts have also applied the qualified privilege against defamation when the interest of a health care provider is not directly affected. Such cases may arise when medical records information is disclosed to employers, insurance companies, litigating parties, news media, etc. For example, an insurance company was sued by one of its insureds after the company had informed an agency subscribed to by other life insurance companies that the insured had a heart condition. The court dismissed the suit, holding that the insurance company's disclosure was shielded by qualified privilege.[13] In a later case based on virtually identical facts, a court found that a qualified privilege to exchange medical information was supported by the insurer's and agency's business interest in the information, as well as the public's interest in the insurance industry.[14] Another court has held that, in an action under that state's privacy statute, a qualified privilege protects parties who disclose medical information where the disclosure is reasonably necessary to protect or further a legitimate business interest.[15]

The qualified privilege may also apply when release of information serves a public duty, such as protecting the community from highly contagious diseases.[16] For example, in an early case, the Nebraska Supreme

---

[13]Mayer v. Northern Life Ins. Co., 119 F. Supp. 536 (N.D. Cal. 1953).

[14]Senogles v. Security Benefit Life Ins., 536 P.2d 1358 (Kan. 1975); *see also* Hauge v. Fidelity Guar. Life Ins. Co., No. 91-C-20033 (N.D. Ill. 1992) (unpublished).

[15]Bratt v. International Bus. Machs. Corp., 467 N.E.2d 126 (Mass. 1984). *See also* Hauge v. Fidelity Guar. Life Ins. Co., No. 91-C-20033 (N.D. Ill. 1992) (unpublished).

[16]Annotation, *Libel and Slander: Privilege of Statements by Physician, Surgeon, or Nurse Concerning Patient*, 73 A.L.R.2d 325.

Court held a physician not liable for disclosing to the owner of a board-inghouse that a patient living there had a venereal disease.[17] In addition to intimating that the diagnosis was incorrect, the court reasoned that the rules of qualified privilege, under the law of defamation, would govern this case. The physician was held to have had a moral or legal duty to disclose his diagnosis to those persons who might be endangered by this contagious disease. In a more recent decision, a physician who misdiagnosed a patient's pelvic inflammatory disease and told the patient's husband that she had gonorrhea was protected by privilege.[18] In spite of the holding in these cases, health care providers should be wary of revealing information regarding a patient's contagious status to third parties. Many states now have statutes specifying when and to whom such information may be revealed (see examples in Chapter 9, HIV/AIDS: MANDATORY REPORTING AND CONFIDENTIALITY). Further, other legal theories, such as those discussed later in this chapter, may serve as a basis for liability.

A request for information by a totally disinterested party, however, never can create a qualified privilege. For a disclosure to be privileged, the party to whom it is made must have a valid interest in obtaining the information. Whether or not the information was requested or volunteered will help to determine whether the publisher acted in good faith or had a moral duty to communicate. Moreover, it is important to remember that the qualified privilege can be lost if the publisher

- knows the statement is false or recklessly disregards its falsity,
- publishes the statement for an improper purpose,
- excessively publishes the statement, or
- lacks reasonable belief that the publication is necessary to protect the interest.[19]

For example, in one case a physician's notation in a medical record that the patient's wife may have abused her children was protected by qualified privilege. The patient's wife could proceed with a defamation suit, however, because she produced evidence that the physician abused the privilege by acting with malice.[20] She alleged that there was a heated telephone

---

[17]Simonsen v. Swenson, 177 N.W. 831 (Neb. 1920); *see also* Shoemaker v. Friedburg, 183 P.2d 318 (Cal. Ct. App. 1947).

[18]Thomas v. Hillson, 361 S.E.2d 278 (Ga. Ct. App. 1987).

[19]RESTATEMENT (SECOND) OF TORTS § 594.

[20]Strauss v. Thorne, 490 N.W.2d 908 (Minn. Ct. App. 1992).

conversation between herself and the physician prior to the notation, that the physician said he made the notation to get back at her, and that the physician refused to remove the notation when he learned his concerns were not reportable to social services.

Consent as a Defense

Even in the absence of a privilege, a health care provider will not be liable for the release of medical information if the patient has consented to the release. A person who knowingly consents to the release of medical records is barred from bringing a defamation suit when those records subsequently are released. In a Minnesota case, for example, a pilot submitted to a chemical dependency evaluation at the request of his employer.[21] Before the analysis, the pilot had consented to the release of information relating to his evaluation and treatment. The records, which contained the diagnosis of alcoholism, were released to the pilot's employer and the employer's insurance company. The pilot sued the facility where the test was performed and the chemical dependency counselor, alleging that they had defamed him with the diagnosis. Although the pilot admitted that he had signed release forms, he contended that he did not consent to the release of the defamatory statements because they did not exist at the time he signed the forms. However, the court found no indication that the pilot did not know the implications of the forms that he signed, and no evidence of fraud or malice on the part of those who prepared the reports. The court concluded that the pilot could not sue for defamation.

Health care providers should take care, however, not to exceed the scope of a patient's consent to release medical records information. If the disclosure of the record exceeds the scope of the authorization given by the patient or other appropriate person, the disclosure will be unauthorized and therefore unprotected in the event of a defamation suit.

To avoid defamation cases, health care personnel are well advised to take the conservative approach and withhold medical records information unless they find exceptionally good reasons to disclose it. They should establish appropriate reasons for disclosure with the help of their legal counsel and should set forth those reasons in their medical records policies.

---

[21]Williamson v. Stocker, No. 4-79-335 slip op. (D. Minn. Dec. 21, 1982) (unpublished); *see also* Clark v. Geraci, 208 N.Y.S.2d 564 (Sup. Ct. 1960).

Invasion of Privacy

A second legal theory upon which a patient could base a suit for improper release of medical information is invasion of privacy. Because health information is highly personal, improper disclosure of patient information to unauthorized individuals, agencies, or news media may make a hospital liable to the patient for an invasion of privacy. A cause of action for invasion of privacy can be based on state common law, state or federal constitutional law, or state statutory law. The purpose of the right is to protect against mass dissemination of information concerning private, personal matters. A claim for invasion of privacy will be successful only if the challenged publication is not a matter of legitimate public concern and would be highly offensive to a reasonable person.[22] Some courts have held that an oral publication alone cannot constitute an invasion of privacy, although others have allowed recovery, especially where the plaintiff proved actual damages.[23]

The theories of defamation and invasion of privacy are similar in terms of the circumstances that may create liability. However, several factors distinguish the two causes of action:

- Truth of the information published is not a defense to an invasion of privacy suit, although it is a defense in a defamation suit. Thus, an unauthorized disclosure even of accurate medical information could subject a hospital to liability for invasion of a patient's privacy.
- To recover for an invasion of privacy, the plaintiff need not prove special damages, unlike the plaintiff in a defamation action, who often must prove that the disclosure actually harmed him or her.
- The two theories provide redress for different types of injury. A cause of action for invasion of privacy focuses on the harm a disclosure has caused to the plaintiff's feelings. Thus, a plaintiff in an action for invasion of privacy may recover even for the disclosure of favorable information. Defamation, on the other hand, focuses on the injury to the plaintiff's reputation.
- Although an action for invasion of privacy often involves publication, it is not a necessary element for recovery. Thus discovery of private information by a single person can invade an individual's privacy. The law of defamation normally requires publication to a second person.

---

[22]RESTATEMENT (SECOND) OF TORTS § 652D.

[23]I.J. Schiffres, Annotation, *Invasion of Right of Privacy by Merely Oral Declarations*, 19 A.L.R.3d 1318.

The common law has established several types of invasion of privacy claims:

- unreasonable intrusion upon the seclusion of another
- appropriation of another's name or likeness
- unreasonable publicity of another's private life
- unreasonable publicity that places another in a false light[24]

Invasion of privacy claims based on state or federal constitutions, as opposed to those rooted in common law, occur less frequently. A patient who brings a claim for improper disclosure of medical information based on the federal or state constitution typically must show that the individual had a "reasonable expectation of privacy" concerning the information that was disclosed.[25] Courts will consider factors such as the content of the disclosure and the circumstances under which the patient provided the information to the health care worker. A patient may also sue a health care provider under a state statute creating a right to sue for certain invasions of privacy. For example, the Massachusetts statute states that "[a] person shall have a right against unreasonable, substantial, or serious interference with his privacy."[26]

If a patient consents to disclosure of patient information, the patient cannot later successfully claim that the disclosure was an invasion of privacy, if the disclosure was within the scope of the consent.[27] Thus, health care providers should obtain a patient's written consent before releasing medical information. If a patient verbally authorizes a disclosure but refuses to sign an authorization form, health care personnel should note the verbal consent, properly sign and date the note, and insert it in the patient's medical record.

Health care institutions, organizations, and providers should protect against invasion of privacy claims by developing and implementing policies and procedures that address problematic circumstances. Confidentiality policies should be written clearly, avoiding vague language.[28] The following discussion illustrates some problematic circumstances where

---

[24]RESTATEMENT (SECOND) OF TORTS § 652A.

[25]*See, e.g.*, Urbaniak v. Newton, 226 Cal. App. 3d 1128 (Ct. App. 1991).

[26]MASS. ANN. LAWS ch. 214, § 1B.

[27]*See, e.g.*, Clark v. Geraci, 208 N.Y.S.2d 564 (Sup. Ct. 1960). Patient had authorized physician to disclose incomplete information about his illness; plaintiff therefore could not claim that he had not consented to the disclosure of the underlying cause of the illness—alcoholism.

[28]*See, e.g.*, Group Health Plan, Inc. v. Lopez, 341 N.W.2d 294 (Minn. Ct. App. 1983).

clear and widely disseminated policies can reduce invasion of privacy liability risks.

Photographs

The use of photographs in medical care creates a potential for invasion of privacy actions, under more than one type of claim. Courts have held health care providers liable for the *appropriation of likeness* type of invasion of privacy primarily where the provider exploited the patient for commercial benefit. However, courts also have imposed liability where a health care provider used a patient's name or likeness for a noncommercial benefit under the *intrusion upon seclusion* type of invasion of privacy. This theory can lead to liability even if the photographs were not published. In an early Pennsylvania case, for example, the court prohibited a physician from using photographs of a patient's facial development in connection with medical instruction.[29] The court found that even taking the picture without the patient's express consent was an invasion of privacy; it was not necessary to show that the physician had used the photographs improperly or shown them to others to establish liability. A court in Maine reached a similar conclusion in a case where a physician photographed a terminally ill patient shortly before his death.[30] The court rejected the physician's argument that his scientific interest in the photograph justified taking the picture. The court held that unauthorized photography under such circumstances would constitute an invasion of privacy, whether or not the photographs were published.[31]

Publication of photographs also may subject health care providers to liability under the type of invasion of privacy known as *unreasonable publicity of private life*. For example, a court ruled that a physician had invaded a patient's privacy by using "before-and-after" photos of her face to demonstrate the effects of a face lift on television and at a department store presentation.[32] The use of the photographs publicized the fact that the patient had had a face lift, which she found embarrassing and distress-

---

[29]Clayman v. Bernstein, 38 Pa. D. & C. 543 (1940).

[30]Estate of Berthiaume v. Pratt, 365 A.2d 792 (Me. 1976).

[31]*See also* Bazemore v. Savannah Hosp., 155 S.E. 194 (Ga. 1930). For a discussion of taking unauthorized photographs as invasion of privacy in this and other contexts, *see* Phillip E. Hassman, Annotation, *Taking Unauthorized Photographs as Invasion of Privacy*, 86 A.L.R.3d 374.

[32]Vassiliades v. Garfinckel's, 492 A.2d 580 (D.C. 1985).

ing. The court held that the patient's right to privacy outweighed the public's general interest in plastic surgery and held the physician liable.[33]

Medical record information policies should establish the circumstances under which a patient may be photographed. Photographs taken in connection with scientific research should be part of a research protocol approved by appropriate committees of the medical staff. All other photographs of patients should be taken in accordance with institutional or organizational policies and procedures. In general, these policies should require approval of such photography by an appropriate health care administrator.

Invasion of Privacy within the Health Care Setting

Courts have found an unwarranted intrusion upon the plaintiff's seclusion or private concerns where the defendant monitored the plaintiff's telephone calls or bedroom, invaded the plaintiff's house, or in other ways intruded in an objectionable manner into the plaintiff's concerns. Monitoring a patient's telephone conversations from the hospital may subject an institution not only to liability for invasion of privacy, but also to liability under federal statutes prohibiting the interception of private communications.[34] Also, in allowing nonmedical personnel to witness medical procedures or to examine a patient without the patient's consent, the invasion of the patient's privacy may lead to litigation.[35] Teaching hospitals, especially, should be certain their patients understand that they will be participating in the education and training of medical, nursing, and other students who may observe or assist in treatment.

Payment-Related Disclosures

It is unlikely that a health care institution, organization, individual provider, or other personnel will be held liable for invasion of privacy upon releasing medical records information for the purpose of obtaining

---

[33]When an individual's name or likeness is published in connection with a newsworthy event, the person does not have an action for invasion of privacy. *See also* Gilbert v. Medical Econs. Co., 665 F.2d 305 (10th Cir. 1981) (newsworthiness of physician's psychiatric history precludes liability for disclosure). *See* discussion under "Disclosure to the News Media," in this chapter.

[34]Gerrard v. Blackman, 401 F. Supp. 1189 (N.D. Ill. 1975).

[35]*See* Knight v. Penobscot Bay Med. Ctr., 420 A.2d 915 (Me. 1980). The viewing of plaintiff's delivery of child by nurse's husband was found, under the circumstances, not to be an invasion of privacy.

reimbursement. Court decisions have established that publication of information to an extent reasonably calculated to serve the legitimate interests of the publisher does not constitute a common law invasion of privacy.[36] This restriction is similar to the qualified privilege in defamation actions. Thus, release or disclosure of information in the medical record to individuals such as insurance company representatives and utilization reviewers for purposes of reimbursement ordinarily would not constitute an invasion of the common law right of privacy.[37] At least one court has extended this type of privilege to provide a shield from liability for even constitutional invasion of privacy.[38] The court held that an employer who reviewed prescription drug benefit records for the purpose of controlling costs did not violate an employee's constitutional right to privacy. The prescription drug records, obtained by the employer's drug benefit vendor, linked employee names with specific medications, revealing that the employee was HIV-positive. The court concluded that the employer's interest in controlling costs outweighed the employee's right to privacy.

Statutory provisions may also protect providers from actions based on payment-related disclosures. In Massachusetts, for example, an exception in the patient bill of rights statute says that confidentiality of records provisions shall not prevent any third-party reimburser from inspecting and copying all records relating to diagnosis, treatment, or other services to determine benefits, as long as the patient's insurance policy permits access to the records.[39]

Disclosure to the News Media

The circumstance most likely to create invasion of privacy questions may be the release of patient information to news entities. (For a related discussion on protecting the confidentiality of celebrity patients, see Chapter 8, DOCUMENTATION AND DISCLOSURE: SPECIAL AREAS OF CONCERN.) A

---

[36]*See generally* Voneye v. Turner, 240 S.W.2d 588 (Ky. Ct. App. 1951); Patton v. Jacobs, 78 N.E.2d 789 (Ind. Ct. App. 1948); Lewis v. Physicians & Dentists Credit Bureau, 177 P.2d 896 (Wash. 1947).

[37]Pennison v. Provident Life & Accident Ins. Co., 154 So. 2d 617 (La. Ct. App. 1963) (disclosure to plaintiff's insurance company not an invasion of privacy); Edwards v. University of Chicago Hosp., 484 N.E.2d 1100 (Ill. App. Ct. 1985) (no liability where hospital publishes diagnosis in standard insurance claim form to obtain payment); Joel E. Smith, Annotation, *Exchange Among Insurers of Medical Information Concerning Insured or Applicant for Insurance as Invasion of Privacy*, 98 A.L.R.3d 561.

[38]Doe v. SEPTA, 72 F.3d 1133 (3d Cir. 1995).

[39]MASS. ANN. LAWS ch. 111, § 70E.

health care provider has no legal obligation to disclose medical records information to news media. In some states, statutes limit the dissemination of medical records information to certain entities or individuals that the state has deemed to have a legitimate interest in the information, such as courts, arbitrators, government and private commissions, insurers, employee benefit plans, and medical staffs.[40]

Where not prohibited by statute, health care institutions and organizations may release patient information to the media under certain circumstances. Announcements of patient admissions, discharges, or births may pose no problem, for example, unless a facility specializes in the care of patients with specific diseases that are considered shameful or embarrassing.[41] A drug or alcohol addiction rehabilitation center, for example, should not release the names of patients. Even where releasing general information is permissible, the scope of the information should be considered carefully. To publicize the fact that a particular patient gave birth to a normal healthy baby may not be considered an invasion of privacy, for instance, but to publicize the fact that the baby was conceived through artificial insemination might be actionable.

A health care entity that discloses medical records information to the news media may be sued for common law invasion of privacy under two theories: (1) unreasonable publicity of another's private life or (2) unreasonable publicity that places another in a false light. However, a health care provider will not be liable for invasion of privacy if the information disclosed to the news media is newsworthy or a matter of legitimate public interest. If the patient is a public figure, the person's prominence, in itself, makes virtually all of the patient's doings of interest to the public and therefore not subject to invasion of privacy actions.[42] Relatively obscure people voluntarily may take certain actions that bring them before the public, or they may be victims of newsworthy occurrences, such as accidents, crimes, etc., thus making them of interest to the public.[43] The

---

[40]*See, e.g.*, Cal. Civ. Code § 56.10.

[41]*See* Koudsi v. Hennepin County Med. Ctr., 317 N.W.2d 705 (Minn. 1982).

[42]*See, e.g.*, Cason v. Baskin, 30 So. 2d 635 (Fla. 1947); Jeffrey F. Ghent, Annotation, Waiver or Loss of Privacy, 57 A.L.R.3d 16.

[43]For example, in Estate of Hemingway v. Random House, Inc., 244 N.E.2d 250 (N.Y. 1968), Ernest Hemingway's widow was unable to recover for invasion of privacy against an author for a memoir describing the widow's personal feelings and relationship with her husband. In Howell v. New York Post Co., 612 N.E.2d 699 (N.Y. 1993), a patient whose photo, showing her walking alongside a public figure on the grounds of a psychiatric facility, was published on the front page of the newspaper could not recover for invasion of privacy.

latitude extended to the publication of the personal matters, names, photographs, etc., of public figures varies.

Ordinary citizens who voluntarily adopt a course of action that is newsworthy cannot complain if their names and pictures are published. For example, a patient who filed a $38 million malpractice lawsuit against a physician was not entitled to sue the physician later for invasion of privacy when the physician informed a newspaper reporter that the patient was HIV positive.[44] The court held that medical malpractice lawsuits, particularly those for large monetary sums, were a matter of legitimate public interest. By filing such a suit, the patient was precluded from later claiming that his privacy had been invaded by the physician's public comments regarding the suit. The physician revealed the HIV status to explain why the patient had not been diagnosed accurately. In another case, HIV-positive individuals who revealed their identities in numerous panel discussions, publications, and meetings could not later sue when their names were published in a "living with HIV" government program guide.[45] By revealing their names in other contexts, they had waived their right to privacy.

An illness or an accident also may be newsworthy.[46] Courts have held that the name and photograph of the victim of a circumstance that itself is newsworthy may be published.[47] However, the court may distinguish between the newsworthiness of the event and the newsworthiness of the identity of the individual involved. One court has ruled that, even when a particular medical condition is of interest to the public, hospitals that reveal the identity of individuals with that condition are subject to invasion of privacy actions.[48] In that case, a married couple who participated in a hospital's in vitro fertilization program sued the hospital for invasion of privacy. The couple attended the hospital's private social function for in vitro participants. Although they refused to be interviewed and avoided a news crew attending the event, the couple appeared on a televised news

[44]Lee v. Calhoun, 948 F.2d 1162 (10th Cir. 1991), *cert. denied*, 504 U.S. 973 (1992).

[45]Doe v. Marsh, No. 96-7453 (2d Cir. Oct. 7. 1996) (unpublished).

[46]*See, e.g.,* The Home News v. New Jersey, 677 A.2d 195 (N.J. 1996)) (newspaper may receive cause of death information about boy who died under suspicious circumstances).

[47]Bremmer v. Journal-Tribune Publ'g Co., 76 N.W.2d 762 (Iowa 1956) (publication of mutilated dead boy's picture); Kelley v. Post Publ'g Co., 98 N.E.2d 286 (Mass. 1951) (publication of automobile accident victim's picture); Jones v. Herald Post Co., 18 S.W.2d 972 (Ky. 1929) (publication of picture of murder victim's wife who had struggled with her husband's assailants); Metter v. Los Angeles Examiner, 95 P.2d 491 (Cal. Ct. App. 1939) (publication of picture of one who committed suicide). *See also* Irwin J. Schiffres, Annotation, *Invasion of Privacy by Use of Plaintiff's Name or Likeness for Nonadvertising Purposes*, 30 A.L.R.3d 203.

[48]Y.G. v. Jewish Hosp. of St. Louis, 795 S.W.2d 488 (Mo. Ct. App. 1990).

report. The court ruled that the couple could sue the hospital, reasoning that although in vitro fertilization may be of interest to the general public, individual involvement in such a program is a private matter.

Similarly, a Missouri court held that a magazine could be liable for invasion of privacy when it published the name and picture of a patient in a story titled "Starving Glutton" concerning the patient's hospitalization to treat her constant desire to eat, possibly caused by pancreatic dysfunction.[49] The magazine's employees had obtained the patient's picture by surreptitious means and over her express objections. Holding that the patient was entitled to recover, the court said, "certainly if there is any right of privacy at all, it should include the right to obtain medical treatment at home or in a hospital for an individual personal condition (at least if it is not contagious or dangerous to others) without personal publicity. . . ." The court found that while the patient's ailment was of some interest to the public, her identity was not. Publishing her name and picture, which conveyed no medical information, thus was an invasion of her privacy.[50]

Further, as time passes, the identity of the participant in such an event loses importance and action for invasion of privacy becomes more likely. However, the publisher need not prove that the event was "currently newsworthy" or published contemporaneously. Courts will consider the length of time that has passed between the "event" and publication, along with other factors such as community standards and the importance of the matter published in determining whether the matter publicized is of legitimate public interest.[51]

Although health care providers should be reluctant to release patient information to the news media, in some cases release of information of legitimate news value may be appropriate. In such circumstances, the risk of liability is dependent on the specific nature of the disclosure. The fact that a patient is newsworthy does not require the release of information; it simply may protect the provider who chooses to disclose the information. The patient's condition may not create liability exposure, but disclosing more detailed information or a photograph without the individual's consent should be avoided. While the patient's participation in a newsworthy

---

[49]Barber v. Time, Inc., 159 S.W.2d 291 (Mo. 1942).

[50]*See also* Vassiliades v. Garfinckel's, Brooks Bros., 492 A.2d 580 (D.C. 1985) (plastic surgery patient entitled to expect that photos would not be published, even though plastic surgery is matter of general public interest).

[51]*See* Montesano v. Donrey Media Group, 668 P.2d 1081 (Nev. 1983), *cert. denied*, 466 U.S. 959 (1984); Romaine v. Kallinger, 537 A.2d 284 (N.J. 1988).

event may protect the health care organization or institution that releases specific information about the person from an invasion of privacy action, the best policy health care administrators can adopt is to refuse to release any information (other than the status of the patient) without the patient's consent.

Breach of Confidentiality

Yet another legal theory under which a patient may sue a health care provider who improperly discloses medical records information is breach of confidentiality, also known as breach of physician-patient privilege. The general rule is that a physician who violates the physician-patient privilege is liable to the patient.[52] A patient who successfully sues for breach of the physician-patient privilege is entitled to damages to compensate for harm caused by the disclosure, such as deterioration of a marriage, the loss of a job, and emotional distress.[53]

In some states, the scope, application, and waiver of the privilege are governed by statute.[54] In other states, the privilege was developed in common law, by court decisions. Some courts recognizing the privilege have relied on a public policy that favors the protection of the confidential relationship between doctor and patient. These courts have typically pointed to professional conduct statutes, physician licensing statutes, and medical records confidentiality statutes as evidence of the social importance of the physician-patient privilege.[55]

---

[52]*See, e.g.*, Anker v. Brodnitz, 413 N.Y.S.2d 582 (Sup. Ct. 1979); Alberts v. Devine, 479 N.E.2d 113 (Mass. 1985); Horne v. Patton, 287 So. 2d 824 (Ala. 1973); Stempler v. Speidell, 495 A.2d 857 (N.J. 1985). For an overview of which states have recognized this cause of action, *see* Judy E. Zelin, Annotation, *Physician's Tort Liability for Unauthorized Disclosure of Confidential Information*, 48 A.L.R.4th 668.

[53]*See* MacDonald v. Clinger, 446 N.Y.S.2d 801 (App. Div. 1982).

[54]J.R. Kemper, Annotation, *Commencing Action Involving Physical Condition of Plaintiff or Decedent as Waiving Physician-Patient Privilege as to Discovery Proceedings*, 21 A.L.R.3d 912.

[55]*See, e.g.*, Bryson v. Tillinghast, 749 P.2d 110 (Okla. 1988); Stempler v. Speidell, 495 A.2d 857 (N.J. 1985); Geisberger v. Willuhn, 390 N.E.2d 945 (Ill. App. Ct. 1979); Schaffer v. Spicer, 215 N.W.2d 134 (S.D. 1974); Horne v. Patton, 287 So. 2d 824 (Ala. 1973); Hammonds v. Aetna Cas. and Surety Co., 243 F. Supp. 793 (N.D. Ohio 1965); Hague v. Williams, 181 A.2d 345 (N.J. 1962); Clark v. Geraci, 208 N.Y.S.2d 564 (Sup. Ct. 1960); Berry v. Moench, 331 P.2d 814 (Utah 1958).

A Nebraska court has described what a patient must prove to invoke the physician-patient privilege.[56] The patient must show the following elements:

1. A physician-patient relationship existed
2. The information was acquired during the relationship
3. The information was necessary for the physician's treatment of the patient in a professional capacity

Which categories of health care providers have a duty of confidentiality to their patients has not been definitively established and varies from state to state. In South Carolina, for example, a court held that a pharmacy patient could sue the pharmacy for defamation, but not for breach of confidentiality.[57] A pharmacy employee had falsely told others that the patient was being treated for venereal disease. The court determined that pharmacists have no duty of confidentiality toward their patients. A Rhode Island court ruled that prescription drug information is confidential health information, however.[58] In Indiana, an appeals court rejected a patient's claim that there is a nurse-patient privilege.[59] State statutes may be helpful in identifying the health care providers who owe a duty of confidentiality. In Mississippi, for example, all communications made to a physician, osteopath, dentist, hospital, nurse, pharmacist, podiatrist, optometrist, or chiropractor by a patient under his or her charge or by one seeking professional advice are privileged.[60]

The scope of the information protected by the physician-patient privilege also may be a subject of dispute. In some cases, even a physician's list of patients may be protected. The Nevada Supreme Court, for example, refused to order a plastic surgeon to reveal his patient list, because to do so would have violated the physician-patient privilege.[61] The court ruled that, although disclosure of a patient's name does not always violate the physician-patient privilege, the names are protected if the nature of the treatment is disclosed. To avoid liability for breaching the physician-patient privilege, health care providers and facilities providing specialized

---

[56]Branch v. Wilkinson, 256 N.W.2d 307 (Neb. 1977). *See also* State v. Randle, 484 N.W.2d 220 (Iowa Ct. App. 1992).

[57]Evans v. Rite Aid Corp., 478 S.E.2d 846 (S.C. 1996).

[58]Washburn v. Rite Aid Corp., 695 A.2d 495 (R.I. 1997).

[59]Darnell v. Indiana, 674 N.E.2d 19 (Ind. Ct. App. 1996).

[60]MISS. CODE ANN. § 13-1-21.

[61]Hetter v. Sanchez, 874 P.2d 762 (Nev. 1994).

treatment, such as drug rehabilitation centers, should take care to protect the confidentiality of the identity of their patients.

Defenses against Breach of Confidentiality

As in defamation and invasion of privacy cases, a privilege may serve as a defense to a breach of confidentiality claim against a health care provider. For example, a disclosure is typically privileged if failure to divulge medical record information would jeopardize the health or safety of the patient or others.[62] In one case, the Supreme Court of Oklahoma held that a patient could not sue for breach of the physician-patient privilege when a physician revealed medical information to police, leading to the patient's arrest for rape.[63] A patient sought treatment at a hospital for a bite wound on his genitals. A physician who treated the patient later learned that police were looking for a suspected rapist with that injury. The physician told the police about the patient, leading to his arrest. The patient sued the physician for breaching the doctor-patient privilege. The court dismissed the suit, holding that the physician-patient privilege was not designed to protect criminals from apprehension. The court also ruled that a public policy exception allows physicians to reveal otherwise confidential medical information when the information will benefit the public.[64]

In several jurisdictions, a patient waives the physician-patient privilege, foreclosing claims for breach of the privilege, by putting information exchanged within the privilege at issue in a lawsuit—for example, a medical malpractice lawsuit.[65] However, courts disagree as to the scope of the waiver. This issue is discussed in detail in Chapter 10, DISCOVERY AND ADMISSIBILITY OF HEALTH CARE RECORDS.

Patient consent to disclosure is another defense to a breach of confidentiality suit, although the disclosure must be carefully tailored to remain within the scope of the patient's consent. In an interesting case involving the newspaper publication of a patient's photograph that was taken in a hospital's AIDS clinic waiting room, a New York appeals court ruled that

---

[62]*See, e.g.*, Horne v. Patton, 287 So. 2d 824 (Ala. 1973).

[63]Bryson v. Tillinghast, 749 P.2d 110 (Okla. 1988).

[64]*See also* Mull v. String, 448 So. 2d 952 (Ala. 1984).

[65]*See, e.g.*, Fedell v. Wierzbieniec, 485 N.Y.S.2d 460 (Sup. Ct. 1985). For a discussion of which jurisdictions have adopted this view, *see* J.R. Kemper, Annotation, *Commencing Action Involving Physical Condition of Plaintiff or Decedent as Waiving Physician-Patient Privilege as to Discovery Proceedings*, 21 A.L.R.3d 912.

a patient could sue the hospital and a treating physician for breach of privilege because he had consented to the picture only after they had assured him that he would not be recognizable.[66] When the photograph was published, a friend recognized the patient. Although the court ruled that the hospital had not violated the privilege simply by allowing the media to be present in the waiting room of its infectious disease unit, it held that the physician-patient privilege protects the identity of a patient, as well as the treatment provided. The court concluded that the hospital and physician had possibly breached the privilege by making such assurances and by not informing the patient that the photographer was with the local media.

The same advice for reducing liability for defamation and invasion of privacy applies to breach of confidentiality. Clearly written and widely disseminated policies and procedures concerning the confidentiality of patient information will decrease the likelihood that confidential information will be released in breach of the physician-patient privilege. Health care administrators should implement guidelines that health care and health information professionals can understand and follow.

---

[66]Anderson v. Strong Mem'l Hosp., 542 N.Y.S.2d 96 (App. Div. 1989).

12

Risk Management and Quality Review

Chapter Objectives

- Compare and contrast risk management and quality review.
- Describe the four steps in the risk management process.
- List some of the data, documents, and records a risk manager relies on to identify risks.
- List the activities that are part of the quality improvement process.
- Describe the seven items that must be part of an effective compliance program according to the federal sentencing guidelines.
- List the laws that a health care organization might want to consider when creating a corporate compliance program.

INTRODUCTION

Risk management and quality review programs depend in large measure on medical records and health information managers for information necessary to identify potential risks. Health information managers, therefore, can contribute significantly to the success of risk management and quality review programs; but to do so, they must have a good working knowledge of risk management principles, risk management and quality review program objectives, and the effect of medical records information on the management of potential risk. Corporate compliance programs also are an important part of a health care organization's risk management and quality review programs. A compliance program can reduce the risk of criminal prosecution or civil suits, reduce criminal fines, establish a way to communicate legal and organizational requirements to all staff, and monitor compliance with legal and organizational requirements.

This chapter discusses generally the relationship between quality review and risk management; the definition and components of risk management, quality review, and corporate compliance programs; and the use of medical records in these programs.

RELATIONSHIP BETWEEN RISK MANAGEMENT AND QUALITY REVIEW

The purposes of risk management and quality review often are viewed as complementary. The patient-safety aspect of risk management—preventing events most likely to lead to patient injury—is the area of greatest interaction between quality review and risk management. Poor quality care that creates a risk of injury to patients poses financial risks both to health care practitioners and to health care facilities. Identification and resolution of problems in patient care—the cornerstones of quality review—ultimately prevent events that may result in patient injury and, consequently, reduce the potential risk of liability to the health care provider. Quality review and risk management use similar methodologies to achieve their common aim of ensuring patient safety. Both depend on the establishment of screening criteria, collection and analysis of data pertaining to those criteria, and correction of identified problems through improvements in the individual practices and the overall health care delivery system.

Nevertheless, quality review and risk management differ in at least one significant respect related to the perspective each brings to the analysis of data. Quality review generally approaches the identification and analysis of patient care problems and issues from the perspective of goals for what should occur in the health care organization, whereas risk management tends to approach these tasks from the perspective of what should not occur in that organization. Accordingly, quality review monitors patient care on an ongoing basis and aims to improve quality of care and prevent adverse outcomes, while risk management focuses on risk identifications, protecting the organization's financial and personnel assets, and investigating specific incidents that may result in liability for the organization. Because the sources of data relied on by each of these disciplines are substantially similar, the data may be obtained in a more cost-effective manner if coordinated properly.[1]

In its accreditation manuals, the Joint Commission requires that health care organizations demonstrate integration of quality review and risk management functions by showing an appropriate sharing of information between established quality review and risk management committees and a coordinated approach to resolving identified problems. For example, information obtained through the monitoring and evaluation process conducted in relation to policies and procedures on hospital safety must be shared by quality review and risk management committees, although each committee ultimately reviews such information and conducts further investigation from different perspectives.

RISK MANAGEMENT

Risk management can be described as a four-step process designed to identify, evaluate, and resolve the actual and possible sources of loss.

1. *Risk identification* is the process of identifying activities that potentially expose the organization to the risk of liability or financial loss. Risk management committees and risk managers rely on many data sources to identify risks, including incident reports and occurrence screening systems, verbal communication, safety and quality improvement committee reports, and patient complaints. Risk identification is most commonly accomplished retrospectively (based on information on past events or incidents), but is often combined with other approaches, including prospective risk identification (based on an analysis of likely exposures) and concurrent risk identification (based on monitoring of situations and events as they occur).
2. *Risk evaluation* is the process of using analytical skills to determine the potential for risk and the financial impact that the risk could have on the practitioner or organization. Risk managers attempt to predict the expected loss frequency (how often an identified risk will generate a loss) and loss severity (how much the generated loss will cost), so that the organization may be prepared to address the conse-

---

[1]*See* JOINT COMMISSION, 1997 HOSPITAL ACCREDITATION MANUAL, Standard PI.3.3.2.

quences of loss events and can prioritize necessary risk management efforts. Risk evaluation usually entails analysis of incident reports and claims generated by the health care organization, as well as analysis of relevant statistical studies and surveys from industry associations, government agencies, and independent organizations.

3. *Risk handling* is the process of taking steps to respond to the risks that have been identified. Risk managers must analyze available methods for reducing exposure and potential losses and implement an appropriate course of action. The primary approach utilized for risk handling is *risk control* (preventing losses from occurring in the first place and reducing the effect of losses that do occur), which can be further classified into several categories, including *risk elimination* (totally avoiding a particular exposure by limiting or completely eliminating an activity, procedure, or particular service) and *risk reduction* (reducing or preventing loss).

4. *Risk monitoring* is the process of continuously monitoring and evaluating the results of risk management initiatives. Risk managers must modify techniques as appropriate and review risk management processes on an ongoing basis, updating approaches in accordance with changing circumstances or revealed inefficiencies.

To identify risks, a risk manager relies on a wide range of collected data, documents, and records. Some common information sources used for risk identification purposes are:

- incident and accident reports
- data on members who utilize greater than average levels of service
- length of stay data
- unexpected patient returns for acute care
- variations from clinical practice guidelines and outcome indicators
- patient complaints and patient satisfaction surveys
- accreditation and federal/state inspection reports
- credentialing, recredentialing, and clinical privileges files
- audit reports of internal committees or insurance surveyors[2]

---

[2]*See* C. Benda and F. Rozovsky, *Liability and Risk Management in Managed Care* (Gaithersburg, Md.: Aspen Publishers, Inc., 1998), 15:3.

The health information management department plays a crucial role in the risk management function. The health information management department can perform the following tasks:

- Supervising data gathering, with documentation of the data produced at all levels.
- Training clerical personnel engaged in locating the most useful sources of required information.
- Determining the incidence of relevant data requested for the use of committees and individuals.
- Screening medical records for compliance with established clinical criteria and designated exceptions or equivalents as established by the medical staff.
- Participating in the selection and design of forms used in the medical record and in the determination of the sequence and format of the contents of the medical record.
- Suggesting to the professional staff methods of improving the collection and organization of primary source data so as to facilitate retrieval, analysis, tabulation, and display.
- Performing continuing informational surveillance of practice indicators or monitors for medical staff review.
- Ensuring the provision of a mechanism to protect the privacy of patients and practitioners whose records are involved in quality assessment activities.
- Reviewing all requests for access to or copies of medical records by patients and third parties to determine their validity under applicable state law.
- Reviewing all medical records for which requests for access or copies have been received, particularly from patients, attorneys, and court orders or subpoenas, to determine whether it is apparent from the medical record that the hospital or health care organization has potential exposure to liability. Department personnel should confer closely with the organization's risk manager and legal counsel in this function, as the early identification of potential claims can greatly enhance and facilitate the defense to any claim that may be brought against it.

Each of these components of a risk management program in the health information management department should be evaluated with respect to the needs of the institution and the available personnel and resources so that the most effective program may be implemented in the hospital or health care organization.

QUALITY REVIEW

The health care industry has long recognized the importance of monitoring health care services with the goal of improving patient care. In recent years, the terminology and methodology of quality review has changed. Today, continuous quality improvement and total quality management have become predominant terms in the language of health care quality review. These two terms, and several others, are frequently interchanged, making the vocabulary used to describe new quality review concepts confusing. For the basic overview of quality review contained in this chapter, "quality improvement" and "quality review" are meant to encompass the numerous labels applied to the quality improvement philosophy and process.

The concept of quality improvement, as applied in the health care organization, focuses on all key organizational functions, including governance, management, and support functions as well as direct patient care. Implementation of quality improvement efforts involves education at all levels, from top executives to employees paid by the hour, such that the entire organization is following the flow of provided health care services from beginning to end, continuously working together to improve quality at every stage of patient care.

Quality improvement relies on statistical evaluation of data collected during review activities for the purpose of improving processes, as opposed to individual performance. Quality review can include the following activities:

- Review of surgical and other invasive procedures.
- Evaluation of drug usage.
- Review of medical records.
- Review of blood utilization.
- Evaluation of pharmacy and therapeutics.
- Review of risk management activities.

During the past decade, quality review has started to include outcome research, comparative research, measurement of illness severity, patient satisfaction surveys, and benchmarking. With the advent of managed care, quality review has become more involved in the business needs of health care by compiling data for managed care contracting, report cards, and physician profiling.[3]

Quality improvement is a multidisciplinary process and can involve many departments, such as the health information management, medical staff, and nursing departments. Some facilities may create multidisciplinary committees to perform quality review activities. Other facilities may have a separate quality improvement department or place the responsibility of quality improvement within the health information management department.

In its various accreditation manuals, the Joint Commission requires accredited health care organizations (i.e., hospitals, ambulatory health care facilities, and other health care networks) to improve organizational performance on a continuous and ongoing basis. The Joint Commission defines improvement as activities undertaken by leaders and support staff for the purpose of continuously measuring, assessing, and improving performance of clinical and other processes, and ultimately improving patient health outcomes.[4] While there are many approaches to improving organization performance, the Joint Commission's standards indicate that all quality improvement programs should contain these elements:

- *Plan.* There is a planned, systematic, organizationwide approach to designing, measuring, assessing, and improving performance.
- *Design.* New processes that are implemented must be designed well.
- *Measure.* There must be in place a systematic process to collect data needed to design and assess new processes.
- *Assess.* There must be a systematic process for assessing collected data to determine whether design specifications for new processes were met.
- *Improve.* The hospital or health care organization must systematically improve its performance.[5]

The National Committee for Quality Assurance (NCQA), an organization that accredits managed care organizations (MCOs), also focuses on clinical and administrative mechanisms for quality management and im-

---

[3]B.J. Youngberg and D.R. Weber, "Integrating Risk Management, Utilization Management, and Quality Management: Maximizing Benefit through Integration," in B.J. Youngberg, ed., *The Risk Manager's Desk Reference* (Gaithersburg, Md.: Aspen Publishers, Inc., 1998), 29.

[4]*See, e.g.,* JOINT COMMISSION, 1997 HOSPITAL ACCREDITATION MANUAL, Standard PI.

[5]*See, e.g.,* JOINT COMMISSION, 1997 HOSPITAL ACCREDITATION MANUAL, Standards PI.1 through PI.5.

provement, and on the communication process for problem identification, analysis, and follow-up. With respect to quality improvement, the NCQA requires that the MCO have a well-organized, comprehensive quality review program accountable to its highest organizational levels. The NCQA measures quality improvement through review of quality improvement program structure, accountability, coordination with management, content, and delegation. The NCQA attempts to answer the following in the course of its review:

- Does the plan fully examine the quality of care given to its members?
- How well does the plan coordinate all parts of its delivery system?
- What steps does it take to make sure members have access to care in a reasonable amount of time?
- What improvements in care and service can the plan demonstrate?[6]

During the evaluation process, the NCQA focuses on the tracking of issues uncovered by the MCO's quality improvement process, including whether that process follows problems through to their resolution, and assesses quality review/quality improvement studies, projects, and monitoring activities; quality review/quality improvement committees; and governing body reports and meeting minutes.[7]

COMPLIANCE PROGRAMS

In response to the proliferation of fraud and abuse legislation and enforcement activities directed at the health care industry, many health care organizations are developing corporate compliance programs. Compliance programs can not only prevent violations of the law but also can reduce the potential for liability should violations occur. Health care providers in all segments of the industry are implementing such programs in response to heightened scrutiny and expectations of compliance and also as part of settlements following health care fraud investigations. An effective compliance program can minimize the consequences resulting from a violation of the law and may, in some cases, convince a prosecutor not to pursue a criminal action. With respect to criminal penalties, the fed-

---

[6]*See* S. Dasco and C. Dasco, *Managed Care Answer Book* (Gaithersburg, Md.: Aspen Publishers, Inc., 1996), 8-13, 8-14 and NATIONAL COMMITTEE FOR QUALITY ASSURANCE, STANDARDS FOR ACCREDITATION OF MANAGED CARE ORGANIZATIONS, Standards for Quality Management and Improvement (1998).

[7]*See* S. Dasco and C. Dasco, *Managed Care Answer Book* (Gaithersburg, Md.: Aspen Publishers, Inc., 1996), 8-13, 8-14.

eral Guidelines, Sentencing for Organizations, which covers every business in the United States including charitable and not-for-profit institutions, specifically mandate lesser criminal sanctions for companies that have effective compliance programs in operation.[8] As far as civil sanctions are concerned, the Department of Justice's Civil Division has implemented a similar philosophy by treating defendants more leniently if they have compliance programs in effect.[9]

In designing a compliance program, a health care organization should begin with the sentencing guidelines' description of the seven minimum steps that a compliance program must include. An effective compliance program must include the following:

1. The organization must establish compliance standards and procedures that are reasonably capable of reducing the prospect of criminal or wrongful conduct.

2. The organization must assign individuals in high-level personnel positions with the overall responsibility to oversee compliance with the standards and procedures that will be developed after completion of a legal audit.

3. In addressing oversight responsibilities, the organization must use due care not to delegate substantial discretionary authority to individuals who the organization knew, or should have known through the exercise of due diligence, had a propensity to engage in illegal activities.

4. Once the organization has developed suitable standards and procedures, they must be communicated effectively to all employees and other agents.

5. The organization must develop a monitoring and auditing system reasonably designed to detect criminal and other wrongful conduct by its employees and other agents.

6. An organization must implement an adequate enforcement and discipline procedure that will ensure consistent enforcement of the compliance standards via an appropriate disciplinary mechanism.

---

[8]United States Sentencing Commission Guidelines, Sentencing for Organizations, 56 Fed. Reg. 22,762 (1991).

[9]Arent et al., *Health Law Trends,* The Dawning of the Age of Compliance, vol. 1, 1996.

7. The organization must take all reasonable steps, including any necessary modifications to its program, to respond to a detected offense
and to prevent further similar offenses.[10]

The precise actions necessary to implement these steps depend on the size
of the organization, the nature of its business, and its history.

An organization's corporate compliance plan should also be targeted to
the needs of the particular health care organization. The health care organization should determine all areas that could be included in a compliance
program by considering every federal, state, and local statute and ordi-
nance that imposes criminal or civil sanctions or liability. The laws that a
health care organization might want to consider when creating a corporate
compliance program include the following:

- Antikickback statute and state or local counterparts
- Antitrust laws
- Civil monetary penalties laws
- Emergency Medical Treatment and Active Labor Act (EMTALA)
- Employment related laws, such as the Americans with Disabilities Act
  (ADA), the Family and Medical Leave Act (FMLA), and the Fair La-
  bor Standards Act (FLSA)
- False Claims Act and state or local counterparts
- Federal fraud statutes, such as mail fraud statute and wire fraud act
- Health Insurance Portability and Accountability Act of 1996 (HIPAA)
- Medical waste management laws
- Medicare and Medicaid Acts
- Patient confidentiality statutes
- Patient Self-Determination Act
- Racketeer Influenced and Corrupt Organizations Act (RICO)
- Safe Medical Devices Act
- Stark law and state or local counterparts
- Tax laws[11]

[10]United States Sentencing Commission Guidelines, Sentencing for Organizations, 56 Fed. Reg. 22,762, § 8A1.3(k) (1991).

[11]M. Hanzal, "Understanding the Need for a Corporate Compliance Program," in B. J. Youngberg, ed., *The Risk Manager's Desk Reference* (Gaithersburg, Md.: Aspen Publishers, Inc., 1998), 112–113.

The health information management department should be integrated with an organization's compliance efforts because documents are crucial to the investigation and enforcement activities of a compliance program. Patient records are an important data source for compliance efforts, particularly for the monitoring and auditing system that must be part of any compliance plan.[12] Health care organizations may choose to conduct a pre-planning audit addressing financial, accounting, billing, transactional, and quality of care issues. Patient records document the treatment provided by a physician and can be used to determine whether the organization complied with all applicable laws, standards, and policies and procedures. Patient records are also crucial to the ongoing monitoring that is part of a corporate compliance program. The health information manager's experience in data collection and analysis, physician documentation practices, billing and coding, and data management is essential to compliance efforts.

The health information management department may want to conduct a medical records audit as part of a compliance program. Some areas that the health information management department might want to review include:

- document retention/destruction and confidentiality policies
- medical record documentation that should be available at the time the record is coded—consider whether all physician documentation and test results must be in the medical record
- procedures that the health information department has in place to ensure that the medical record has adequate documentation and supports the coded diagnoses and procedures
- education and training of physicians, nurses, coders, and other individuals involved in documentation, coding, and billing[13]

---

[12]United States Sentencing Commission Guidelines, Sentencing for Organizations, 56 Fed. Reg. 22,762, § 8A1.3(k) (1991).

[13]*See* L.S. Vincze, "Compliance, Medical Records, and the FBI: Preventing Fraud and Abuse," *Journal of the American Health Information Management Association* 69, no. 1 (1998): 41–42; S. Prophet and C. Hammen, "Coding Compliance: Practical Strategies for Success," *Journal of the American Health Information Management Association* 69, no. 1 (1998): 52–53; S. Prophet, "Fraud and Abuse: What You Can Do," *Journal of the American Health Information Management Association* 69, no. 1 (1998): 68–70.

MEDICAL RECORDS IN RISK MANAGEMENT, QUALITY REVIEW, AND COMPLIANCE ACTIVITIES

Patient records form an essential part of the data used in risk management, quality review, and compliance activities. The health information management department and its personnel occupy an important position in ensuring that staff who have either the authority to make entries in the patient record or the right to examine the record do so in accordance with applicable laws, regulations, and accreditation standards. For Joint Commission-accredited hospitals and health care networks, the accreditation standards recognize several purposes for maintaining medical records, which also are important to the proper functioning of a risk management, quality review, or corporate compliance program.

The Joint Commission standards relating to patient-specific data and information recognize several uses for patient- or member-specific data. The information may be useful to

- facilitate patient or member care;
- serve as a financial and legal record;
- aid in clinical research;
- support decision analysis; and
- guide performance improvement or document outcomes of care.[14]

As is evident from the Joint Commission standards, a complete and accurate medical record is necessary to fulfill several important functions: (1) it chronicles the history of a patient's care and will reveal both the positive and negative aspects, if any, of that patient's dealings with health care providers; (2) it will be used, for both risk management and quality review purposes, to evaluate the quality of the care rendered and to identify potential problems with either the system of delivering care or with the providers who deliver it; and (3) it can be used for compliance purposes, either in an audit or to ensure that the organization has complied with all applicable laws and regulations.

---

[14]JOINT COMMISSION, 1996 COMPREHENSIVE ACCREDITATION MANUAL FOR HEALTH CARE NETWORKS, Intent of Standard IM.6; JOINT COMMISSION, 1997 HOSPITAL ACCREDITATION MANUAL, Intent of Standards IM.7 through IM.7.2.

13

Computerized Medical Records

Chapter Objectives

- Distinguish between a fully computerized patient record system, a fully automated computer-based patient record, and computer-based records.
- Discuss the benefits of computerized patient records.
- Explain the legal concerns that arise from computerization of patient records.
- Identify the sources of law that govern confidentiality of health information, discussing their application to computerized records.
- Explain why security is important to a computerized medical record system, giving examples of safeguards against unauthorized access, including technological, physical, and user access controls.
- Discuss the concerns associated with outside users of computerized medical record information.
- Clarify how durability and accuracy requirements apply to computerized patient records.
- Discuss the legal obstacles to admission of computerized medical records into evidence, and how the obstacles can be overcome.
- Describe the role of federal standards in electronic claims processing.

- List methods of protecting the security of faxed and e-mailed medical information.
- Define telemedicine and give examples of current applications, highlighting medical record concerns.
- Discuss the internet as a method of conveying patient specific information, including risks and safeguards.

EMERGING TRENDS IN COMPUTERIZATION OF MEDICAL RECORDS

Many people would be surprised at just how exposed they are. Millions of individual medical records float around these days in a vast electronic network that serves both commerce and scientific research. The information zips around the country, speeded by computers at every stage. Computers help diagnose disease, monitor patients, organize the data about their conditions and transmit the information to managed care networks, medical research networks, pharmaceutical benefits managers and other outposts of America's increasingly wired health care system.[1]

As the above quote would suggest, hospitals and other health care providers increasingly rely on cutting-edge technology to provide medical treatment to patients, and a growing number also realize the benefits of technological advances in administration and record-keeping. In the recent past, most health care providers maintained patient records in paper files, eventually transferring the completed records to microfilm for safe-keeping. Many providers now, however, use computers and computer networks, microwave technology, facsimile machines, and optical scanning and storage equipment in the creation, transmission, storage, and retrieval of medical records.

A fully computerized patient record system is one that captures, stores, retrieves, and transmits patient health data, including clinical, administrative, and payment data. A fully automated computer-based patient record is one in which all of the data and images collected over the course of a patient's health care are created, authenticated, modified, stored, and retrieved by computer. Computer-based records may be created using a vari-

---

[1] A. Allen, "Exposed," *The Washington Post Magazine* (8 February 1998): 11.

ety of media, including magnetic media such as disks and tapes and digital media such as optical disks.

The trend toward computerization of all types of health care information has accelerated significantly in the past decade. Important strides have been made toward automating exchanges of information in the health care industry, although many of the efforts to date have focused on records containing financial, rather than medical, information. A significant development in this regard occurred with the enactment of the Health Insurance Portability and Accountability Act of 1996 (HIPAA), which enunciates standards and requirements for the electronic transmission of health information.[2] As new advances in technology occur and the value of large databases of clinical data continues to grow, the conversion of medical records from paper to a computerized format will remain a dominating trend in health information management in the decade to come.

Health care reform initiatives and the increasing penetration of managed care into the health care delivery system have further heightened the need for comprehensive automation and the automated exchange of health care information. Whether it is to monitor costs, improve patient care, or evaluate participating health care professionals, the basis of managed care operations is in the gathering and sharing of health care information. In a managed care setting, confidential patient information is frequently linked through databases that allow participating providers to access all the clinical data about a patient who may have received treatment at a variety of points of service within an integrated delivery system. In this environment, paper medical record systems that were provider-based are being replaced with electronic medical record systems centered on the patient.

Computerization of a provider's records can enhance quality of care by permitting quick capture of information in a patient's record and by improving access to a patient's records by the many health professionals who may be involved in his or her care. In addition, quality improvement and quality assurance programs can be strengthened with the help of automated record systems. Automated record systems create the possibility of linking the patient record to expert diagnostic systems and other electronic decision support tools to further enhance the quality of patient care. A fully integrated computer-based record system can also increase effi-

---

[2]Health Insurance Portability and Accountability Act of 1996, Pub. L. No. 104-191, § 262 to be codified at 42 U.S.C. § 1301.

ciency by reducing the volume of paperwork required for admissions, order entry, reporting of the results of radiological examinations and laboratory tests, and pharmacy dispensing. This, in turn, diminishes the overall time spent on updating and filing the records. In addition, a computerized record system can assist with patient scheduling, diagnosis-related group (DRG) and case-mix analysis and other management, staffing, and costing functions.[3]

Increased automation will permit management of health information based on the electronic patient record and the automatic transmission of information required for case and utilization management, claims processing, and other financial transactions. These information exchanges will increasingly be accomplished without the need for significant human intervention. In addition, access to health care information will become more widespread, with health care data networks permitting the exchange of health information concerning individuals by providers, payers, care managers, employers, vendors, support organizations, and others, with the information then stored in distributed or centralized databases.[4]

Although a computer-based patient record system can improve efficiency and the quality of care rendered by a provider, it may also increase a health care facility's exposure to liability under many of the legal theories or causes of action traditionally associated with health information management. The computerization of medical records generates unique confidentiality concerns, for example, with respect to the improper disclosure of personal health information and computer sabotage committed by persons gaining unauthorized access to a computerized record system. Questions also arise as to whether providers with fully computerized record systems satisfy state licensure requirements, and the conditions of participation for Medicare reimbursement.

Moreover, the legal issues associated with the computerization of patient-related data have become increasingly complex as information systems expand beyond the electronic capturing of medical records within a single health care facility. As health care providers integrate to provide a relatively seamless continuum of care across a network of participants, the need to integrate information systems has also arisen, generating complex legal issues about the rights and duties of the provider who originates

---

[3]"Patient bedside system enters the computer age," *Hospitals*, July 1989, p. 76.

[4]*See* B. Broccolo, D. Fulton, and A. Waller, "The Electronic Future of Health Information: Strategies for Coping with the Brave New World," *Journal of the American Health Information Management Association* 64, no. 12 (1993): 38–51.

the data and of the integrated delivery system (IDS) or network that operates the shared information system.

The computerization of health care information, and in particular automated payment systems, also has significant repercussions in the area of health care fraud and abuse prevention. Violations of health care fraud prohibitions are facilitated when a claims payment system is highly automated. Although these systems are designed to accelerate claims processing by catching errors, testing eligibility, matching diagnoses to procedure codes, and returning erroneous claims to the provider, they have also made it possible to identify what combinations of diagnoses, procedures, and charges guarantee payment without any human review. The improved speed and efficiency of automated payment systems also make it possible to augment the volume of these types of claims, and to extend fraudulent activity across multiple patients and payers. As one commentator stated: "... to beat the industry's current defenses, all [health care providers] need to do is bill *correctly*."[5] Electronic data exchange has also opened the door to new kinds of health care fraud, arising from the growing number of computer links to claims information and the addition of electronic fund transfer capabilities.

The law has not kept pace with many of the advances in health information technology, and many of the legal issues discussed above must therefore be addressed without the benefit of formal legal guidance. Nonetheless, a provider who is contemplating installing or modifying a fully automated record system must still ascertain whether the system will comply with applicable licensure laws and regulations, Medicare requirements, and applicable accreditation requirements. In addition, preserving the confidentiality and integrity, accessibility, accuracy, and durability of medical records on an automated system presents special problems. As mentioned, computerized medical records present unique security concerns because of their vulnerability to computer viruses and other sabotage. Courts have not yet dealt with the liability and damages issues relating to patient injuries caused by these and other forms of sabotage committed against a computerized medical record system. Finally, it is vital that computerized patient record systems be designed, installed, and maintained in a manner that preserves the reliability of records created and stored on such systems so that such records will be admissible as evidence in court and will be credible as evidence.

---

[5]M.K. Sparrow, Commentary, "A Criminal's Dream," *Modern Healthcare* (October 6, 1997): 94.

LEGAL ISSUES RAISED BY COMPUTERIZED MEDICAL RECORDS

Electronic patient records raise specific legal concerns, many of which are offshoots of the evolving status of traditional rights and responsibilities associated with ownership and control of patient information. Historically, health care providers owned and maintained the medical records for the patients to whom they delivered care, subject to the patients' rights with respect to the information contained in the records. Although a patient may have been treated by multiple providers, each facility or professional generally kept a separate record on the patient reflecting the services that it had provided. The integration of health care providers into delivery systems and the creation of multi-provider information systems that allow access to patient information gathered by every other provider in the system challenge traditional notions about who has the right to use and the duty to protect medical record information, and about the scope of these rights.

Confidentiality and Integrity Issues

A computerized medical record system must be designed, installed, and maintained to preserve both the confidentiality and the integrity of patient health information. A report issued in 1993 by the Office of Technology Assessment defined confidentiality and integrity as follows:

- *Confidentiality* involves control over who has access to information.
- *Integrity* means that information and programs are changed only in a specified and authorized manner, that the computer resources operate correctly, and that the data in them are not subject to unauthorized changes.[6]

The Joint Commission on Accreditation of Healthcare Organizations (Joint Commission) has promulgated standards relating to patient record information confidentiality and integrity, requiring that hospitals and health care networks safeguard records against loss, destruction, tampering, and unauthorized access or use.[7] Significant legal risks directly asso-

---

[6]U.S. Congress, Office of Technology Assessment, *Protecting Privacy in Computerized Medical Information*, OTA-TCT-576 (Washington, D.C., 1993), 89.

[7]JOINT COMMISSION, 1998 COMPREHENSIVE ACCREDITATION MANUAL FOR HOSPITALS, Standard IM 2.3 and 1998-2000 COMPREHENSIVE ACCREDITATION MANUAL FOR HEALTH CARE NETWORKS, Standards IM 2 and IM 2.3.

ciated with computer-based patient systems relate to the failure to preserve the confidentiality or integrity of data.

The legal obligation to protect the confidentiality of patient health information derives from various sources but is primarily based on state statutes and the common law. Other sources of health care providers' duty to maintain the confidentiality of patient health care information include federal statutes and regulations, such as those concerning alcohol and drug abuse patient records, Medicare regulations, accreditation standards, and ethical standards promulgated by various health care trade and professional associations. (See Chapter 6, ACCESS TO MEDICAL RECORD INFORMATION, for a more complete discussion of these subjects.) In addition, the importance of medical records as evidence in trials and administrative hearings requires a provider to protect its records from unauthorized access.

Legal confidentiality obligations do not vary with the medium on which patient records are stored. The same confidentiality requirements apply to paper records and computer-based patient records, even though special safeguards may be legally mandated to preserve the confidentiality of computer-based patient records.[8] However, the applicability of confidentiality requirements is to a large extent based on whether the health care information can be linked to a specific patient or has been cleansed of all patient-identifiable data. Most of the legislative protections governing the confidentiality of health care information apply only when the medical record data identifies the patient (patient-identified data) or when the patient's identity can be derived or inferred from the data (patient-identifiable data). HIPAA, for example, protects the confidentiality of patient-identifiable information, defined as information "with respect to which there is a reasonable basis to believe that [it] can be used to identify the individual."[9] If the data has been cleansed, there are very few restrictions on its use. The growing sophistication of computer search engines and the large number of nonmedical demographic databases, however, make it more difficult to completely mask identifying elements of a medical record, or to determine whether the information has been sufficiently masked to exempt it from traditional rules governing confidentiality and access.[10]

---

[8]*See, e.g.*, Illinois Hospital Licensing Requirements, ILL. ADMIN. CODE tit. 77, § 250.1510.

[9]Pub. L. No. 104-191, § 262 to be codified at 42 U.S.C. § 1301.

[10]For a comprehensive analysis of this topic, *see* A. Waller and O. Alcantara, "Ownership of Health Information in the Information Age," *Journal of the American Health Information Management Association* 69, no. 3 (1998).

Confidentiality obligations vary from state to state. Many states have general health information confidentiality statutes that apply to specific categories of persons, including health care providers, third-party administrators, and employers.[11] Other general confidentiality requirements are imposed on providers in legislation enunciating patients' rights.[12] For the most part, however, confidentiality provisions are found in statutes and regulations that license or otherwise regulate specific categories of providers and their duty to maintain medical records. These requirements apply to the providers maintaining the patient records, and in some instances also apply to those who receive patient information from a regulated provider.[13] Confidentiality requirements also may vary depending on the type of information recorded or the purpose of a particular disclosure of information.

When medical record data is transmitted across state lines, it may not always be clear which state's law applies or which courts will have jurisdiction if a dispute arises over disclosure of an individual's health information. Several factors determine which state has jurisdiction to resolve such a dispute, including where the medical record entries were made, where patient care was delivered, and the location of the medical records. The consolidation of the health care industry into national networks of providers located in many different states and the increasing availability of electronic medical record data have highlighted the issue of identifying applicable confidentiality requirements.

Computerization of patient data increases the risk of unauthorized disclosure of personal medical information, thereby necessitating special safeguards to keep the data confidential. The ease with which personal health information can be collected, stored, and accessed on a computer-based record system means that, generally, more information is included in a computer-based record than in a paper record. The detailed and sophisticated health information often found in computer-based records and the trend toward use of this data for nonhealth purposes makes computerized patient records attractive targets. A single breach of a computerized record system's security can lead to disclosure of hundreds or even thousands of records and to potentially catastrophic liability for such disclosure, because computers are capable of accessing, copying, and transmitting large numbers of records within a very short time span.

---

[11]*See, e.g.*, MD. CODE ANN., HEALTH-GEN. § 4-301; CAL. CIVIL CODE § 56.

[12]*See, e.g.*, 410 ILL. COMP. STAT. § 50/0.01.

[13]*See, e.g.*, TEX. REV. CIV. STAT. ANN. art. 4495b, sec. 5.08.

Automation of the information distribution process and the integration of computer and telecommunication linkages allow widespread access to patient records, not only by the parties involved in providing care but also by secondary users of the information.[14] Secondary users of patient record information include life, health, and disability insurers, employee health benefit plans and support organizations, educational institutions, both the civil and criminal justice systems, rehabilitation and social welfare programs, credit agencies and banking centers, public health agencies, and researchers. Accordingly, confidentiality must be maintained and unauthorized access to patient records prevented both by inside and outside users of computerized patient record systems and by primary and secondary users of individual health information.

System Security Measures

Because the potential for large-scale breaches of data security is much greater in a computerized medical record system, and because a provider bears the greatest risk of liability for unauthorized disclosure, a provider who implements such a system must be sure that it adequately protects confidentiality with respect to both internal and external users of the system. Computer system security must, therefore, balance the need for ready access to patient information by those involved in patient care with the need to protect against unauthorized access.[15] This may require some delicate balancing between conflicting objectives. A provider may be liable when its records are so highly guarded that medical information is not readily available to those caring for a patient; on the other hand, the provider can be liable for breaches of confidentiality that result from permitting easy access to medical records by unauthorized personnel.

The level of system security required by law for systems containing patient records is not clear. Under general principles of negligence liability, however, it is clear that security must be reasonable at a minimum. Because what is considered reasonable security changes over time, it is important that system security be periodically reviewed and updated.

To comply with legal requirements, a medical record system must provide for both system and data security. Data security exists when data are

---

[14]U.S. Congress, Office of Technology Assessment, *Protecting Privacy in Computerized Medical Information*, OTA-TCT-576 (Washington, D.C., 1993).

[15]*See* A. Waller and D. Fulton, "The Electronic Chart: Keeping It Confidential and Secure," *Journal of Health and Hospital Law* 26, no. 4, 104–107.

protected from improper disclosure or unauthorized or unintended alteration.[16] System security implies that a defined system functions in a defined operational environment, serves a defined set of users, contains prescribed data and operational programs, has defined network connections and interactions with other systems, and incorporates safeguards to protect the system against defined threats to the system and its resources and data.[17]

Appropriate computer security can generally be achieved through a combination of technical measures, system management, and administration and procedures. It is generally preferable to incorporate the technical safeguards into the system application or program (i.e., the medical record system) rather than relying on network infrastructure for security.[18] Technical safeguards include personal identification and user verification techniques, access control software and audit controls, computer architecture, communications linkage safeguards, and encryption.

Personal Identification and User Verification. Personal identification assists in ensuring that a user of a communication or computer system is authorized to do so and may be held accountable for his or her actions. The most common method of verifying the user's identity is through a secret password or code, which must be used to access a system or a particular part of a system. If password identification is used, the passwords should be at least five characters in length, and the system should require the users to change passwords frequently. Relying solely on passwords to identify users often fails to provide adequate security for computer systems. Users may share passwords, leave them at their work stations, or write them on desk blotters, or an unauthorized person attempting to gain access to the system may correctly guess one or more passwords if common words are used as passwords. Tokens, such as a key card or machine-readable badges, are difficult to reproduce but they can be lost or left at home. Biometric identification involves verifying the identity of the user based on a unique physical feature of the user, such as fingerprint, written signature, voice print, typing pattern, retinal scan, or hand geometry. Biometric identification generally provides a high level of security, but may

---

[16]*See* Institute of Medicine, *The Computer-based Patient Record: An Essential Technology for Health Care* (Washington, D.C.: National Academy Press, 1991).

[17]Institute of Medicine, *Health Data in the Information Age* (Washington, D.C.: National Academy Press, 1994).

[18]*See* U.S. Congress, Office of Technology Assessment, *Protecting Privacy in Computerized Medical Information*, OTA-TCT-576 (Washington, D.C., 1993), 91.

be cost-prohibitive for many health care providers. User verification systems frequently involve a combination of identifiers, such as a key card in conjunction with a password or access code or some physical characteristic of the user, e.g., thumbprint.[19]

Access Control Software and Audit Trails. Once a system has identified a user, it is still necessary to limit the user's access to only the resources and data that he or she is authorized to access. Data access control software prevents a user from accessing or modifying a file unless the user has been given prior authorization. Through authorization checking, a system can determine whether a user's access request is valid, based on the permission assigned to the user, and then grant or deny the access request. Auditing access and attempted access by users helps to ensure user accountability. An examination of audit trails may also reveal suspicious patterns of access and lead to detection of improper conduct by both authorized and unauthorized users.

Computer Architecture. The computer itself may be designed to enhance security by monitoring its own activities and preventing users from gaining access to data they are not authorized to see. Additionally, it may have features built in to protect against sophisticated tampering and sabotage.

Communications Linkage Safeguard. Since computer links to telecommunications lines may make the computers vulnerable to improper access through the lines or through taps on the lines, a security system should also include security features designed to limit such improper use or access. One means of limiting access via dial-up lines has been dial-back protection devices. New security modems combine features of a modem with network security features, such as passwords, dial-back, and encryption.[20]

Encryption. Encryption is a method of protecting data vulnerable to unauthorized access or tampering. It is used to encode data for transmission or for storage in a computer. Encryption can provide an electronic

---

[19]U.S. Congress, Office of Technology Assessment, *Protecting Privacy in Computerized Medical Information*, OTA-TCT-576 (Washington, D.C., 1993), 94-95.

[20]For a more detailed discussion of technical safeguards, *see* U.S. Congress, Office of Technology Assessment, *Protecting Privacy in Computerized Medical Information*, OTA-TCT-576 (Washington, D.C., 1993), 89-99.

signature to verify that a message has not been tampered with, and to protect against fraud or repudiation by a sender. Encryption can protect confidentiality by encoding a message so that its meaning is not obvious. An encrypted message is encoded in such a way as to permit interpretation of the message only with the appropriate key, to which only authorized parties have access. Encryption can also protect data integrity through message authentication. Message authentication allows a system to verify that a message arrived in exactly the same form as it was sent, without errors or alterations; that it came from the stated source; and that it was not falsified by an impostor or fraudulently altered by the recipient. Digital signatures also can be created through encryption. Like a handwritten signature, this digital signature can be used to verify that information was not altered after it was signed, thereby ensuring message integrity.

Implementing System Security

With respect to inside users of a system, the security system should permit only authorized users to have access to medical records. Access may be controlled and users may be identified in one or more of the ways discussed above, including passwords, key cards, access codes, and biometric identification. In addition, a system should allow access to the system through only one workstation at a time for each user identifier. It is wise to program a system to log off automatically when a workstation has not been used for a predefined period of time. A user's access to the system should be limited to that portion of the system or record that relates to the user's position and duties. A system can be programmed to lock out an individual who attempts to retrieve files that he or she is not authorized to access or who repeatedly attempts to gain access to the system using an improper access code. In such cases, the system can be programmed to sound an alarm at the workstation or at an operator's console. It is important to strictly limit access to sensitive records and to portions of records containing highly sensitive health information for which the law provides a higher level of confidentiality protection. Such information includes human immunodeficiency virus (HIV) antibody test results, acquired immune deficiency syndrome (AIDS) patient records, alcohol and drug abuse patient records, and records of celebrities. (For a more extensive discussion of these specific confidentiality requirements, see Chapter 8, DOCUMENTATION AND DISCLOSURE: SPECIAL AREAS OF CONCERN.) Because of the intense controversy over abortion, common sense dictates that abortion records be accorded the same level of protection as other highly sensitive health records, whether or not such protection is expressly required under applicable law.[21]

The scope of a user's access should be periodically reviewed and modified as appropriate. It is vital that a user's access to the system be promptly terminated when the person's employment, medical staff membership, or other relationship justifying access to patient records is terminated. When a user's relationship with the provider is to be terminated involuntarily, it may be wise to terminate the user's access to the system just prior to notifying the user of the termination. Access to records by each authorized user should be periodically reviewed to discourage casual browsing through records. Such casual browsing increases the risk that confidentiality will be breached.

Provider policy should specifically prohibit revealing or sharing passwords and other user identifiers and should also prohibit attempting to access records beyond the scope of one's authorization. Hospitals and other institutional providers should require medical staff members to sign confidentiality statements, in which they acknowledge that passwords, access codes, and the like are for personal use only and assume responsibility for any entries made using the medical staff member's identifier. Policies against sharing passwords or other identifiers or permitting another person access to the system should be strictly enforced.

Finally, internal system security should be promoted through ongoing education and training programs that offer a minimum level of knowledge before users are granted access to the system, and through a more general understanding that security is the responsibility of each individual who accesses the system. Medical staff, employees, and other authorized users should be required to attend an orientation session that explains the provider's policy on system security, management of user identification, and access control. Continuing education sessions to update users on amendments to the policy or changes to the system and to periodically stress the importance of maintaining appropriate security measures are also recommended.[22]

---

[21]Some providers have chosen not to store highly sensitive health information on computers, or to encrypt such information or use other techniques to provide a higher level of security for records or the portions of records containing such information.

[22]*See* National Research Council Report, *For the Record: Protecting Electronic Health Information,* 1 October 1997, for recommended security practices and procedures to protect all patient-identifiable health care information.

Implementing External Security

Improper access to computerized medical records must also be prevented with respect to outside users of a medical record system. Controlling access from multiple and sometimes remote locations is more difficult than controlling access from one centralized location. Dial-up access makes it possible for external parties to repeatedly try to gain access to a system without being visible if a system is unmonitored. There are several possible methods to combat external parties' attempts to gain unauthorized access to a patient record system. Such methods include recording and monitoring such attempts to gain access, having the computer system call back users requesting remote access, and requiring remote users to have physicians' "keys," such as encoded disks, in order to gain access.

Regardless of whether providers outsource their patient records to a computer outsource vendor or acquire their own systems, third-party vendors and consultants will usually be involved in some way in developing, installing, operating, and maintaining the patient record system. These third parties may have access to live patient data, either on-site or from remote locations. Such third-party access to patient data may be occasional or ongoing. When a provider outsources its patient records, the outsource vendor will have possession of the patient records. Such vendors and consultants are generally not subject to the same legal or ethical obligations with respect to confidentiality as are providers. If such a third party improperly discloses confidential patient information, the provider permitting the third party access to patient information can expect to be held responsible for any harm resulting from the improper disclosure, unless the provider can demonstrate that all reasonable precautions to prevent such disclosure had been taken.

In many cases, the contract between the provider and the vendor or consultant will disclaim any liability on the part of the latter for damages such as those that would result from a disclosure in breach of a patient's confidentiality, or will limit the amount of damages for which the vendor or consultant may be liable. It is, therefore, advisable to include in all contracts with such third parties obligations for the third party, such as:

- to hold all patient information in strict confidence;
- to use the information only to perform the third party's obligations under the contract;
- to disclose the information only to the third party's employees who need access under the contract and who have signed a confidentiality

agreement obligating them to hold all patient information in confidence;

- to return the records in usable form upon request and/or upon termination of the contract; and
- to indemnify the provider for breaches of these obligations. It may not be possible to obtain such indemnification. However, the contract should not place any limits on the liability of the third party for breaches of its obligations.

Some outside computer services or data organizations analyzing a provider's patient data may wish to obtain the provider's patient data for purposes not in keeping with the provider's duty to preserve patient confidentiality. It is not uncommon for an outside computer service or data organization to attempt to obtain a provider's patient data to create databases or other proprietary information products. Such third parties will seek to own and control the information products and will want the right to distribute them freely. Such distribution will generally not accord with the provider's confidentiality obligations, unless the information has been adequately cleansed of all patient-identifiable data. All contracts with such outside computer and data services should address whether the service will be permitted to use patient data in its information products, and should establish the precautions that the service will be required to observe concerning patient confidentiality if the contract permits the use of patient information in the organization's information products.

When patient information is transmitted over public channels of communication (including telephone lines, radio waves, microwaves, etc.), as in the case of wide-area networks, protecting the information from outside access becomes more difficult and requires additional precautions. As communications protocols become more standard, the potential for unauthorized tapping of such communication channels will increase. One possible response to this confidentiality problem is to encrypt information communicated over public channels of communication.

An additional threat to patient confidentiality results from the computer's vast capacity for storage and copying of records. One possible safeguard against the mass breach of confidentiality that would occur if numerous records were improperly accessed or disclosed is to restrict use of software functions that permit the copying of multiple records at one time.

Computer Sabotage

Computerized patient record systems make possible widescale alteration or destruction of patient data through computer sabotage. Viruses and other forms of sabotage, such as worms, bombs, and Trojan horses, can jeopardize both the integrity and accessibility of information on the system by causing the system to slow or crash. Although both inside and outside users of the system potentially can commit sabotage, the biggest threat to computer security is often internal. Disgruntled employees may pose a substantial threat of sabotage.

The risk of sabotage by outside parties is present whenever there is any networking or electronic datasharing with outside parties, or when disks or other storage media from outside sources are used on the system. It may be impractical to control this risk by eliminating networking and datasharing with outside computers or by not using storage media from outside sources, since connections with outside facilities and with other databases may be essential for clinical, research, or other purposes. Joint Commission standards specifically address the need for hospital information systems to link up with external databases and bodies of clinical, administrative, and research knowledge.[23] Antivirus software, which assists in detecting and/or blocking computer viruses, is a useful means of reducing this risk. It is advisable to check all disks and similar media from outside sources for viruses prior to using them on a patient record system.

Health care organizations should also be sensitive to the risk of sabotage from software vendors. In isolated cases, software vendors have sabotaged or threatened to sabotage a system after a provider withheld payment (as permitted under the system contract when the system failed to meet contractual standards). This form of sabotage involves the insertion of a virus or keylock into system software, which enables the vendor to lock or shut down the system in the event of a payment dispute. Contracts for the purchase, lease, license, or maintenance of a computerized patient record system should obligate the vendor and its agents to refrain from inserting viruses or keylocks into the system. Contracts should also provide that the vendor will indemnify the provider for any and all losses and damages resulting from insertion of viruses or keylocks by the vendor or its agents.

---

[23]*See* Joint Commission, 1998-2000 Comprehensive Accreditation Manual for Health Care Networks, Standard IM 9.1.

While no computer security technology and methods available to the provider can totally protect against breaches of system security, it is important to employ system security technology and techniques that are at least reasonable by current standards. Nevertheless, the need to preserve the confidentiality and ensure the integrity of patient records will have to be balanced against the practical constraints on achieving perfect computer security.

Preserving Access to Computerized Records

Delivering quality patient care requires that medical records be readily available. Federal reimbursement regulations,[24] state licensure requirements,[25] and Joint Commission accreditation standards all require that medical records for current hospital patients be readily accessible and stored so as to be promptly retrievable.[26] Thus, a computerized patient record system must make records readily accessible and provide for prompt retrieval of the records. When a system crashes or experiences downtime, computerized records become inaccessible. It is, therefore, imperative that a system be designed and maintained to minimize downtime and that adequate backup mechanisms be available. Patient record system downtime may hinder patient care and result in negligence liability. Excessive system downtime may also violate applicable licensure requirements and accreditation standards.

There are several precautions that can assist in preserving accessibility of computerized patient records. First, it is important that system hardware be properly maintained and that system software be tested, debugged where necessary, and maintained appropriately. When considering acquisition of a particular system, it may be wise to inquire as to other users' experience with the system relative to downtime and the time required to bring the system back up quickly. Any agreement for acquisition of a computerized record system or any component thereof should contain performance standards, as well as warranties of reliability and covenants to provide ongoing maintenance and support. Second, it is also important to take appropriate precautions against viruses and other forms of sabotage to prevent the system locking up or crashing. Third, a provider should

---

[24] C.F.R. § 482.24 (a) & (b).

[25] See, e.g., Mass. Regs. Code tit. 105, § 130.200; Utah Admin. Code, 432-100-35 (4) (a) & (b).

[26] See Joint Commission, 1998-2000 Comprehensive Accreditation Manual for Health Care Networks, Standard IM 2.2.

create and conduct adequate backup procedures. Fourth, a provider's disaster or emergency plan should include requirements for emergency capabilities in the patient record system.

Durability Concerns

Computerized patient records must be durable to meet state licensure requirements, to be available as evidence in malpractice and other litigation involving the care received by a patient or the medical condition of a patient, and to provide data for research. When medical records are computerized, the problem of durability becomes more complex than is the case with paper records. There are two preconditions for durability of computerized records. The first is that the medium on which the information is stored must last for at least the minimum time a provider is required to retain medical records. The second is that the provider must be able to access old records created or maintained on older, and perhaps obsolete, technology.

Changes in technology can render a computer system obsolete before the need for records stored on the system has ended. Frequently old and new systems do not interact, making the older records inaccessible through the newer system. Equipment may need to be maintained in good working order long after it is obsolete and another record system is in use. If an old and a new system are able to interface, copying patient records from one system to the others can be problematic. Prior to copying such records, providers should check with knowledgeable legal counsel to ascertain whether such copied records will be considered original records for evidentiary purposes and whether retention of the copies in lieu of the originals complies with state licensure requirements. When records are copied from one system to another, it is important to preserve evidence of the chain of copying. When copying records, it is also important to verify that both the medium onto which the record will be copied and the copying process comply with applicable state licensure requirements.

Before selecting a medium for creation and storage of computerized patient records, the long-term durability of the medium should be investigated. Only media with proven durability should be utilized for patient record storage. It is important to note that the durability of some storage media, such as certain types of optical disks, has yet to be proven.[27]

---

[27]*See* P. Zachary, "Compact Disks Aren't Forever, It Turns Out," *Wall Street Journal*, 6 October 1991.

Some state licensure regulations address medical record storage and retention requirements in general terms, stating that hospitals must store records to provide easy retrieval and security.[28] A few states have promulgated more elaborate requirements for record storage.[29] Some states specify acceptable storage media for medical records.[30] A provider that adopts a method for storing computerized records should verify in advance that the method complies with state licensure requirements for record retention. (For a more detailed discussion of retention of medical records, see Chapter 3, MEDICAL RECORD REQUIREMENTS.)

Accuracy Issues

Computerized patient records, like paper records, must be completed in a timely and accurate fashion. Maintaining a complete and accurate record is essential not only for compliance with licensure and accreditation requirements but also to establish that appropriate care was provided to each patient. (For a more extensive discussion of these standards, see Chapter 4, MEDICAL RECORD ENTRIES.)

Errors in computerized medical records can result from defective performance of either the hardware or the software or from human or machine input. In complex systems with open architecture, errors can result from unanticipated interactions among programs. To minimize the risk of error, a provider should have regular maintenance and performance checks conducted, and the results should be documented. The provider should also have a system to review human input for accuracy and should document that such review has occurred. Joint Commission standards require a periodic[31] or ongoing[32] review of the completeness, accuracy, and timeliness of medical record entries. In addition, all laboratory and other types of equipment that generate input for a computerized records system

---

[28]*See, e.g.*, KAN. ADMIN. REGS. 28-34-9a.

[29]*See, e.g.*, CAL. CODE REGS. tit. 22, § 70751.

[30]*See, e.g.*, OR. ADMIN. R. 333-505-0050 (B). (Paper, microfilm, electronic, or other media are acceptable.)

[31]JOINT COMMISSION, 1998-2000 COMPREHENSIVE ACCREDITATION MANUAL FOR HEALTH CARE NETWORKS, Standard IM 3.2.1.

[32]JOINT COMMISSION, 1998 COMPREHENSIVE ACCREDITATION MANUAL FOR HOSPITALS, Standard IM 3.2.1. Scoring guidelines for this standard stipulate that findings from medical record reviews will be available at least quarterly.

should be well maintained and should be tested and calibrated periodically to minimize machine input errors.

The use of bar codes and other programmed codes can also raise accuracy concerns. Optical scanning of bar codes is used to monitor services and supplies provided to patients and to enter clinical data, such as temperature, pulse, blood pressure, and respiration. Bar codes can also be applied to a patient's wrist band and to packages of supplies. The use of such codes allows providers to create medical records much more quickly than is possible if data are charted by hand or entered through a computer keyboard. Optical scanning equipment should be tested periodically and the test results recorded. There should be a mechanism for confirming input generated from bar codes or other programmed codes either visually or otherwise.

COMPUTERIZED MEDICAL RECORDS AS EVIDENCE

In addition to enabling providers to respond properly to the medical needs of patients, medical records serve as a diary of a provider's actions. It is, therefore, important that the information contained in a record be admissible as evidence in court when the care received by the patient or the patient's medical condition is an issue. Because of the widespread computerization of general business records, courts have developed standards for judging the trustworthiness of computerized records.

The Rule against Hearsay

One barrier to introduction of any medical record as evidence in court is the rule against hearsay. Hearsay is generally defined as a statement made out of court by a declarant and proffered as evidence to prove the truth of the matter asserted in that out-of-court statement. Courts exclude hearsay from evidence, unless one of the exceptions to the hearsay rule applies. Since all medical records, regardless of form, are written statements made outside the courtroom, they are classed as hearsay if offered as evidence to prove the truth of any matter asserted in the record.

One important exception to the hearsay rule is the business records exception. Although the wording of this exception may vary from jurisdiction to jurisdiction, the general rule is that to come within the business records exception, records must be kept regularly in the ordinary course of business and must not have been prepared specifically for trial. The business record exception applies only to record entries made at or near the time of the event recorded. In addition, the identity of the person making or recording the entry must be captured in the record, and the record must have been prepared by a person with firsthand knowledge of the event recorded or from information transmitted by such a person. The person making the record or transmitting the information for the record must be acting in an ordinary business capacity at the time the record is made.

A computerized record made in the ordinary course of a provider's business should meet the requirement that the record be kept regularly and in the ordinary course of business. An automated record system should record the date and time of each entry and update to a patient record so that the time of the entry or update and its timeliness can be shown in court. The identity of the person who makes each entry or update should be captured by the system. If employees or health professionals share passwords or make entries under an identifier that is not their own, it will be impossible to ensure that the system's record of the identity of the person making the entry is accurate.

It is important that errors in computerized records be corrected appropriately. The system should preserve both the original entry and the correction and should record the identities of the persons making each original entry or correction so as not to create an appearance that the record has been altered or that records on the system are not reliable and trustworthy as evidence.

Write-once, read-many (WORM) technology or nonerasable compact disk read-only memory (CD-ROM) technology may be attractive in this context, because records cannot be altered once information is recorded. Another method of preserving records in their original form is write-protecting the portions of computer disks on which patient information is stored so that the integrity of records is protected. Nevertheless, if a system uses reliable software and preserves erroneous entries, tracking the history of each entry and correction, the provider should be able to demonstrate the reliability of the record in court.

It is advisable for the provider to have an employee or technical consultant who can testify concerning the reliability of the system's identification and entry-dating features and the trustworthiness of the system as a whole, including system security features and procedures.

Records created and stored on a properly designed and maintained computer-based record system should come within the business record exception to the hearsay rule (or a similar exception applicable to medical records) if the procedures described above are followed. Under the business record exception to the hearsay rule, statements contained in such computerized records may also be admissible if made by providers or staff acting in the ordinary course of business. Statements contained in such computerized records may also be admissible if made by the declarant for "purposes of medical diagnosis or treatment and describing medical history, or past or present symptoms, pain, or sensations, or the inception or general character of the cause or external source thereof insofar as reasonably pertinent to diagnosis or treatment."[33]

Best Evidence Rule

Another evidentiary rule relevant to the admissibility of computerized medical records is the best evidence rule. The best evidence rule expresses a judicial preference for the original of a writing if the contents of a writing are in dispute. In the context of computerized records, a question arises as to whether a hard copy of the contents of the record is an "original" for purposes of the best evidence rule. The Federal Rules of Evidence state the requirements for data stored on a computer or similar device. Rule 1001(3) states that "[i]f data are stored in a computer or similar device, any printout or other output readable by sight, shown to reflect the data accurately, is an 'original.' "[34] The Federal Rules of Evidence also provide that duplicates are admissible to the same extent as originals, unless a genuine issue of authenticity or unfairness arises.[35] Some states' evidentiary rules also provide that computerized documents shall be accepted as originals.[36] Other states permit admission of reproductions into evidence when the reproductions are made in the regular course of business and satisfy other criteria for trustworthiness.[37] The trustworthiness of a record created on a computerized system refers to the reliability of system hardware and software, the use of proper procedures for creating and storing records, the assurance that entries are made by adequately trained personnel, and the prevention of unauthorized access to the records and of tampering with the system.

---

[33]FED. R. EVID. 803(4). This exception to the rule against hearsay is known as the medical records exception.

[34]FED. R. EVID. 1001(3).

[35]FED. R. EVID. 1003.

[36]*See, e.g.*, FLA. STAT. ANN. § 90.951.

[37]*See, e.g.*, CAL. EVID. CODE § 1270-1272.

SPECIFIC ELECTRONIC PATIENT INFORMATION SECURITY ISSUES

Facsimile Transmission of Medical Records

The widespread use of facsimile (fax) machines to transmit information, including medical records, from one location to another has created a new threat to confidentiality and may, in some circumstances, call into question the integrity or authenticity of orders and other medical record entries transmitted by fax. Both paper and computerized records can be sent via fax machines; in addition, the use of a fax modem on a computer makes possible transmission of computerized records from one computer to another without generating any hard copy of the record as a necessary byproduct of the transmission. In either case, fax transmissions to external parties generally travel over telephone networks or other public channels of communication. Because there is a significant risk that fax transmissions will be misdirected, use of facsimile machines to transmit confidential medical record information is risky, and is extremely risky if highly sensitive patient information is involved.

These risks can be reduced, however, if proper maintenance and security techniques are used and if proper procedures are followed in transmitting medical records by fax. Nevertheless, it is probably never prudent to send via fax highly sensitive health information, except in encrypted form or over nonpublic channels of communication that are highly secure (e.g., a local area network within a facility). The American Health Information Management Association (AHIMA) recommends use of the fax machine to transmit patient health information only when the original document or mail-delivered photocopies will not serve.[38] A provider sending confidential information by fax off-site should verify that the recipient is authorized to receive it. Some, but by no means total, protection against unauthorized access to a fax transmission can be obtained by calling the recipient before sending the transmission, alerting the recipient to stand by for the transmission, and verifying that the fax number to which the transmission will be directed is the correct number. The cover sheet on the

---

[38]American Health Information Management Association, Practice Brief, "Facsimile Transmission of Health Information," *Journal of the American Health Information Management Association* 67, no.7, (1996).

document should also include a confidentiality legend, emphasizing the nature of the information contained in the transmission and requesting that the person receiving the fax, if other than the recipient shown on the cover sheet, contact the sender immediately.

Encrypting faxed information is another method of protecting its confidentiality. However, this process generally requires that the receiving fax machine or computer be equipped to decode the encrypted information, and this will often not be the case. When sending faxes off-site, a provider should retain a record of each fax transmission (including the phone number of the receiving fax machine) and the contents of the fax.

When receiving orders or other medical record information from outside the facility, a provider should also take special precautions. If caller identification is available, the receiving fax machine should be equipped with a mechanism for recording the number of the telephone from which the fax transmission originated. The personnel operating the fax machine should have a list of telephone numbers from which medical staff members transmit orders and should verify that the telephone number identified on the fax machine appears on that list.[39] A hospital may also treat faxed orders like verbal orders and require authentication of the order by the appropriate medical staff member within the time period permitted for authentication of verbal orders. Nevertheless, the advent of computer fax boards, with their attendant opportunities for electronic manipulation, may make it difficult to establish the accuracy and authenticity of a faxed order in court, if either is disputed by the originating practitioner.[40] In the context of computer fax boards and fax modems, use of cryptography for message authentication may be advisable.

Providers should refer to state rules of evidence to determine if, and under what circumstances, facsimile transmissions that become part of a patient record are admissible in court.[41] Fax machines used to transmit orders internally should also be equipped to print the date, time, and address of the originating fax machine to help support the authenticity of

---

[39]*See* Practice Brief, "Guidelines for Faxing Patient Health Information," *Journal of the American Health Information Management Association* 62, no. 46, (1991).

[40]For a discussion of the possibility of such manipulation, *see* F. Sommers, "Is a Fax a Legal Document?" *Banking Law Review*, Fall 1991.

[41]It is important to note that a number generated by the fax machine originating the transmission and printed on the fax may not be a correct number, since some fax machines can be programmed to transmit a number other than that of the originating telephone.

internally faxed documents. The original of each such fax transmission should be retained.[42]

Electronic Claims Processing

The Health Insurance Portability and Accountability Act of 1996 contained important provisions relating to the establishment of standards for electronic claims processing that could eventually lay the framework for formal standards regarding electronic medical records.[43] In particular, the statute charges the Secretary of Health and Human Services to establish standards to enable electronic exchanges appropriate for financial and administrative transactions. These transactions include health claims or equivalent encounter information, enrollment and disenrollment in a health plan, eligibility for a health plan, health care payment and remittance advice, health plan premium payments, first reports of injury, and health claim status and referral certification. The Secretary is also mandated under the law to establish standards in other areas. Standards to be established by the Secretary include the provision of a unique health identifier for each patient, employer, health plan, and health care provider. The Secretary is also charged with setting up security standards for health information, which take into account the technical capabilities of record systems used to maintain health information, the cost of security measures, training needs, and the value of audit trails in computerized record systems. Finally, the Secretary must adopt standards specifying procedures for the electronic transmission and authentication of signatures.

Under the law, health care providers are not required to process their claims electronically, but those who do so will have to comply with the standards enunciated under the law within two to three years after the standards are finalized. The law also creates a sanction to enforce privacy concerns, with fines up to $250,000 and imprisonment for up to ten years for anyone who wrongfully discloses or uses "individually identifiable" health information.

---

[42]A number of states has adopted legislation that authorizes the admissibility of reproductions made in the regular course of business without need to account for the original.

[43]Health Insurance Portability and Accountability Act of 1996, Pub. L. No. 104-191 § 262, to be codified at 42 U.S.C. § 1301.

Telemedical Records

Telemedicine is the delivery of health care services at a distance with the use of interactive telecommunications and computer technology. Using this technology, for example, a physician in one location can interview a patient, listen to his heart, examine lesions on his skin, examine his X-rays, read his EKG, diagnose conditions, and prescribe treatment. Because the practice of telemedicine relies on electronic signals to communicate medical information from one location to another, it raises significant legal issues with respect to the accuracy, confidentiality, and security of health care data that is transmitted this way.

The clinical applications of telemedicine are varied and differ technologically. Currently, it is applied in several settings, including in communications between emergency medical technicians providing care to a patient in an ambulance and a hospital emergency department, and in data-linking systems for remote evaluations of CT scans and radiology tests. Another application of telemedicine is the development of databases of patient records and the provision of distributed access to these databases in community health information networks (CHINs). Some of the data in CHIN databases include multimedia information collected and communicated through sophisticated telemedicine technologies. CHIN databases also include patient data from laboratories, pharmacies, medical instrument readings, and other sources. CHIN databases allow health care providers at different hospitals within a community to directly access all of a patient's medical information.

Telemedicine applications rely on a variety of technologies, many of which require a bandwidth. Although the practice of telemedicine can require different amounts of bandwidth depending on the circumstances, it generally requires the transmission of a large amount of data in a short period of time and the use of a large amount of bandwidth. Through the use of a coder-decoder, the analog signal produced by audio and video equipment can be converted to a digital signal for transmission to another location and converted back at the location receiving the broadcast, so as to compress the data, use less bandwidth, and reduce the costs of the communication.

Distortion of data can occur when it is compressed, raising concerns that the medical information a provider receives via telemedicine is inaccurate and will lead to misdiagnoses. In addition, the potential for breach of confidentiality is significant, for many of the same reasons discussed above with respect to computerized patient records and also because telemedicine involves not only collecting and storing patient data electronically, but also broadcasting it off-site. The airwaves are not secure, and the confidentiality of a patient's medical history may not be guaranteed when using telemedicine for video consultation. Individuals may intentionally or unintentionally intercept video broadcasts, leading some telemedicine locations to scramble their broadcasts to protect confidentiality. Technical personnel must be present at both ends of the transmission during a consultation broadcast, requiring that these individuals be included in institutional policies and training that relate to patient confidentiality. Finally, patients should receive specific information about telemedicine as part of the informed consent process, and understand that confidentiality may not be guaranteed. A consent form should be tailored to include this type of disclaimer for video consultations.

There are very few legislative or accreditation requirements that govern the creation or maintenance of telemedical records. AHIMA has addressed these topics in a Practice Brief, recommending minimum content standards for telemedical records and suggesting specific actions to protect confidentiality and security.[44] Accreditation standards do not specifically address telemedical records, but the Joint Commission has specified that a facility using telemedical information in patient treatment decisions must comply with all relevant standards.[45]

Electronic Mail

The trend toward integrated health care delivery systems has prompted hospitals and other health care facilities to develop various forms of information linkages, among which perhaps the most commonly used is electronic mail, or "e-mail." Communications via e-mail may be transmitted through direct modem-to-modem links, in-house routers, servers and bulletin boards, commercial third-party host services, and the Internet. (For a more detailed description of security risks related to Internet e-mail, see "The Internet" later in this chapter.) As people become more accustomed to the benefits of e-mail, they use e-mail to transmit a wide variety of sensitive information, including patient data, large documents for research

---

[44]American Health Information Management Association, Practice Brief, "Telemedical Records," *Journal of the American Health Information Management Association* 68, no.4, (1997).

[45]*See, e.g.,* American Health Information Management Association, Practice Brief, "Telemedical Records," *Journal of the American Health Information Management Association* 68, no. 4 (1997).

projects, budgets, and other confidential time-critical information. At many health care organizations, e-mail is used as a communication vehicle between patients and their caregivers.

The development of e-mail technologies (i.e., modes of e-mail communication) has been occurring at such a rapid pace, however, that, at times, the related implementation of technological safeguards has lagged behind; this raises confidentiality and security challenges for health care facilities in relation to the transmission of patient health care information via e-mail. Health care facilities must provide their staffs with training to ensure organization-wide recognition of the security risks associated with e-mail; at the very least, all health care professionals using e-mail to transmit patient health care information should understand that e-mail affords individuals no more confidentiality than written memoranda or letters and may in fact offer less privacy and security in the absence of adequate technological safeguards. Health care professionals who send electronic transmissions must recognize the necessity of exercising caution when transmitting patient information, and should be trained about the importance and means of sending e-mail messages that neither compromise the integrity of data nor give rise to a breach of patient confidentiality.

Before outlining recommended safeguards that health care facilities may want to consider in addressing e-mail security risks, it is worth briefly noting relevant federal law (and corresponding state laws in some states) enacted with the legislative intent to provide enhanced protection for the privacy of electronic communications. Title III of the Omnibus Crime Control and Safe Streets Act of 1968, also known as the federal wiretapping law, was amended by the Electronic Communications Privacy Act of 1986 (ECPA) to provide protection against improper interception of new forms of electronic communications such as e-mail and to thereby increase acceptance of e-mail and other electronic data transmissions as a secure means of communication.[46] In addition, some states have adopted wiretapping statutes modeled after the ECPA.[47] The ECPA imposes civil and criminal liability on individuals who intentionally (i) intercept any wire, oral, or electronic communication; (ii) disclose or use the contents of such communication with knowledge or reason to know that it was unlawfully

---

[46]18 U.S.C. §§ 2510 through 2711.

[47]*See, e.g.,* MINN. STAT. § 626A.01; VA. CODE ANN. § 19.2-61; UTAH CODE ANN. § 77-230-1.

intercepted;[48] or (iii) access without authorization an electronic communications facility and thereby obtain, alter, or prevent authorized access to stored communications.[49] The ECPA provides several exceptions to these prohibitions for certain access to messages by the communications service provider and the government (e.g., law enforcement agencies).

Although these federal and state wiretapping laws generally indicate what types of e-mail communications activity may lead to liability, they provide little guidance on how to protect the privacy of such communications. In the health care realm, this practical information regarding steps to be taken for the protection of patient-related e-mail communications is of utmost importance. The health care organization must ensure that adequate security technology is being used, and that confidentiality standards (set forth in its policies and procedures) are being met on an organization-wide basis. Staff training is also a crucial element for effective e-mail information security programs in the workplace.

Implementing security technology that adequately protects the confidentiality of e-mail communications involves setting up a well-managed system of access controls. All e-mail users should be required to have user IDs and passwords to access their electronic mailboxes, and should be informed as to the importance of adherence to user personal identification procedures. Users should also periodically be reminded not to leave e-mail messages on their screens when they are away from their computers. Without such controls and training, e-mail messages may be forged and may be retrieved by unauthorized persons. Moreover, to minimize the risk of misdirected messages, users should be trained to verify the address of an e-mail account and confirm that the message has been received by the intended recipient. The health care organization's policies and procedures also should address ways to ensure the confidential handling of messages within both the sender's and receiver's organizations; a policy may require that a sender take certain steps to verify that the recipient has sole access to his or her electronic mailbox prior to sending a confidential e-mail communication.

In addition, systems controls (such as encryption methods, discussed next) should be used to prevent unauthorized review of e-mail messages by systems and network support personnel. A very significant security risk in relation to patient health care information may well be posed by a health care organization's network administrator who, in monitoring traf-

---

[48]18 U.S.C. § 2511(1).

[49]18 U.S.C. § 2701(a)(1) & (2).

fic on certain parts of the network to ensure proper functionality, is tempted to read e-mail that contains information about an individual with whom he or she is acquainted, or about a public figure. Moreover, if e-mail messages are stored off-line (e.g., on backup tapes), then access to such storage facilities should be restricted.

With respect to developing policies and procedures on the use and retention of e-mail communications, the health care organization should first take into consideration any existing policies regarding the security of patient health care information. Many health care organizations have successful information security policies in place but need to develop additional policies specifically directed at strengthening the security of e-mail communications. Because the content of an e-mail communication can range from a request for a consultation to a detailed report on the patient's current medical status, health care organizations should adopt specific standards with respect to the use and retention of e-mail for patient care-related purposes.

These standards should prohibit the use of e-mail for transmitting sensitive patient information (such as HIV infection status and AIDS records, alcohol and drug abuse diagnosis and treatment records, mental health and developmental disability records, and genetic screening and test results) unless such e-mail messages are encrypted. In health care settings, unencrypted e-mail messages can be an unnecessary temptation to breach patient confidentiality. For example, one individual may send an unencrypted e-mail message containing patient information to another individual external to the organization, and later find that the message has been widely disseminated through a forwarding mechanism or some other means to other individuals. Even an inadvertent disclosure can result in a breach of patient confidentiality and consequent liability, statutory penalties, and licensure sanctions for the health care organization. Accordingly, policies regarding sensitive e-mail communications should include a prohibition against the forwarding of such messages to others without the prior permission of the sender.

As an additional safeguard, health care organizations may want to consider displaying a warning notice on its e-mail system reminding users that electronic mail should not contain information that could identify any patient, directly or indirectly, unless the message is secured via encryption.[50] According to AHIMA, some information management specialists

---

[50]Such warning may appear as a flashing dialogue box on the computer screen, or as an interactive message that requires the user's response before the e-mail is sent.

who advocate caution with respect to protecting confidentiality of information transmitted via e-mail recommend that such encryption techniques be used on a regular basis, even when the content of a message does not warrant secrecy.[51]

A health care organization's information security policies should also address e-mail retention issues; these policies should address whether all or certain e-mail communications should be archived and, if so, for what period of time. The organization's document retention and destruction policy should cover treatment of e-mail communications, including messages saved on the central computer system, backup tapes, and individual computer hard disk drives. Many health care organizations require that e-mail communications be included in the patient's medical record, in which case retention of these communications will be subject to medical record retention requirements. The health care organization may want to consider a policy encouraging individual health care providers to read sensitive e-mail messages immediately upon receipt and then, to avoid being retained in the system's nightly back-up tape, to promptly delete such messages.

In addition to access controls and specific policies covering the use and handling of e-mail communications, health care organizations must provide adequate staff training and education in this area. Individual health care providers should understand how e-mail communications regarding patient care are to be recorded, and the risks of conveying information in an e-mail message. It is particularly important that health care professionals who use e-mail to transmit patient health care information are informed that any e-mail communication containing information relevant to the patient's diagnosis and treatment should be included in the patient's medical record in hard copy or, in the alternative, linked to any existing electronic medical record. This procedure follows the same rule that applies under circumstances when the health care provider transmits patient information over the telephone; these phone calls typically are recorded in a patient's chart or medical record, and e-mail communications should also appear in the patient's medical record. The health care organization's policies should identify the individual(s) responsible for including the communication in the patient's medical record (e.g., sender, receiver, or both).

---

[51]*See, e.g.*, M. Hanken, "E-Mail Security," *Journal of the American Health Information Management Association* 67, no. 10 (1996), *citing* B. Schneier, *E-mail Security: How to Keep Your Electronic Messages Private* (New York: John Wiley & Sons, 1995).

With respect to the content of e-mail messages, health care profession-als should be trained to understand that e-mail communications pertaining to patient care must be checked for accuracy and appropriate language. A training program should emphasize the importance of drafting e-mail messages with the same caution that users would exercise in writing a for-mal memorandum because e-mail messages may ultimately be forwarded to numerous individuals other than the original recipient. A point that bears repeating in training e-mail users is that e-mail communications are not private and may be discoverable in litigation,[52] external investigation by law enforcement personnel, and internal security investigations.

Moreover, many health care organizations have decided to formally support e-mail communications with patients, and in these settings, physi-cians and other health care professionals must be trained as to the risks of electronically relaying health information to the patient. For example, a physician may create a physician-patient relationship without realizing it simply by engaging in e-mail communications with an unknown individ-ual. Perhaps a more common occurrence is that patients may perceive a physician's e-mail messages to be impersonal, and thus become dissatis-fied with the care they are receiving when no such complaints would have arisen in a person-to-person exchange where emotions are more effec-tively communicated. As a risk management strategy, the health care organization may want to consider providing patients with written mater-ial describing the risks of breaches of confidentiality and adopting a pol-icy that requires patients requesting e-mail communications from their physicians to submit signed forms that acknowledge such risks.

Health care professionals should be trained to handle a number of other content-related problems that may arise in using e-mail for patient care purposes. For example, e-mail messages may be ambiguous to the recipi-ent and, in such instances, health care professionals must recognize the need for follow-up with a telephone call to the sender. Also, if e-mail is used by health care professionals to update a patient's status, an unan-swered e-mail can trigger liability concerns. Where the recipient of an e-mail fails to respond to a message requesting an urgent consultation, for

---

[52]*See, e.g.,* United Air Lines, Inc. v. Hewins Travel Consultants, Inc., 622 A.2d 1163 (Me. 1993) (computer printouts of system data were admissible as evidence in breach of contract action); Boone v. Federal Express Corp., 59 F.3d 84 (8th Cir. 1995) (e-mail messages offered as evidence of a con-spiracy); Strauss v. Microsoft Corp., 856 F. Supp. 821 (S.D.N.Y. 1994) (defendant's motion in limine to exclude e-mail messages into evidence denied).

example, the sender who fails to take appropriate steps to treat the patient in the absence of such response may encounter liability in a negligence action. In addition, e-mail communications containing patient information are increasingly common between the health care organization and third-party payers with authorized access to such information; if an e-mail contains incorrect information in these circumstances, the result may be denial or delay of reimbursement, and potential liability or other sanctions. Health care organizations should also have protocols in place regarding approved uses of e-mail and procedures to follow under all of these circumstances.

Health care organizations should consider developing and implementing an information security program for the purposes of informing its staff and/or participating providers about the relevant policies and providing training on e-mail use and necessary security measures. AHIMA has published recommended topics to be covered by such a program, including:

- any policies in place pertaining to e-mail and the types of information that may be sent by e-mail
- the level of protection that is afforded to e-mail communications (e.g., encryption, if available, and other access controls)
- guidelines for personal use of e-mail
- guidelines for forwarding e-mail, including when it is necessary to get the originator's permission before forwarding a message
- guidelines for protecting e-mail messages that are printed from or stored on personal computers
- guidelines regarding potential disclosure of confidential information in response to list servers and chat rooms via Internet e-mail access.[53]

The Internet

As the health care industry continues its transition from hospital-based organizations to integrated health care delivery systems comprising widely dispersed referral networks, health care facilities have shown greater interest in making use of the Internet for transmitting patient health information over substantial distances. In recent years, use of the Internet as a medium for delivery of clinical information has increased

---

[53]*See, e.g.*, American Health Information Management Association, Practice Brief, "E-mail Security," *Journal of the American Health Information Management Association* 68, no.6 (1997).

dramatically, and has shown significant potential for facilitating information transfer among geographically dispersed members of a health care team. For example, the University of Virginia Medical Center, the Virginia Neurological Institute, and Hewlett-Packard have collaborated on a project to enable the viewing of patient records using an application called the Virtual Electronic Medical Record.[54] Another electronic medical record system developed by the Kansas University Medical Center links the medical center's e-mail and radiology systems so that an attending physician can automatically receive a radiologist's dictation, and the physician can then log on to the World Wide Web (WWW)[55] to view a patient's X-ray and download it to a local computer.[56]

Maintaining adequate confidentiality and security of patient data while still facilitating patient care should be every health care organization's primary objective in using the WWW to transmit patient-identifiable health care information and/or medical records to other locations. Each organization must ensure that the appropriate security technology (secured commerce servers, encryption standards, authentication mechanisms, etc.) is implemented and confidentiality standards are enforced through policy and procedure development. Training and education are also effective in minimizing an organization's risk in this area.

Two significant security risks related to Internet access are (1) unauthorized access to the health care organization's computer systems and networks and (2) unauthorized disclosure of confidential patient information. To address these concerns, health care information managers should consider the following necessary elements of a secure electronic medical records system involving the Internet:

- authentication of users to ensure that patient information is accessed only by authorized users

---

[54] J. Kazmer, A. Crosby, and K. Oliver, The Creation of a Virtual Electronic Medical Record (Paper presented in *Proceedings of the 1996 Annual HIMSS Conference*, Atlanta, Georgia, March 1996.

[55] The WWW is a client-server application that uses data transfer standards known as hypertext transfer protocol ("http") to transmit information. The linkage of documents made possible by means of "http" provides a universal naming scheme for information on all computers accessible through the Internet, and allows users to navigate the WWW by following one hypertext link to another.

[56] *See* W. Hardin, D. Masys, C. McDonald, and D. Voran, Medicine Across the Internet (Paper presented in *Proceedings of the 1997 Annual HIMSS Conference*, San Diego, California, March 1997.

- access control mechanisms to limit each user's access to patient information in the system to data that the individual has a legitimate need to know
- data integrity to ensure that patient information is not altered during transmission
- reliability of the network to ensure the continued availability of clinical information

Moreover, if the health care organization makes use of the Internet to exchange patient-identifiable information, health care information managers should devote special attention to security weaknesses associated with a publicly accessible network such as the WWW. Finally, one other concern related to Internet use is the potential for introducing computer viruses and other computer contaminants into the organization's computer systems and networks.

The need for network security does not apply to the health care industry alone, however; many industries now rely on the Internet for commercial purposes, and thus there is a growing demand for techniques to secure information relayed in transactions over the Internet. Accordingly, health care information managers should become knowledgeable about such techniques, including the establishment of standards for encryption of documents as well as choices of software and hardware for user authentication.

The health care organization must implement measures to ensure network security and the confidentiality of patient medical records, especially where transmitted information may include particularly sensitive patient health data (e.g., HIV infection status, genetic screening and test results). Many health care organizations already have implemented a comprehensive information security program, in which case many of the policies, training procedures, and controls will be in place to address Internet information security risks. Because the Internet is changing so rapidly, however, health care information managers should continually review information security measures to ensure sufficient protection of health care information; an organization-wide information security program may facilitate ongoing attention to this objective.

AHIMA has outlined steps for developing and/or enhancing policies and procedures related to Internet security.[57] A starting point, according to

---

[57]D. Miller, "Internet Security: What Health Information Managers Should Know," *Journal of the American Health Information Management Association* 67, no. 8, (1996).

AHIMA, is to determine how the Internet is being used within the health care organization. For health care professionals, use of the Internet usually falls within one or more of the following categories:

- using the WWW to access the vast amount of available information through online libraries or other sites
- extending an organization's network by connecting with other health care providers (e.g., linking an employee's computer to another organization's computer system to participate in a joint research project; providing remote access for staff members; or transferring files to other organizations)
- using electronic communications, such as sending and receiving e-mail and participating in mailing lists and discussion groups

After evaluating how the Internet is used by the health care organizations, health care information managers should determine how the Internet connection is actually made. Some means of connection present far greater security risk than others; according to AHIMA, high-speed connections to the health care organization's networked computer systems create far greater risk than a dial-up connection from a personal computer solely for browsing the WWW. In either case, however, AHIMA recommends that health care organizations have an organization-wide information security program and an information systems department specifically responsible for establishing and maintaining the organization's links to the Internet and for developing related policies and procedures.

One important security-related responsibility of the information systems department is ensuring that the organization's connections to the Internet are protected by a "firewall," which is the computer hardware, software, and network equipment used to control the link to the Internet. The department also should be responsible for ongoing monitoring of the firewall and, as necessary, updating its functions to protect against new security threats. The department may also want to recommend that an organization-wide information security program include policies specifically prohibiting (i) the establishment of other connections to the Internet from the organization's computer and (ii) dialing into the Internet from personally owned computers while those computers are on the organization's premises (if those computers are also connected to the organization's network at the same time).

Access to the organization's systems and network from the Internet also should be totally prevented or stringently controlled. The information systems department should be responsible for implementing and maintaining strong system access controls and firewalls to prevent unauthorized access from outside the organization. Remote log-ins, Telnet, remote procedure calls, and other functions that permit accessing the organization's computers from the Internet should be blocked by the firewall. Moreover, any staff education undertaken by the information systems department should Include a recommendation that file transmissions using File Transfer Protocol (FTP) be done with caution.[58] As AHIMA has explained, using FTP to transfer files into the organization may result in downloading software in violation of copyright laws or infecting the organization's computers with viruses, while FTP used for file transfers outside the organization may result in disclosing confidential patient information.[59]

In developing policies regarding the use of the Internet to send e-mail to other Internet users, the health care organization in conjunction with the information systems department should emphasize that the Internet is not secure as a communications mode. E-mail messages sent over the Internet have the potential for being read by many persons and stored on many different systems prior to delivery, and for easily being copied and forwarded by the recipient to many other people. As a safeguard in this area, health care organizations that intend to use e-mail for communication with patients should require the patient to request in writing that e-mail be used and to acknowledge the potential for breaches of confidentiality. Other policies governing the use of Internet e-mail should be implemented and made known to all Internet users in the organization. (For a more detailed description of policies in this area, see "Electronic Mail" earlier in this chapter.)

A health information systems department may also want to develop policies regarding the use of Internet e-mail in relation to mailing lists, discussion groups, or bulletin boards. Internet users who subscribe to mailing lists and who send e-mail messages to the list should know that the e-mails usually are available to all subscribers. Although these groups can be a valuable source of information, they may also be the cause of inadvertent disclosure of confidential or proprietary information. Aside from areas involving confidential patient information, staff members should be educated as to other restrictions on e-mail sent to mailing lists.

---

[58]FTP allows files to be transferred from one computer to another via the Internet, often without verifying the identity of the requestor.

[59]D. Miller, "Internet Security: What Health Information Managers Should Know," *Journal of the American Health Information Management Association* 67, no. 8, (1996).

For example, a typical message to a mailing list might be a request from one health care organization interested in developing specific policies for a copy of another organization's established policies. Some health care organizations do not permit such distribution of proprietary materials, and thus, staff members should be informed about the organization's policy for participating in mailing lists, the type of information subscribers can post, and whether or not they are permitted to provide comments on behalf of the organization. Staff members also should be informed that patient-identifiable information must never be posted to these lists in order to illustrate procedures or methods.

While use of the Internet gives rise to significant information security risks, the benefits of the Internet when used properly as a research and information source and a communications tool are probably more significant. Use of the Internet will likely continue to increase at a rapid pace, and health information managers therefore must keep abreast of the latest developments in this area. Health information managers who have not already explored Internet opportunities should consider becoming Internet users to more fully understand the issues. It is likely that the future will bring increased Internet-related responsibility for health information managers as they face the challenges of ensuring that their organizations have established formal information security programs that include policies, training, and controls specific to Internet use, while also ensuring that all systems and networks storing and processing patient information with links to the Internet are protected with firewalls.

Appendix A _____

Glossary: Acronyms and Definitions

ADA:	Americans with Disabilities Act
Advanced Directive:	A written instruction, such as a living will or durable power of attorney for health care, recognized under state law that expresses an individual's wishes regarding future medical treatment should the individual become incompetent.
AHIMA:	American Health Information Management Association
Authentication:	The process that requires the physician or other medical practitioner to sign the medical record(s) or a portion thereof. A handwritten signature, a rubber stamp or computer key are acceptable authentication methods.
Auto-authentication:	The process by which a physician authenticates a report by computer code before the report is transcribed.
Bill of Rights:	The first ten amendments to the Constitution.
Breach of Confidentiality:	A legal theory under which a patient may sue a health care provider for the improper disclosure of medical records information, also known as breach of physician-patient privilege.
Business Records:	Documents that are made in the regular course of business at or within a reasonable time after the event recorded occurred and under circumstances that reasonably might be assured to reflect the actual event accurately.
CDC:	Centers for Disease Control and Prevention
CHIN:	Community Health Information Network

Common Law: The principles of law that evolve from court decisions resolving controversies.

Computerized Patient Record System: A system that captures, stores, retrieves, and transmits patient health data including clinical, administrative and payment data. A fully automated computer-based patient record is one in which all the data images collected over the course of a patient's health care are created, authenticated, modified, stored and retrieved by the computer.

Confidential Intermediary: A person authorized to contact one or both of the biological parents of an adopted person and to request information sought by the adoptee.

Constitution: The supreme law of the land, establishing the general organization of the federal government, granting certain powers to the federal government, and placing certain limits on what the federal and state governments may do.

Corporate Compliance Programs: A document that outlines standards and procedures to be followed by an organization's employees and agents for the purpose of preventing and detecting criminal or illegal conduct with the organization.

Data Security: A process or mechanism that protects data from improper disclosure or alteration.

Defamation: A legal theory under which patients my file civil lawsuits for unauthorized disclosure of medical information. Libel is the written form of defamation, while slander is the oral form.

DNR: Do Not Resuscitate

Due Process of Law: A legal concept that requires that the rules being applied are reasonable—not vague or arbitrary and that fair procedures are followed in enforcing the rules.

ECPA: Electronic Communications Privacy Act of 1986

Emancipated Minors: A term describing the legal status of minors when they are married or otherwise are no longer subject to parental control or regulation and are not supported by their parents. The specific factors necessary to establish emancipation usually are established by statutes and vary from state to state.

EMTALA: Emergency Medical Treatment and Active Labor Act

Encryption:	A method of encoding data to protect it from unauthorized access or tampering when the data is transmitted or stored in a computer.
Entry errors:	Minor errors in transcription (spelling, etc.) or more significant errors involving test results, physician orders, inadvertently omitted information and similar substantive errors.
EPO:	Exclusive Provider Organization
Equal Protection:	A legal concept utilized to ensure that like persons are treated in like fashion, and applied by analyzing the legitimacy of the classification used to distinguish persons for various legal purposes.
ERISA:	Employee Retirement Income Security Act of 1974
Express Consent:	The consent given by direct words, whether orally or in writing.
FDA:	Food and Drug Administration
FOIA:	Freedom of Information Act
Fraud and Abuse:	A term referring to a complex and expanding array of legislative restrictions on the way health care providers conduct business and structure relationships amongst themselves. Provisions governing this conduct are primarily found in the Medicare/Medicaid statute, Stark legislation, and the civil False Claims Act. Violations of these provisions generally consist of executing a scheme or artifices to defraud a health care benefit program or obtaining through false representations money from a health care benefit program. Other federal offenses relating to health care fraud include theft or embezzlement, false statements and obstructions of criminal investigations.
Freedom of Information Laws:	The laws which grant the public access to records maintained by state agencies. In some states, the statute is called the "public records" or "open records" law.
GPWW:	Group Practice Without Walls
HCFA:	Health Care Financing Administration
HIPAA:	Health Care Insurance Portability and Accountability Act
HMO:	Health Maintenance Organization
IDS:	Integrated Delivery System

Implied Consent:	The consent inferred from the patient's conduct and consent presumed in certain emergencies.
Informed Consent:	The process by which a patient is apprised of a procedure's risks and benefits, and freely agrees to undergo the proposed treatment.
IPA:	Independent Practice Association
IRB:	Institutional Review Board
IRS:	Internal Revenue Service
JCAHO:	Joint Commission on Accreditation of Healthcare Organizations
Legal Process:	Refers to all writs issued by a court during a legal action or by an attorney in the name of the court but without court review. There are two types of legal process—the subpoena and the court order.
Living Will:	A document providing direction as to medical care, if the adult becomes incapacitated or otherwise unable to make decisions personally.
Long Consent Form:	A form with a detailed description of a patient's medical condition, proposed procedure, consequences, risks and alternatives to treatment, also called a detail or special consent form.
Managed Care:	Any method of health care delivery designed to reduce unnecessary utilization of services, and provide for cost containment while ensuring that high quality of care or performance is maintained; a system to minimize cost of care and "churning" while still delivering good access to high-quality health care; arrangements made by payers to promote cost-effective health care through establishing selective relationships with health care providers, developing coordinated or integrated delivery systems, and conducting medical management activities
MCO:	Managed Health Care Organization
Medical Group Practice:	A traditional practice structure, in which physicians combine their resources to be a medial group practice. Also known as a "consolidated medical group.
Medical Record:	A collection of data relating to the medical and health care services, a patient receives from a health care professional or other licensed health care provider, also known as "patient records.
MSO:	Management Service Organization

NAIC:	National Association of Insurance Commissioners
NCQA:	National Committee for Quality Assurance
NLRB:	National Labor Relations Board
NRC:	Nuclear Regulatory Commission
OIG HHS:	Office of the Inspector General of the Department of Health and Human Services
PHO:	Physician/Hospital Organization
Physician Ownership Model Integrated Delivery System:	A vertically integrated system, in which the physicians hold a significant portion of ownership interest of the health care entities that comprise the system.
Physician-Patient Privilege:	A legal privilege, often created by statute, that protects the communications between a patient and a physician from disclosure in judicial or quasi-judicial proceedings under specified circumstances. The purpose of this privilege is to encourage the patient to tell the physician all the information necessary for treatment, no matter how embarrassing.
Power of Attorney:	A written document that authorizes an individual, as an agent, to perform certain acts on behalf of and according to the written directives of another—the person executing the document—from whom the agent obtains authority. The agent is called the attorney-in-fact and the person executing the document is called the principal.
PPO:	Preferred Provider Organization
PSDA:	Patient Self-Determination Act
Quality Improvement:	A management engineering theory for obtaining continuous and incremental improvements, identifies problems in health care delivery, test solutions to those problems and tracks implemented solutions.
Reasonable Patient Standard:	One of the two standards used to determine the adequacy of the information the physician has given the patient during the informed consent process. Most states have adopted this standard whereby the physician's duty to provide information is determined by the information needs of the patient, rather than by customary professional practice.
Reasonable Physician Standard:	One of the two standards used to determine the adequacy of the information the physician has given

the patient during the informed consent process. This standard requires the physician to provide the information that a reasonable medical practitioner would offer under same or similar circumstances.

Risk Management: A four step process designed to identify, evaluate and resolve the actual and possible sources of loss. The four steps are risk identification, risk evaluation, risk handling, and risk monitoring.

Short Consent Form: A form that provides space for patient name and description of the specific procedure and states (1) the person signed has been told about the medical condition, consequences, risks, and alternative treatments; and (2) all the person's questions have been answered to the individual's satisfaction. The short form does not list the particular risks and benefits that were described to the patient. Also called a general or battery consent form.

Stare Decisis: A legal doctrine, imposing the requirement to follow the precedents of higher courts in the same court system that has jurisdiction over the geographic area where the court is located. For example, each appellate court, including the highest court, generally is bound to follow the precedents of its own decisions, unless it decides to overrule the precedent due to changing conditions.

Statute of Limitations: A period of time established by statute, usually measured in years, during which a party may bring a lawsuit.

Statutes: A source of law enacted by a legislature.

Subpoena ad testificandum: A written order commanding a person to appear and to testify at a trial or other judicial or investigative proceeding. These orders are used to obtain documents during pre-trial discovery and to obtain testimony during trial.

Subpoena duces tecum: A written order commanding a person to appear, give testimony, and bring all documents, papers, books, and records described in the subpoena. These orders are used to obtain documents during pre-trial discovery and to obtain testimony during trial.

System Security: A process in which a specified system functions in a defined operational environment, serves a defined set of users, contains prescribed data and operational reports, and defines network connections and interactions with other systems and incorporates safeguards to protect the system against

	defined threats to the system and its resources and data.
Telemedicine:	The delivery of health care services at a distance with the use of interactive telecommunications and computer technology.
Therapeutic Privilege:	An exception to the informed consent doctrine, which permits a physician to withhold information when disclosure of the information poses a significant threat of detriment to the patient.
UHCIA:	Uniform Health Care Information Act
URO:	Utilization Review Organization
Utilization Review:	The function of evaluating the medical necessity of non-emergency care.

Index

N